Community Health and Wellness

Principles of Primary Health Care

7e

Community Health and Wellness

Principles of Primary Health Care

7e

Jill Clendon and Ailsa Munns

ELSEVIER

ELSEVIER

Elsevier Australia. ACN 001 002 357
(a division of Reed International Books Australia Pty Ltd)
Tower 1, 475 Victoria Avenue, Chatswood, NSW 2067

ISBN: 978-0-7295-4394-1

Notice

National Library of Australia Cataloguing-in-Publication Data

NATIONAL
LIBRARY
OF AUSTRALIA

A catalogue record for this book is available from the National Library of Australia

Senior Content Strategist: Melinda McEvoy
Content Project Manager: Kritika Kaushik
Copy edited by Leanne Peters
Proofread by Tim Learner
Cover and internal design by Natalie Bowra
Index by SPi Global
Typeset by GW Tech
Printed in Singapore by KHL Printing Co Pte Ltd

Last digit is the print number: 9 8 7 6 5 4 3 2 1

Contents

Preface

This book is intended to guide the way nurses and other health practitioners work with people as they seek to maintain health and wellbeing in the context of living their normal lives, connected to their families, communities and social worlds. Life is lived in a wide range of communities, some defined by sociocultural factors such as ethnicity or Indigenous status, some defined by geography of 'place', others by affiliation or interest and some by relational networks such as social media. Because most people live within multiple communities, it is important to understand how their lives are affected by the combination of circumstances that promote or compromise their health and wellbeing. Knowing a person's age, stage, family and cultural affiliations, employment, education, health history and recreational and health preferences has an enormous effect on the way we, as health practitioners, interact with them. Likewise, our guidance and support are heavily influenced by the environments of their lives: the physical, social and virtual environments that contribute to the multilayered aspects of people's lives. Knowing how, why and where people live, work, play, worship, shop, study, socialise and seek healthcare, and understanding their needs in these different contexts, underpins our ability to develop strong partnerships with people and communities to work together as full participants, in vibrant, sustainable and equitable circumstances to achieve and enable community health and wellness.

This edition of the text represents contemporary thinking in community health and wellness from local, trans-Tasman and global communities. As access to comprehensive online sources of information grow and develop, our focus remains on the fundamental principles of *primary health care* that underpin community health and wellness. Using these principles as a foundation, the reader can then use the internet to investigate other, specific areas of interest while maintaining a core understanding of what comprises community health and wellness. We have signposted many areas that readers may want to explore further and we encourage you to also access any supplementary material available online.

Despite a lack of definitional consensus between *primary health care* and primary care in contemporary policy in both Australia and New Zealand, primary health care continues to be an integral approach to promoting health and wellness throughout the world and remains a focus in this edition. We encourage readers to use this text to fully understand the principles of primary health care and how a primary health care approach can be applied to any practice context regardless of setting. The principles of primary health care are outlined in Chapter 1 and elaborated on throughout the book.

A primary health care approach revolves around considering the social determinants of health (SDH) as we work in partnership with individuals, families and communities. The text examines the inter-relatedness of the SDH throughout the various chapters, to examine where such things as biological factors, employment, education, family issues and other social factors influence health and the way we approach our role in health promotion and illness prevention. As partners our role is to act as enablers and facilitators of community health, encouraging community participation in all aspects of community life. Incorporating the principles of primary health care into our practice enables us to facilitate these approaches.

Another foundational element that guides our consideration of community health is the notion that health is a socio-ecological construct. As social creatures, we are all influenced by others and by our environments, sometimes with significant health outcomes. The relationship between health and place and the growing impact of climate change are therefore crucial to the opportunities people have to create and maintain health. Interactions between people and their environments are reciprocal; that is, when people interact with their environments, the environments themselves are often changed. Further, achieving health and wellness must be sustainable and equitable. Analysing these relationships is therefore integral to the process of assessing community strengths and needs as a basis for health promotion planning. The first two sections of the text focus on these principles and the practice of primary health care. In this edition we continue to grow the repository of primary health care practice skills practitioners need to work effectively with individuals, families and communities. This includes community assessment, project planning, health informatics, health promotion and education, working in groups, motivational interviewing, difficult conversations and approaches to quality improvement activities. New for this edition is increased content on communicable disease, contact tracing and community infection prevention.

Our knowledge base for helping communities become and stay healthy is based on understanding the structural and social determinants of health that operate in both global and local contexts. We also know that what occurs in early life can set the stage for whether or not a person will become a healthy adult and experience good health during the pathways to ageing. Along a person's life pathway, it is helpful to know the points of critical development and age-appropriate interventions, particularly in light of intergenerational influences on health and wellbeing. We outline some of these influences and risks in Section 3 of the book, which addresses healthy families, healthy children, adolescents, adults and older people. We provide a set of goals in each chapter for achieving health and wellbeing and how these influence professional practice.

Maintaining an attitude of inclusiveness is the main focus of Section 4. Within the chapters of this section, we suggest approaches that promote cultural safety and inclusiveness in working with Indigenous people and others disadvantaged or discriminated against. To enable capacity development within communities, we need to use knowledge wisely, which means that we need evidence and innovation for all of our activities. Clearly, our professional expertise rests on becoming research literate and developing leadership skills for both personal and community capacities to reach towards greater levels of health, vibrancy, equity and sustainability for the future.

As you read through the chapters you will encounter the Mason family in Australia and the Smith family in New Zealand. Their home lives revolve around their respective communities and the everydayness of busy families. Throughout the chapters you will see how each family deals with their lifestyle challenges and opportunities as they experience childcare, adult health issues and some of the characteristics of their communities that could potentially compromise their health and wellbeing. We hope you enjoy working with them and develop a deeper sense of their family and community development and how nurses and other health practitioners can help enable health and wellness.

Throughout the text, we have included boxes that will encourage you to stop and think on the content (Key points and Points to ponder) and direct you to find further information (Where to find more ...). We have also included group exercises and questions that can be used in practice or tutorial groups to help add depth to your conversations on how to improve community health and wellness. You will also find a number of practice profiles of nurses and other health practitioners who use a primary health care approach in their practice to contextualise the varying theoretical concepts that are presented. We hope you enjoy this new edition of *Community Health and Wellness: A Primary Health Care Approach.*

About the Authors

JILL CLENDON is a registered nurse and Fellow of the College of Nurses, Aotearoa. She is currently associate director of nursing and operations manager for ambulatory care at Nelson Marlborough Health in New Zealand. She is also an adjunct professor in the School of Nursing, Midwifery and Health at Victoria University of Wellington and chair of the College of Primary Health Care Nurses, New Zealand Nurses Organisation (NZNO). Jill spent the 24 years previous to her current position in nursing policy, research and child and family health. Jill's research has examined issues with contemporary nursing workforces, the efficacy of community-based nurse-led clinics and nursing history. Jill has taught at both undergraduate and postgraduate levels with a specific interest in primary health and the contemporary context of community-based well child care in New Zealand. Jill's qualifications include a PhD in Nursing and a Masters of Philosophy in Nursing from Massey University, and a Bachelor of Arts in Political Studies from Auckland University. She also holds a Diploma in Career Guidance and Certificate of Adult Teaching from the Nelson Marlborough Institute of Technology. She has held a range of community positions including chairperson of Victory Community Health in Nelson and president of the Nelson Orienteering Club. Jill has a clinical background in public health nursing and paediatrics. She has been actively engaged in the New Zealand COVID-19 vaccination program as a vaccinator and quality lead.

AILSA MUNNS is a registered nurse, registered midwife and child and adolescent health nurse. Ailsa has practised in a range of hospital and community health settings in metropolitan, rural and remote areas of Western Australia. She works at Curtin University as a senior lecturer at the School of Nursing and coordinator of the Community Mothers Program (Western Australia), and at Child and Adolescent Health Services in Western Australia as a senior research fellow. Ailsa's current research interests include exploration of current practice for child and school health nurses, early years peer-led support for a range of population groups, community nurse-led strategies to support students transitioning to secondary school, and prevention of childhood iron deficiency anaemia in rural and remote Aboriginal communities. Her academic qualifications include a PhD in Nursing from Curtin University, Master of Nursing from Edith Cowan University and a Bachelor of Applied Science (Nursing) from Curtin University.

Acknowledgements

We offer our sincere appreciation to our colleagues, clients, students and friends who encouraged us in the creation and development of this book; sharing their practice insights, thought-provoking recommendations, stories, profiles and photos which have highlighted the motivation and impact of community health. We express our thanks to the reviewers whose feedback strengthened the book and to the team at Elsevier who supported us in crafting this work.

Reviewers

Sally Bristow BN, Grad Dip Mid, MN, PhD
Nursing Academic University of New England

Genevieve Edwards RN, BN, MN
Lecturer in Nursing, School of Nursing, Midwifery & Paramedicine (Ballarat), Australian Catholic University
Course Coordinator, Program for Nurse Immunisers, Australian Catholic University
Course Coordinator, National Immunisation Education Program for Health Professionals, Australian Catholic University

Angela Sheedy RN, BHSc, MPH, GCUTL
Senior Research Officer, School of Medicine, Charles Darwin University

Patricia (Trish) Thomson RN, Med(merit), CTLT
Member of College of Nurses Aotearoa
Department of Nursing, Midwifery and Allied Health, Ara Institute of Canterbury, Christchurch

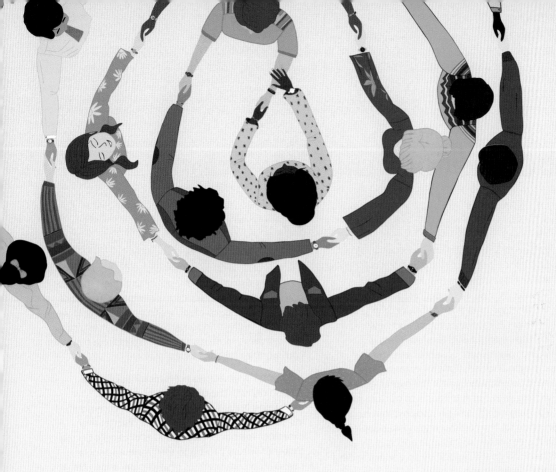

Section 1

Principles of primary health care

Introduction to the section

The three chapters that introduce this text provide a foundation to help frame what we understand about communities in contemporary society, and how community health and wellness is achieved and maintained. Chapter 1 explores the principles and foundations for creating and maintaining community health. The overall goal for those working with communities is to nurture health within a *primary health care* philosophy; that is, providing care for the community and its people in a way that is equitable, sustainable and socially just. This overarching goal is guided by an understanding of the social determinants of health (SDH). The SDH outlined in Chapter 1 explain that health is a product of social and environmental factors, which underlines the importance of *place* in health.

Chapter 2 provides an overview of the health systems in Australia and New Zealand, providing the context within which primary health care is provided. The chapter also discusses the way policy is formed and how nurses and other health practitioners can be involved in developing policy to achieve healthy communities. Our discussion culminates in a list of characteristics of an ideal health system, so that we can all strive beyond today to create a better policy environment, more responsive systems and healthier communities for tomorrow.

In Chapter 3 we address communities of place, beginning with the global community and examining features of urban and rural communities in Australia and New Zealand. The chapter then examines relational communities of people bound together virtually through electronic and social media, and communities of affiliation, which create a bond based on occupation, religious or cultural characteristics. We examine impacts of the COVID-19 pandemic on health and wellbeing, and primary health care management strategies developed in response to these stressors. At the end of each chapter, we revisit the Smith and Mason families introduced in Chapter 1, demonstrating how many of the concepts we have learned are played out in the realities of their lives.

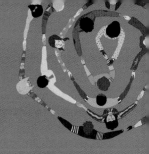

CHAPTER 1

Fundamentals of creating and maintaining a healthy community

Introduction

For most people, 'community' is a friendly term, conjuring up a sense of place, a sense of belonging. Communities are social systems where people's participation in community activities encourages this sense of belonging. Healthy communities are where people are empowered to work together to enhance the health and wellbeing of individuals and families through local action (Taylor et al 2021). This is essentially an ecological relationship. *Ecology* embodies the idea that everything is connected to everything else. Health is both a social and an ecological phenomenon, in that it is created and maintained in the context of community life. Although as individuals we can experience relative states of health or ill health because of our biological make-up, these are manifest within the supporting or challenging social ecology of a community. Health is therefore dynamic, changing as a function of the myriad interactions between biology and our genetic predispositions, and the psychological, social, cultural, spiritual, physical and political environments that surround us. The socio-ecological model of health underpins models of care that are discussed in Chapter 6.

As health practitioners, our role in working with communities is quite different from that of working within a healthcare institution. Whereas institutional care is focused on an episode of illness, the community role ranges from preventing illness to protecting people from harm or worsening health once they have

OBJECTIVES

By the end of this chapter you will be able to:

1 explain health, wellness and community health in socio-ecological terms

2 identify the social determinants of health and discuss how they impact on individuals, families and communities

3 define the principles of primary health care and explain how they guide community health practice

4 explain the concept of health literacy and how it enhances health capacity for individuals, families and communities

5 describe the differences between health education and health promotion and the significance of each in community health practice.

experienced illness, to recovery and rehabilitation, or sometimes a good death. Undertaking this type of role requires extensive knowledge of people in the many contexts of their lives. Community practice also revolves around caring for the community itself. It is *multilayered* in that it can include protecting communities from harm or stagnation, helping its citizens to enhance their existing capacity for future development by fostering *health literacy* (i.e. knowledge that contributes to health and wellbeing) and working in partnership with them to become *empowered* to make decisions that will maintain the community's viability and capability to cope with any future challenges.

This chapter starts by exploring concepts of health and wellness, and the principles and foundations for maintaining healthy communities. We examine social determinants of health and how they influence people's lives, including the emerging importance of climate change. We further introduce readers to the fundamental principles underpinning primary health care, with profiles of nurses and other health professionals who use primary health care approaches in their practice being presented to contextualise the varying theoretical concepts.

The ecological multilayered perspective of community health

WHAT IS HEALTH?

The concept of health can be varied and interpreted differently between individuals, communities and governments. The World Health Organization's (WHO) definition of health encompasses a holistic approach where health is seen not only as a lack of disease or infirmity, but as a state of overall physical, mental and social wellbeing. Further to this position, the WHO recognises the fundamental right of all people to attain the highest standard of health without divisions related to race, religion, political beliefs or economic or social conditions (WHO 2020a, p. 1). Over time, there has been ongoing debate on people's capabilities to cope with and to manage their health, particularly with

long-term impacts of chronic disease. As such, a more contemporary view of health may be the capacity of individuals, families and communities to have appropriate emotional, cognitive and behavioural responses in order to respond to a range of environmental impacts (Huber et al 2011, Huber et al 2016, Leonardi 2018).

Health itself is multifaceted. Each of us brings a number of factors influencing our health which are unique to us alone, including:

- a personal history
- our biology as it has been established by heredity and moulded by early environments
- previous events that have affected our health, including past illnesses or injuries
- our nutritional status as it is currently, and its adequacy in pregnancy and early infancy
- stressors; that is, both good and bad events in our lives that may have caused us to respond in various ways.

Biological factors provide the foundation for an individual to develop into a healthy person, but these are shaped by the environments or conditions of their lives. Becoming and staying healthy depends on our ability to reduce the environmental risks to health. In 2019, an estimated 5.2 million children under 5 years of age died from predominantly modifiable and preventative causes, which could potentially be treated with access to simple, affordable primary health care interventions (WHO 2020b).

Biological factors provide the foundation for an individual to develop as a relatively healthy person, which is an adaptive process. Development and wellbeing occurs when individuals and population groups are positively engaged with their physical, social, political, economic and structural environments (Office of Disease Prevention and Health Promotion [ODPHP] 2020a). Reciprocal exchanges between people and their environments, therefore, build the capacity for individual, family and community health.

Concepts of health are not uniform, with contrasting understandings between groups and individuals. People's understandings of health are influenced by a wide range of experiences, social norms and contexts. As health practitioners, we need to be aware of these different cultural interpretations and what it means for individuals, families and communities to be ill or well (Australian Institute of Health and Welfare [AIHW] 2018). For example, Indigenous Australian and New Zealand people have very holistic definitions reflecting the importance of social, emotional, spiritual and cultural wellbeing of individuals and whole communities, along with their physical environment, dignity, self-esteem and justice (Durie 1999, National Aboriginal Health Strategy Working Party 1989). It is also important to recognise that these meanings may vary between specific Indigenous environments. This differs from the Western mainstream biomedical approach, emphasising a community perspective.

The inclusion of cultural perspectives within health frameworks highlights issues of health governance for the delivery of services. Supportive government policies for resources and models of care are essential for health service provision across a wide domain (AIHW 2018), which will be explored more extensively in the following chapter.

THE SOCIAL MODEL OF HEALTH

Recognising the social determinants of health and their impact on health inequalities highlights the need to have a primary health care approach to care rather than a traditional biomedical model of health for individuals, families and communities. A social model of health incorporates primary health care responses to complex psychosocial issues and socio-ecological inequalities occurring in societies, acknowledging a broad range of impacts such as the effects of early life development, cultural environments and, more recently, climate change (Guzys 2021a, Taylor et al 2021).

The World Meteorological Organization (2021) has highlighted the effects of climate change on human health through high-impact events such as extreme heat, drought, bushfires, floods and cyclones. These are in addition to disruptions to infrastructure and economic stability. A noted consequence is a rise in food insecurity. The ongoing health and social impacts of climate change disproportionately affect vulnerable people, such as children, women in the antenatal period, those with chronic diseases and socioeconomic disadvantage (Taylor et al 2021). It is imperative that interdisciplinary primary health care approaches are undertaken at local, national and international levels to plan, develop and advocate for integrated action for prevention and active intervention for climate change.

The social determinants of health (SDH)

From birth, individuals are programmed through experiences to develop certain biologically preset behaviours at critical and sensitive developmental periods. This is called 'biological embedding', and it is influenced by how people interact with the genetic, social and economic contexts of their lives. Early life adversity within these environments increases the risk for a range of physical and psychosocial health problems later in life (Ehrlich 2020). Health outcomes can be influenced by social conditions such as family, cultural, community and economic and political determinants. These social determinants of health (SDH) have a direct influence on the immediate and long-term health and wellbeing of individuals, families and entire communities, with a particular focus on health and social inequities (Keleher 2020a).

A WHO report (Wilkinson & Marmot 2003) identified 10 SDH which impact on people's ability to adopt healthy lifestyles.

1   The social gradient
2   Stress
3   Early life
4   Social exclusion
5   Work
6   Unemployment
7   Social support
8   Addiction
9   Food
10 Transport

Figure 1.1 demonstrates examples of contemporary social determinants of health that impact globally on the health and wellbeing of individuals, families and communities. This figure shows the

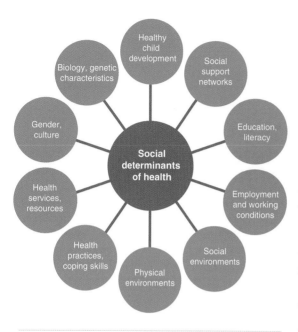

Figure 1.1 Examples of the social determinants of health

SDH as we use them in this text and forms the basis of the SDH assessment circle which we will introduce to you in Chapter 4.

The WHO (2021a) and ODPHP (2020a) have also recognised the influence of genetics and access to and use of health services as being further determinants influencing health. Within the SDH are a number of structural conditions. For example, improving a community's development requires employment opportunities and working life opportunities, in addition to housing and environments that support healthy physical and psychosocial development. Food security in relation to affordable, accessible and nutritious foods is an ongoing issue within and between countries. Other structures within the community supporting the maintenance of health and wellbeing include a wide range of stakeholders within and outside the health sector. The impacts of organisations indirectly involved with health have been found to surpass the contribution of established health sectors (WHO 2021b). It is important that all services are accessible where and when they are needed.

SDH strongly influence healthy child development, with healthy early child development being the most crucial stage within the lifespan (WHO 2021a). Parenting support and skills, family stability and adequate physical and socioeconomic resources are integral to health and wellbeing. Interactions between individuals, families and communities, such as having healthy and supportive neighbourhoods and accessible child health and childcare services, are additional supports for families and children. Employment conditions such as parental leave without loss of promotional opportunities, flexible working hours and income protection in the case of unemployment all support healthy growth and development. On-site and out-of-hours child care underpin contemporary working conditions that facilitate economic and family security.

THE SOCIAL GRADIENT

The SDH create advantages and disadvantages for individuals, families and groups, with some members of society having reduced chances of reaching their full health potential due to a range of physical, psychosocial, spiritual and cultural factors (Taylor et al 2021). Those who earn income at successively higher levels have better health than those who are unemployed or have lower levels of income. Research studies have shown there is a 'social gradient' in health where key social determinants, such as employment, income and poverty, affect health inequalities. This gradient can lead to earlier physical, psychosocial and mental health disabilities, along with shorter life spans (Kendall et al 2019; Marmot et al 2020). This inequity creates disadvantage from birth for some children. A child born into a lower socioeconomic family, for example, may be destined for an impoverished life, creating intergenerational ill health. This child lives in a situation of 'double-jeopardy', where interactions between the SDH conspire against good health and access to support. Without these community supports, the family may spiral into worsening circumstances, affecting their child's opportunities for the future. This is the case for many Indigenous people, whose parents have not had access to adequate employment or community supports that would sustain their own health, much less that of their children. They become caught in a cycle of vulnerability where the SDH interact in a way that creates disempowerment across generations. Political decisions governing employment opportunities may hamper the parents' ability to improve finances. A less than optimal physical environment may deprive both the parents and the child of a chance to access culturally important social groups or gatherings. There may be few opportunities for education, healthcare or transportation to access services. Parenting skills may be absent for a range of reasons, including younger age, a lack of role modelling, geographical disadvantage or acute and chronic illness.

Reducing the impact of inequities requires people, communities and governments to take action on the SDH. As stated earlier, many of these determinants are influenced by the social, political and economic environments in which people live. As people may have very limited opportunities to exert control over their SDH, attributing blame or a lack of commitment to personal decision-making in relation to these particular situations further disadvantages people. Global, national and local policy decisions such as employment strategies and public health priority setting affect the ability of people and communities to influence their own health decisions. Any marginalisation of individuals and families through adverse SDH prevents them from fully interacting with community assets, leading to social exclusion. Social exclusion leaves many members of society disadvantaged and without the support and resources they need for health and wellbeing (Marmot 2019). In contrast, social inclusion creates social capital, trust, norms of reciprocity and cohesion: the essence of a healthy community.

WELLNESS

Health influences the sense of wellness of individuals and communities. Healthy people's lives are characterised by balance and potential. A wellness perspective reduces the focus on illness prevention alone. There are differing viewpoints on the understanding of wellness. An established definition from the National Wellness Institute (2020) highlights wellness as a conscious and self-directed process through which people make choices towards achieving their full potential. This addresses social, emotional, mental and environmental dimensions of their lives, demonstrating multidimensional and holistic considerations. When these dimensions are part of a healthy community there are opportunities for the community as a whole to develop high levels of health or wellness, thereby supporting individuals and families. This socio-ecological connectivity between people and their environments embodies community health and wellness in that people feel supported and able to develop health capacity. For example, they may feel they have lifestyle choices if these are accessible and affordable; and if they choose, they will be able to exercise or relax in safe spaces. They have access to nutritious foods; students balance study with recreation; young families immunise their children and have time out from work to socialise. Older people are valued for their contribution to the community and inclusive policies promote opportunities for all citizens to participate fully in the community and lead a high-quality, happy life.

> **KEY POINT**
>
> Health and wellness are ecological. Biological factors provide the foundation for an individual to develop into a healthy person, but these are shaped by the environments or conditions of their lives.

WHAT DO WE MEAN BY COMMUNITY?

The meaning of 'community' can vary. It is usually explained as being geographical or functional, where members interact and share both a sense of identity and resources. Communities can also be defined by culture, beliefs or issues of interest around a shared perspective, accommodating a dynamic diversity of ethnicities, strengths and needs (Taylor et al 2021). Of growing interest across age groups is the emergence of virtual communities, which involve members using a range of communication technologies to interact as groups, with the potential for collective empowerment (Atanasova & Petric 2019).

Feelings of connectedness have been positively associated with higher levels of physical and mental health, social support and having control over issues affecting a person's life (Taylor et al 2021). A community is often seen as a context for action, particularly in the areas of health and social wellbeing. These are impacted by members' varying beliefs, traditions, feelings of collective identity and determinants of health. There are many contextual meanings for community, and its influence on the capacity of individuals and families to interact meaningfully will be explored throughout this text.

POINTS TO PONDER

What is 'community'?

- A place we share with others?
- A network of like-minded people?
- A group who lives, works and plays together?
- An interdependent group of people inhabiting a common space?
- A context for action?
- An online group?
- All of the above?

COMMUNITY, PUBLIC AND POPULATION HEALTH

SDH help determine strengths and challenges in community health. When people are asked to define community health, their responses usually reflect a blending of community, public health and population health characteristics. Public health focuses on promoting and sustaining the health of whole populations or subpopulation groups (Fleming 2019, Guzys 2021a), with programs involving measurement and surveillance with development of evidence-based strategies to prevent or overcome diseases. A wide range of disciplines contribute to public health, including those from traditional health professions, social science, education and epidemiology fields (Keleher 2020a). Community health nursing may have elements of public health practice, but has a

prime focus on individuals, families and their communities, rather than whole populations, using a primary health care approach to address the impact of SDH on client care (Guzys 2021a). Population health is similar to public health in that its focus is risk of health and disease in the community, but population health programs tend to address multiple disparities and determinants in health status between different groups. It is also proposed that this approach also needs to include integrated health systems that enhance intersectoral collaborations across health and non-health sectors, thereby encouraging gains in social engagement and growth (Keleher 2020a).

KEY POINTS

Public health focuses on promoting and sustaining the health of populations.

Population health aims to address disparities in health status between different groups.

Healthy communities are the *synthesis* or product of individual people interacting with their environments with their unique understandings of what it is to be healthy, working collaboratively to shape and develop the community in a way that will help them achieve positive health outcomes.

Our definition of community health is as follows:

Community health is characterised by the presence of: strong social capital; engaged and empowered community members; a dynamic and healthy physical, social and spiritual environment; accessible, affordable and equitable services and resources; and a system of governance that is inclusive and responsive to community members in addressing the SDH.

This and other definitions of community health embody an ideal where all community members strive towards a common state of health. Of course, in real life, communities and societies are neither consistent nor stable, which reflects the variability among individuals and the dynamic social and environmental changes that occur in people's lives.

Social conditions are particularly important to community health, because social environments provide the context for interactions in all other environments. Social support fostering positive connections for people to take part in society, thereby enhancing feelings of dignity and security, enables people to feel *empowered*, and have greater control over their lives and their health and life opportunities (World Bank 2021). We call this *social inclusion*. On the other hand, if their social situation is plagued by civil strife, an oppressive political regime, crime, poverty, unemployment, violence, discrimination, food insecurity, diseases or a lack of access to health and social support services they may be *disempowered*, leaving them less likely to become healthy or recover from illness when it occurs. As Taylor and colleagues explain, 'empowerment is a process which enables people to participate in a way that improves their lives and achieves social justice' (2021, pp. 18–19) and needs to occur through community development activities. This is underpinned by the Declaration of Alma-Ata where the concepts of equity, social justice and empowerment were identified as key principles of primary health care (Taylor et al 2021, WHO & UNICEF 1978). The community health practitioner can be an advocate for community empowerment, facilitating and encouraging transforming strategies that take SDH into account (Fleming et al 2019). When people live in situations of disadvantage or disempowerment, they are unable to access the same resources for health as those who live in more privileged situations, and their lives and potential for the future are compromised. This is called *social exclusion*. Chapter 9 explores these themes in more detail.

The role of health practitioners in community health is to recognise enabling and challenging features within a range of cultural, economic, social and health environments, working with individuals, families, groups and political entities to collectively identify issues and strategies to enhance health and wellbeing. One of the challenges is the development of relevant, acceptable and sustainable approaches that take into account the complexities and impacts of social determinants of communities (ODPHP 2020b). Community health practitioners need to step outside traditional models of practice and work within an increasingly recognised social model of health, incorporating a primary health care approach.

> ## KEY POINTS
>
> The characteristics of an enabling community health practitioner include:
>
> - promoting health and providing care where people live, work and play
> - advocating for the community, its people and its physical, social and spiritual environments
> - promoting equity, access, social inclusion and adequate resources by assessing community needs and disadvantage and then lobbying for change where required
> - encouraging empowerment and health literacy to promote citizen participation in decisions for health and wellbeing
> - generating the evidence base relative to community health needs.

Primary health care

When working with communities, nurses are aware of the need to address goals for social justice, along with promoting equity and access to health resources. The 'social determinants' approach to health resonates with the notion of human rights and social justice, which underpins the social model of health. As such, nurses have an obligation to identify disadvantaged individuals, families and communities, their health inequities and predisposing social determinants, facilitating equitable distribution of resources and assistance (Guzys 2021a).

Primary health care is a set of principles and an organising framework to guide nurses and other health practitioners in facilitating socially just, equitable conditions for good health. The International Conference on Primary Health Care was held in Alma-Ata in 1978, where a resolution was passed calling on the international community to protect and promote the health of all people (WHO & UNICEF 1978). Primary health care is defined in the 1978 Declaration of Alma-Ata as:

> Essential healthcare based on practical, scientifically sound and socially acceptable methods and technology made universally accessible to individuals and families in the community through their full participation and at a cost that the community and country can afford to maintain at every stage of their development in the spirit of self-reliance and self-determination. It is the first level of contact of individuals, the family and community with the national health system bringing healthcare as close as possible to where people live and work and constitutes the first element of a continuing care process.
>
> *World Health Organization 1978*

Primary health care activities that are limited to a particular group are considered 'selective' rather than 'comprehensive' primary health care. Selective primary health care does not focus on SDH and equity, tending to adopt an individualised health practitioner-led medical technology approach, addressing specific illnesses and diseases. Comprehensive primary health care focuses on health and wellbeing priorities that have been identified through partnerships between health professionals and community members within their psychosocial and ecological contexts (Taylor et al 2021). An important aspect of this approach for community health nurses is the focus on strength-based care which is client-centred and community directed. Individuals and families are encouraged to develop self-determination in their own health and wellbeing pathways, enhancing trust and reliable relationships between people, their communities and nurses (McKillop & Munns 2021). Table 1.1 captures the differences between selective and comprehensive primary health care.

PRIMARY HEALTH CARE PRINCIPLES

The principles of primary health care guide our activities in illness prevention, health promotion

and structural and environmental modifications that support health and wellness. These are identified as:

- accessible healthcare
- appropriate technology
- health promotion
- cultural safety
- intersectoral collaboration
- community participation.

These principles are a framework to guide us to work towards equitable social circumstances, equal access to healthcare and community empowerment through public participation in all aspects of life. The literature on primary health care includes cultural inclusiveness as a common thread in each of these principles. However, we include cultural safety as a separate principle. Being culturally safe and enabling culturally appropriate healthcare is one of the most important factors in achieving primary healthcare. The principles are interconnected, but they are examined separately below to underline the importance of each to the overall philosophy of primary health care (see Fig 1.2).

Accessible healthcare

In many countries of the world, including those considered highly developed, there is a widening gap in access to health services between population groups such as Indigenous and non-Indigenous people, and those living in urban and rural or remote areas (Taylor et al 2021). These factors cause disparity between rich and poor, which is inequitable and socially unjust. The major objective of providing equity of access is to eliminate disadvantage, whether it is related to social, economic or environmental factors. Barriers to access include areas such as unemployment, lack of education and health literacy, racial discrimination, age, gender, functional capacity and cultural or language difficulties. These factors inhibit the development of capacity for individuals and families. Barriers to community capacity include geographical features that isolate people from services or opportunities, civil conflict or inadequate supporting structures and services.

TABLE 1.1 **Selective and comprehensive PHC**

Characteristic	Selective primary health care	Comprehensive primary health care
Main aim	Reduction of specific disease	Improvement in overall health of the community and individuals
Strategies	Focus on curative care, with some attention to prevention and promotion	Comprehensive strategy with curative, rehabilitative, preventive and health promotion that seeks to remove root causes of ill health
Planning and strategy development	External, often 'global', programs with little tailoring to local circumstances	Local and reflecting community priorities: professional 'on tap not on top'
Participation	Limited engagement, based on terms of outside experts and tending to be sporadic	Engaged participation that starts with community strengths and the community's assessment of health issues, is ongoing and aims for community control
Engagement with politics	Professional and claims to be apolitical	Acknowledges that primary health care is inevitably political and engages with local political structures
Forms of evidence	Limited to assessment of disease-prevention strategy based on traditional epidemiological methods, usually conducted out of context and extrapolated to situation	Complex and varied research methods including epidemiology and qualitative and participatory methods

Source: Reproduced with permission of Taylor & Francis Ltd. From Baum, F. 2003. 'PHC: can the dream be revived?' Development in Practice 13(5), 515–519.

KEY POINTS

Inequity means unfair distribution of resources and support (e.g. lack of health practitioners in rural areas) arising from poor governance, corruption or cultural exclusion.

Inequality means disparity in health status or capacity (e.g. poorer health among Indigenous people than non-Indigenous people).

Evidence has shown that in any country, the greater the income gap between rich and poor, the worse the health status of all its citizens. Poverty reduces people's access to healthcare services and lifestyle choices (WHO 2021c). This occurs unevenly, as health is distributed differently among different groups. Poor social determinants of health influence the stark differences in the health of communities and the ways in which populations can enhance their social and physical environments (Centers for Disease Control and Prevention [CDC] 2021). Local, national and global impacts on health need to be considered by health professionals working in partnership with communities. Creation of sustainable environments and social conditions are priority areas in order to build capacity for improving health and wellness (Baldwin & Fleming 2019). Decisions for community health should therefore be based on simultaneous assessments of the impact on individuals, families and communities, future generations and the global community. Social justice, or equitable access for all, needs to ensure the least advantaged people in a community receive equal opportunity, education, care

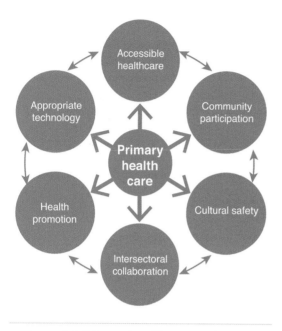

Figure 1.2 Primary health care principles

and service as those who are advantaged by virtue of both tangible (finances) and intangible (knowledge) resources. This may sometimes mean prioritising care for those most disadvantaged to achieve equity.

Appropriate technology

The failure of healthcare systems to address inequities in health is due, in part, to the use of inappropriate technologies in healthcare. Primary health care requires efficiency, effectiveness and acceptability using sustainable technologies and systems (Guzys 2021a). Although progress has been made in community management of health and wellbeing, health systems continue to revolve around services with a medical-technical focus rather than those that support community empowerment and 'distributional equity' (Taylor et al 2021). Not all communities can afford the latest and most expensive technologies, so health expenditure on technological supports can sometimes be a barrier to less expensive but adequate, sustainable care for more people.

Health promotion

Health promotion is a capacity-building process, focusing on broad social, environmental and cultural

impacts of health, with a primary health care approach being a key requirement (Taylor et al 2021). Health promotion activities guide advocacy, mediation and enablement, with global and local strategies incorporating a capacity-building, enabling and supportive framework as outlined in the Ottawa Charter (WHO 2021d). These will be discussed in more detail later in the chapter.

Cultural safety

Culture is the shared patterns of social behaviours and interactions, ideas and mutual understandings of particular groups that are acquired through a process of socialisation (Center for Advanced Research on Language Acquisition 2019). SDH and health practitioner cultural reflexivity have an impact on the development of culturally safe practice. Ramsden (1993) first developed the concept of cultural safety within the New Zealand healthcare system. Cultural awareness is the first step, where health practitioners learn about cultural diversity. Self-reflection on knowledge and clinical practice relates to attainment of cultural sensitivity, becoming more responsive to the way an individual or group's cultural mores shape health and health behaviours. Cultural safety is where health professionals and their organisations promote health equity and accountability in healthcare delivery for individuals and families. Importantly, it is not the nurse, midwife or other health practitioner who determines whether practice is culturally safe, but the recipient of care (Curtis et al 2019). We will explore these concepts further in Chapter 9.

Intersectoral collaboration

Intersectoral collaboration requires cooperation between different community sectors, including (but not limited to) those managing health, education, social services, housing, transportation, environmental planning and local government. Tapping into the expertise of different sectors and different alliances enables more holistic, flexible and collaborative responses to certain needs, enabling multi-focused strategies in addressing SDH. Another advantage of intersectoral collaboration is promoting acceptance of the need for a health initiative when all parties involved work together for its success. Collaborative alliances encourage efficient and effective use of resources, with economies achieved from less duplication, improved quality and continuity of health and wellbeing activities (Taylor et al 2021). However, in addressing the allocation of economic resources to health budgets it is important to lobby for national primary health care policies that support decentralised control so that communities themselves can participate in health planning. These concepts are explored more fully in Chapters 2 and 6.

Community participation

Community participation is a central tenet of a primary health care approach with improved health outcomes as the result. Effective partnerships see healthcare practitioners and community members having equal status, both actively working to plan and implement health and wellness activities (Guzys 2021a). Community partnerships are not only empowering but they enhance capacity for developing social capital with mutual trust and reciprocity as well as cooperative networks for better health. However, it is imperative that funding policies support development of equitable health services, particularly in remote areas, and facilitation of sustainable primary health care services, especially in relation to employment of Aboriginal health practitioners, in Aboriginal Community Controlled Health Services which are grounded in a community participation approach (Wakerman et al 2019). The major goal of community participation is empowerment, which facilitates more socially just, inclusive environments (Taylor et al 2021).

Primary health care is focused on redressing social disadvantage by promoting healthy social and structural conditions for good health. We achieve this within an *enabling* role, acting in partnership with people who are empowered to make informed choices to develop their personal and community capacity. The aim of these community partnerships is to enable better health, equity, justice and governance in health services, including appropriate, effective and efficient use of available technologies. However, these outcomes are only achievable where there is the political will to support and sustain good health for all members of the community, which is integral to the notion of social capital.

KEY POINTS

. . . .

Primary health care in practice

Accessible healthcare: working to alleviate the barriers that prevent equal access to health for all members of the community—identifying any disparities in access to education, health services, employment or other SDH.

Appropriate technology: advocating for the right care for the right person or community at the right time, to maximise efficiency and equity rather than the most expensive technologies for all communities.

Health promotion: encouraging community capacity through comprehensive promotion of health for the whole-of-community; promoting selective care for those most in need of specific care.

Cultural safety: being aware of your own and others' cultural beliefs, values and knowledge and how these shape health and health decisions.

Intersectoral collaboration: working in partnership with health, disability services, transportation, education, environment and other sectors to respond to all the SDH.

Public participation: ensuring that community members are able to participate fully in making decisions for their health and wellbeing.

Primary care is a term which is often used instead of primary health care; however, there are several differences. Primary care typically relates to medical and allied health management of conditions, being a defined occasion of care through a range of private and public health providers. There is an established primary care sector in Australia and New Zealand in general practice settings. However, in terms of improving overall health outcomes, a broader primary health care approach that addresses SDH such as housing, employment and food security is necessarily more encompassing and more likely to address the inequities that leave some population groups disadvantaged. Primary care, while an important aspect of care provided within the health sector, comprises part of a primary health care system, not the entirety of the system (Keleher 2020b).

Equity and sustainability

The social model of health promotes equity for individuals, families and communities, addressing SDH to enhance access to empowering health and wellbeing support. Community health nurses need to facilitate strategies addressing equity and equality and, as such, have an appreciation of both approaches. Equality ensures each person, family or group is given the same resources or opportunities, while equity recognises that they may have different circumstances, with more resources and opportunities needed to reach an equal outcome (Milken Institute School of Public Health, George Washington University 2020). Comprehensive primary health care is fundamental for the development of sustainable and equitable approaches across a range of population groups. Health activities need to be meaningful, realistic, culturally appropriate and responsibly sustainable before they can be actioned by clients (Munns 2021).

Planning equitable health services to meet the needs of people in diverse population and socioeconomic groups requires primary health care innovation with sustainable strategies for the future. Community health professionals, particularly community health nurses, can only achieve this by working in partnership with clients and communities to identify and co-design acceptable strategies for their health and wellbeing. Practice nurses are one example of a community health nurse who works in partnership with clients and communities to improve health. Box 1.1 includes a practice profile of a practice nurse demonstrating this work in action. You will find more practice profiles in Chapter 6.

BOX 1.1

PRACTICE PROFILE: PRACTICE NURSE

Hi. My name is Carter and I'm a practice nurse.

What the role entails:

The role of a practice nurse involves working closely with patients to support them with their health needs, whatever these may be. A typical day may include immunising a baby, working through a diet plan with a person newly diagnosed with diabetes, managing an acute asthma attack, following up on lab results or removing a set of stitches. I work hard to improve population health, meet my responsibilities under the Treaty of Waitangi and address inequity in a community-based way.

How I came to be in the role:

I came to practice nursing within a year of graduating from my education. Practice nursing is not a traditional place for male nurses to find themselves but I wanted to work closely with people in the community and I have an active interest in healthy living and lifestyle. Practice nursing seemed an ideal place to be able to support people to achieve healthy lives.

What I find most interesting about the role:

I enjoy the ongoing interaction and relationship development with my patients that a general practice allows. It is rewarding to help people of all ages maintain good health and successfully manage chronic conditions. The generalist setting and multidisciplinary team approach helps me advocate for patients and guide them through the system. Sometimes, it is simply the honour of listening to people share their fears and to help them find context, meaning and acceptance.

Advice for anyone wanting to become a practice nurse:

Build your skills and knowledge of working in the community by taking relevant courses on smoking cessation, cardiovascular risk assessment and immunisations. Consider courses on motivational interviewing,

Where to find out more on ...

Equity and equality

Review the YouTube video 'Jill Clendon on improving health equity' at www.youtube.com/watch?v=6xKYqOn2Uo8. This is a short overview of health equity in New Zealand.

Please note: Aotearoa is the Māori name for New Zealand. Māori are the Indigenous peoples of New Zealand. Pacific refers to the well-established Pacific communities who have migrated from Pacific Islands to New Zealand.

Social capital

When the health of the community is defined from a social perspective, we acknowledge its *social capital*. Social capital relates to the quality of the social norms and values and how these associations link and benefit people within different types of communities. Health and wellbeing are enhanced through strong social capital (Taylor et al 2021).

Internationally, social capital can have different concepts and dimensions, such as bonding, bridging and linking approaches, and has definitive evidence-based links with health and wellbeing outcomes. A current exemplar is the relationship of social capital on the effects of COVID-19 on individuals, families and communities across differing global socioeconomic and geographical locations, and their ability to develop prevention strategies. Please review the article relating to this issue in the United States (Makridis & Wu 2021): https://journals.plos.org/plosone/article?id=10.1371/journal.pone.0245135.

The importance of understanding social capital in a community is in knowing where and how to implement health promotion programs that will have a greater chance of success. For example, where communities have developed a sense of coherence and commitment to one another there is a greater likelihood of mutual support in achieving health goals.

KEY POINT

....

Involving community members in activities or projects to pursue common goals will help build social capital.

RESEARCH TO PRACTICE: SOCIAL CAPITAL AND HEALTH

Communities with high social capital have a better chance of coping with adversity and limitations, as well as being able to build a positive sense of place. Social capital is reflective of the social norms and values between individuals and families within their communities, reflecting mutuality, respect and trust, all of which enhance collective health benefits. These links significantly enhance health benefits, quality of life and a sense of wellbeing. Importantly, social capital enhances a range of health promotion strategies for sustaining communities (Taylor et al 2021).

Community health capacity can be supported or weakened by the presence or lack of organisational structures, such as schools, workplaces and community planning mechanisms that include participatory decision-making. When such organisational structures are present, communities can work together to respond to the SDH, sharing common attitudes, goals and activities to address inequalities and work towards a more inclusive society (Taylor et al 2021).

Health literacy

Health literacy offers the ability for individuals, families and communities to make sound health decisions in everyday life and is influenced by contextual SDH (Sykes & Wills 2018). Some decisions may be related to healthcare, but others may be lifestyle choices, decisions that improve quality of life or that help in understanding civic responsibilities or opportunities. Health literacy is an important element in addressing health inequities, as those at the lower levels of health literacy are often the ones who live in socioeconomically disadvantaged communities. Health literacy offers the potential for individuals, families and communities to have significant influence over their health, with building of literacy being more effective when learned in the context of people's unique lifestyles (Sykes & Wills 2018). However, people experiencing psychological distress have reported difficulties in navigating healthcare systems (Australian Bureau of Statistics [ABS] 2018). The COVID-19 pandemic has also drawn attention to the value of health literacy, with families and communities needing to understand the implications for themselves and society. Being aware of how to manage their new health environments relating to prevention and active management of the new virus has been dependent on health messaging from health professionals that is clear and easily understood (AIHW 2020a). This emphasises the need for health practitioners to work in partnership with individuals, families and communities to facilitate effective health communication and decision-making.

KEY POINT

There are three levels of health literacy: functional, communicative (or interactive) and critical

Three levels of health literacy have been identified by Nutbeam and Lloyd (2021) and are shown in Table 1.2. *Functional health literacy* means that individuals have received sufficient factual information on health risks and health services, which they also understand, and which allows them to apply the knowledge to a range of relevant health risks, and clearly defined goals and specific contexts such as prevention and early intervention activities (Nutbeam & Lloyd

2021). Individuals need to be able to read essential materials such as medication administration labels, particularly for children, and when to cease medications. They also need to be able to understand and act on test results, know how to complete health-related forms and participate in shared decision-making. It also needs to be remembered that health literacy can be variable, depending on a person's psychological state, the impacts of illnesses and psychosocial, environmental and cultural stressors (Patient Safety Network & Agency for Healthcare Research and Quality [AHRQ] 2019).

At a second level, *communicative* or *interactive health literacy* develops personal skills to the extent that community members are able to derive meaning from and distinguish between information from a range of health communication and health education strategies such as mobile apps and interactive websites. They are able to participate in community life, influencing social norms and helping others develop their personal health capacity through avenues including self-help and peer-led support groups.

The third level of literacy, *critical health literacy*, describes the most advanced literacy skills where people use cognitive skills to improve individual capabilities and resilience to exert greater influence over life events that impact on health. This paves the way for community leadership structures to support community action and to facilitate community development. This type of health literacy can enhance health benefits for individuals, whole communities and populations (Nutbeam & Lloyd 2021). Examples of outcomes include workers exerting pressure on workplaces to reduce hazardous risks, lobby groups gathering support for environmental preservation or supportive resources for parenting practices or health services.

A further consideration is cultural literacy, which encourages health professionals to identify and use appropriate cultural understandings within

TABLE 1.2 Health literacy: a continuum of knowledge and skill development

Functional	Communicative/interactive	Critical
Knowledge to choose	Ability to influence	Skills for action

Source: Adapted from Nutbeam, D., Lloyd, J.E., 2021. Understanding and responding to health literacy as a social determinant of health. Annu. Rev. Public Health, 42, 159–173. Online. Available: https://doi.org/10.1146/annurev-publhealth-090419-102529.

their health information that is communicated to individuals, families and communities (CDC 2019). This is particularly important in Indigenous communities where understanding of the holistic nature of health is often already embedded and intertwined with a range of cultural practices that need to be included in discussions about health.

For health practitioners, the focus of promoting health literacy is to provide information, education and advocacy to ensure consumers' understanding of health information and shared decision-making in a supportive environment. This is in addition to health systems providing services to accommodate consumer needs and abilities, and enhance support for navigating differing health situations (Network & AHRQ 2019). To help people read, understand, evaluate and use health information requires an understanding of how people learn. This varies according to age, class, cultural group, gender, beliefs, preferences and coping strategies and experience with the health system. These individual and group differences draw into clear focus how communities differ in their populations, resources and capacity to support health and wellness, which is the subject of chapters to follow.

Health literacy has a multifaceted relationship with health promotion and health education. It can be seen as an outcome, as well as a foundational factor for health promotion activities, facilitating the impact of health education on health behaviour changes. As such, health literacy has a positive link between health promotion, health education and these changes (Gugglberger 2019).

Health promotion

Health promotion is a significant feature of comprehensive primary health care (Guzys 2021a) and is described by the WHO (2021e, p. 1) as:

> the process of enabling people to increase control over, and to improve, their health. It moves beyond a focus on individual behaviour towards a wide range of social and environmental interventions.

Historically, health promotion has had a narrow focus on individual behaviour, with contemporary practice supporting a broad interplay of social and structural determinants of health influencing people's ability to maintain their health and wellbeing. Health promotion is essentially a political, ecological and capacity-building process, aimed at arranging these determinants in a way that facilitates health and reduces inequality which is evident in both high- and low-income nations. To help people build health capacity requires awareness of global, national and local conditions that affect health. As such, health promotion actions achieve the best outcomes for health when they involve intersectoral collaboration (Green et al 2019).

A key health promotion concern is how individuals, families and communities can develop empowerment and control over their health and wellbeing when they lack the power to do so. Their relationships between their physical and psychosocial environments is not unidimensional, and can be influenced by issues such as poverty, environmental factors, famine, war, lack of access to facilities, social inequality and poor health literacy (Green et al 2019), all of which relate to primary health care principles and SDH.

Specific health promotion actions begin with community assessment. From this basis of knowledge, plans are developed in partnership with community members to maximise assets, reduce risks to health and plan for a sustainable future for current and future generations. The role of nurses and other health practitioners in promoting community health includes advocating for, teaching and enabling good health based on local knowledge and understanding of the community's health literacy and health goals. Central to this type of analysis is assessing the relationships within SDH, how these are interacting with the environment in the local context and what influences are exerting pressures on the community and its residents along their social, cultural and developmental pathways. This is a more inclusive, comprehensive view of health promotion than simply seeing the community in terms of a single issue or health problem at a discrete moment in time. Community assessment is discussed in Chapter 4.

Health promotion should be focused on the community's assets and strengths with a focus on people's values, attitudes and beliefs to facilitate improved health and wellbeing outcomes (Taylor et al 2021). Health promotion actions may be aimed at different population subgroups, such as creating daycare centres for the elderly to prevent them from being socially isolated or working with new parents to ensure they have the information and the support systems they need. What these have in common is a commitment to enabling capacity through participation, empowerment and health literacy.

The historical context of health promotion is closely aligned with the historical phases of the public health movement. The old public health movement (1975 to mid-1980s) was based on the biomedical model of health, focusing on factors impacting on individual health and environmental issues. The new public health approach (early 1980s to late 1990s) recognised the need for health promotion, highlighting the need to focus on collective factors influencing health and wellbeing, rather than the traditional focus on individual responsibility (Green et al 2019). During this period, the WHO's Health for All by the Year 2000 statement was published (WHO 1981), influenced by the Lalonde Report (Lalonde 1974), which highlighted the need for health promotion. The WHO's Ottawa Charter, developed in 1986, has been one of the most influential frameworks for health promotion and primary health care. The ecological public health movement emerged from the year 2000, recognising ecological and environmental issues, along with the necessity for sustainable use of resources. Multidisciplinary strategies have been highlighted to deal with health promotion in these areas due to complexity of health issues, including ongoing chronic diseases (Fleming et al 2019). In 2012, Health 2020: the European Policy for Health and Well-being was developed (WHO 2021f), complemented by the global health-promoting Sustainable Development Goals in 2015 (United Nations 2021).

Where to find out more on …

Health promotion charters and declarations

The five key strategies for the Ottawa Charter for Health Promotion are:

- build public health policy
- create supportive environments
- strengthen community action
- develop personal skills
- re-orient health services.

Source: Reprinted from World Health Organization (1986) The Ottawa Charter for Health Promotion, http://www.who.int/healthpromotion/conferences/previous/ottawa/en/

These can be compared with the Health 2000 key components and strategies (www.euro.who.int/en/health-topics/health-policy/health-2020-the-european-policy-for-health-and-well-being/about-health-2020) and the Sustainable Development Goals where each of the 17 goals is interconnected and challenged by ecological and environmental factors (www.undp.org/content/undp/en/home/sustainable-development-goals.html). See also Chapter 3.

All WHO health promotion charters and declarations will be further outlined in Table 1.3.

Health education

Health education is an integral strategy within health promotion. It can be described as assisting individuals, families and communities to develop skills through planned or opportunistic learning experiences to improve their health and wellbeing. Prevention, maintenance and restoring health is typically achieved through behavioural change which presents challenges due to complex SDH (Parker & Baldwin 2019a). Traditionally, health education has focused on individual behaviour change and not recognising wider influences of SDH. A more contemporary recognition of health education acknowledges its contribution to equity and empowerment, which are foundational objectives of health promotion (Green et al 2019).

The process of health education begins by building the knowledge base, then working with community members to identify strengths, weaknesses, assets, inequities, vulnerabilities or other aspects of community life that may impinge on health. This knowledge is gained through assessment, and maintaining a receptive and resourceful attitude towards new ideas and local approaches to thinking about problems or areas that need to be strengthened.

People's ability to interpret their health literacy skills to make positive decisions is impacted by complex situational pressures such as instructions on how to manage chronic diseases and hospital discharge information for culturally and linguistically diverse clients. This has confirmed the need for taking into account social, economic and environmental contexts when planning health education strategies (Nutbeam 2019). Building effective and sustainable health literacy is an important aspect of practice, as people need to understand how activities and processes affect their health. As such, health professionals need to appreciate the abilities of their clients to fully understand health information and health education, with health literacy being integral to effective health practices and behaviour change (Guzys 2021b). Health education facilitates empowerment by showing people where to access appropriate, relevant information on health and how to use it to enhance their health literacy and capacity.

The approach of knowledge plus capacity is the contemporary approach to health education. This approach is oriented towards improving self-efficacy and individual capacity to change (Guzys 2021b), which is essential for developing and using health literacy. Health education can provide people with substantive information and processes for accessing health knowledge, including the structures and processes that help them use this knowledge for self-management (functional health literacy), helpful techniques for influencing determinants in their local community and society (communicative health literacy), skills and mechanisms for developing coalitions and networks for change (critical health literacy), and political skills to engage in community action and work with others for health capacity building. Partnership approaches with health practitioners such as shared decision-making, client-centred care and self-management enhances people's capacity to be well informed and take an active part in decision-making about their healthcare. It is also vital for healthcare providers to develop effective health communication through a range of contemporary strategies including social marketing, digital and non-digital media and eHealth resources (Guzys 2021b).

Enabling approaches when working with culturally and linguistically diverse clients are of particular importance. To help reduce the impact of ill health, understanding the key concepts of cultural safety, cultural competence, cultural humility and cultural intelligence in health education helps to reduce the impacts of health inequity across diverse settings. These concepts facilitate understandings of the nuances of different cultures, and adaptations of health education practice to develop appropriate strategies that engage with a range of health knowledge, learning, motivations and behaviours (Luquis 2021).

Models of health education and health promotion

Improving health is complex, due to the underpinning SDH which need to be recognised within health education activities. Commonly used evidence-based health education and health promotion models that support individuals with planning their health behaviours are:

- Pender's health promotion model which is a socio-educational health educational model incorporating SDH and a nursing focus (Pender et al 2015, Whitehead 2021)
- Whitehead's effect planning model for health promotion that has a socio-ecological community development approach (Whitehead 2003, 2021)
- the PRECEDE-PROCEED model which uses a socio-ecological approach (Green & Kreuter 2005, Whitehead 2021)
- the health belief model where the focus is on social contexts of people's personal health behaviours (Taylor et al 2021, Becker 1974)
- the theory of planned behaviour model explains people's personal health seeking behaviours (Bastable 2014, Taylor et al 2021)
- the transtheoretical (stages of change) model which recognises personal challenges influencing people's health behaviours (Taylor et al 2021).

You can see there is an extensive theoretical base for health education and health promotion activities; however, the PRECEDE-PROCEED model is regarded as the most interdisciplinary and evidence-based health promotion program model (Whitehead 2021).

Health promotion evaluation

Evaluation of the effectiveness of health promotion activities is an essential step to ensure effectiveness and appropriateness of interventions. The principles of primary health care guide the evaluation. Where change is expected, evaluation strategies help to provide mutual feedback to all involved so that barriers and facilitating factors are identified and lessons learned can be taken away from one situation and applied to another.

Evaluation continues to be problematic in developing the evidence base for practice. Challenges include difficulties in measuring complex issues with contributing SDH. Change in health behaviour can be difficult to measure, especially in the short term. Some programs and projects simply conduct an internal review of general and immediate outcomes, while others may have large data sets to analyse. Whichever type of evaluation you are developing, it is imperative that you clarify sustainability indicators and social or cultural demographic population characteristics (Parker & Baldwin 2019b). Careful, thorough

evaluative information on processes and outcomes can be invaluable to future planning by indicating which groups or contexts are receptive to various health education strategies, how best to access community resources and how partnerships can be developed to help build community capacity. Evaluation is being increasingly mandated by funding bodies and should be integral to all health promotion practice.

When developing evaluation plans, it is important to remember to use multiple research methods, including the voices of participants. Different types of evaluation include:

- process evaluation, which is a formative evaluation reviewing ways in which strategies were implemented
- impact evaluation, where the program's objectives are assessed to see if the primary effects have been achieved
- outcome evaluation, where the long-term program effects are reviewed to ensure the project aim has been achieved (Taylor et al 2021, Parker & Baldwin 2019b).

WHAT'S THE POINT?

The Declaration of Alma-Ata, the Ottawa Charter and other health promotion and health education statements since that time are aimed at overcoming inequalities (bias and disadvantage) and inequities (unfair distribution of healthcare and other resources) through action on the SDH at all levels of society. The ultimate goal is social justice for health and wellbeing.

In 2008 the WHO and the Commission on the SDH commemorated the 30th anniversary of the Declaration of Alma-Ata by recommitting to the primary health care agenda in the report: 'Primary health care—now more than ever'. 'Now more than ever' referred to the state of global healthcare, which continues to this day to be plagued by inequitable access, impoverishing costs and erosion of people's trust in governments. Together, these factors constitute a threat to social stability. The primary health care approach challenged the presiding biomedical view of health, setting new contexts for health as a human right, ensuring equity and community participation. The WHO and Commission on the SDH statement refocused attention on how primary health care can be implemented in times of fiscal restraint and neoliberalism to improve health and wellbeing for individuals and families, and for communities as a whole, particularly for those impacted by vulnerabilities (Rifkin 2018). Since the development of the Ottawa Charter, there have been profound global changes such as: globalisation of trade; improved internet communication; epidemics and pandemics such as severe acute respiratory syndrome (SARS), Ebola and COVID-19; migration due to conflict; and changes to the burden of disease, most notably the rise of non-communicable diseases. These provide continuing challenges to the meaning, relevance and adaptation of the Ottawa Charter's strategies (Nutbeam 2019).

All of the declarations and charters (Table 1.3) have highlighted causal pathways linking social factors to health and wellbeing, in addition to health effects of widespread inequalities (bias and disadvantage) and inequities (the moral aspect of health inequality, in terms of policies and decisions taken on healthcare and the distribution of resources)

(Rifkin 2018). These important statements and the declarations from subsequent international meetings and policy deliberations have been unequivocal in their goal to address SDH, and they have been extremely powerful in shaping primary health care thinking today. Contemporary mainstream thinking in the promotion of health takes the view that without equal access to education, healthcare, transportation, nutritious food and social support, the world will never have health for all. In 2012, Professor Ilona Kickbusch, who convened the group that developed the original Ottawa Charter for Health Promotion, declared that all societies need to address 'the political, the commercial, the social, the environmental and the behavioural determinants of health' (Kickbusch 2012, p. 427), emphasising a global primary health care approach. This remains an ongoing challenge globally.

Promoting global health

There are major challenges to the management of contemporary health risks internationally, with health promotion requiring cooperation and coordination within and between countries. The maintenance and promotion of global delivery of the Sustainable Development Goals (Chapter 3) is a core government responsibility, with emerging impetus towards international legal commitments and obligations to ensure every person and community has the right to equitable health outcomes (Gostin et al 2019). Legal, policy and regulatory environments underpinned by evidence and human rights enhance accessibility to universal health coverage, thereby reducing risks for populations and enhancing sustainable, empowering health outcomes. Without supportive structures, resources and governance, many countries are not able to develop capacity to deliver essential health programs (Webb et al 2019).

Holst (2020) further highlights global health as a rights-based, universal good, recognising the impact of disproportionate availability of resources and how these are managed. It is noted that international public–private partnerships are tending to promote biomedical and technocratic approaches to health issues, without taking into

TABLE 1.3 Global health promotion conferences and charters

Year	Place	Outcomes	Conference document
1986	Ottawa, Canada	Confirmation of social justice and equity from Declaration of Alma-Ata with advocacy and mediation as the processes for enabling health promotion.	The Ottawa Charter for Health Promotion
1988	Adelaide, Australia	Confirmation of Ottawa Charter strategies and call for collaboration across all public policy levels. Support for developing counties recommended.	Adelaide Recommendations on Public Health Policy
1991	Sundsvall, Sweden	Call for the international community to create sustainable health and ecological environments.	Sundsvall Statement on Supportive Environments for Health
1997	Jakarta, Indonesia	Endorsement of a global health promotion alliance to advance priorities for action in health promotion, recognising changing SDH, need for collaborative health networks, shared learning and accountability and transparency in health promotion.	Jakarta Declaration on Leading Health Promotion into the 21st Century
2000	Mexico City, Mexico	Calling for promotion of health as a fundamental priority in all sectors and public policies in member countries.	Mexico Ministerial Statement for the Promotion of Health: From Ideas to Action
2005	Bangkok, Thailand	Identification of a need to close an implementation gap for Ottawa Charter resolutions. Recommendation for worldwide partnerships with global and local initiatives to promote health.	Bangkok Charter for Health Promotion in a Globalised World
2009	Nairobi, Kenya	Identified need for health promotion strategies to close the implementation gap in health and development.	Nairobi Call to Action
2013	Helsinki, Finland	Confirmed health and health equity as core government responsibilities. Call for effective public policies and resources to enable Health in All Policies across all government and non-government sectors.	The Helsinki Statement on Health in All Policies
2016	Shanghai, China	Commitment to enhance implementation of the Sustainable Development Goals through political and financial priorities in promoting health.	Shanghai Declaration on promoting health in the 2030 Agenda for Sustainable Development

Sources: World Health Organization (WHO), 2009. Milestones in health promotion. Statements from global conferences. WHO, Geneva; World Health Organization (WHO), 2014. Health in all policies: Helsinki statement. Framework for country action. WHO, Geneva; World Health Organization (WHO), 2017. Promoting health in the SDGs. Report on the 9th global conference for health promotion: All for Health, Health for All, 21–24 November 2016. WHO, Geneva; World Health Organization (WHO), 2021g. Nairobi call to action. WHO, Geneva.

account their complexities and contributing SDH, thereby leading to selective healthcare access. The ability to reduce health inequalities throughout the world is dependent on a human rights approach to health for all.

These features of global health promotion are supported by Labonté & Ruckert (2019), who recognise that promoting health at the global level requires not only major economic changes but consideration of communicative, cultural and cognitive factors in order to address an ever-increasing imbalance between people holding the majority of the world's health, resources and political power. Many crises are created by global forces and affect the most vulnerable disproportionately. In particular, global transport and trade has historically been a path for transmission of infectious diseases, epidemics and pandemics. Global market commodities create risks for development of non-communicable diseases with tobacco, alcohol and nutrition being global issues of concern. A further major issue has seen globalisation impacting on the world's labour markets, creating opportunities for a selection of people and families, while causing employment displacement and lack of opportunities for others (Taylor et al 2021, Labonté & Ruckert 2019).

Global strategies to promote sustainable development have been hindered by climate change crises, environmental degradation through unregulated activities such as excessive logging, overpopulation, geopolitical changes and destruction of biodiversity which have impacted low-socioeconomic populations, most notably Indigenous peoples. Environmental protection is embedded in the SDGs, with the ultimate aim of enhancing health and wellbeing. Global, national and local intersectoral activities are required, recognising interdependence of individual, community and political policies and actions to maintain livable, healthy environments (Raphael et al 2020, Taylor et al 2021). International aid granted by wealthier countries to support improved health, economic and social outcomes in poorer nations has frequently been underpinned by the eight Millennium Development Goals which preceded the current SDGs. However, increasing disagreement on the aims and intended impacts of these strategies has raised questions as to future sustainability of these approaches (Labonté & Ruckert 2019).

All the global health factors discussed can be viewed as SDH, influencing health and wellbeing beyond an individual level and capability. Globalisation has facilitated positive changes in population health status within a number of countries. However, contemporary globalisation has limited the governance of governments to sustain healthy living conditions through restructuring and manipulation of political and economic policies and regulations. As such, significant inequities remain in many populations across the world (Raphael et al 2020, Taylor et al 2021).

The political orientation of a country can also determine the outcomes of health promotion rhetoric. Raphael and colleagues (2020) have found that despite a country's explicit commitment to health promotion in public policy, governments at the local and national levels create policies and laws that do not necessarily result in implementation of such concepts in practice. Liberal welfare states such as Canada, Australia, New Zealand and the United Kingdom have all been seen to provide leadership in health promotion, but have favoured market-based approaches which have led to increasing individual responsibility and people's capacity to contribute financially to their healthcare. This emphasis has placed less focus on the impacts of SDH and providing the prerequisites for health than in social democratic nations such as Finland, Norway and Sweden who have achieved the greatest success in articulating health promotion concepts in policy, implementing these in communities and improving health outcomes. These examples demonstrate the importance for those involved in health promotion to understand that health promotion is inherently a political activity where social policy has an important influence on health outcomes. As such, gaining knowledge of broad policymaking processes is essential, as they impact a great deal on standards of living and quality of life (Marston 2019). Advocacy is required in many different places within the health system and other sectors.

Promoting global health clearly requires both diplomatic and evidence-based persuasive advocacy, based on social justice which affects how people live and their risks of ill health, chronic disease, disability and premature death. Addressing the need for ethical, equitable healthcare, including prevention and early intervention, includes a range of social, environmental, housing and employment factors, all of which promote security for all people (Marston 2019). Previously under-recognised SDH include union density and the presence of collective employment agreements that help reduce income inequality and improve human rights in the workplace, such as racial disparities in wages. Additionally, union influence has been able to negotiate safe crisis responses for workers through the COVID-19 pandemic (Economic Policy Institute [EPI] 2021, McNicholas et al 2020). Countries that have employment policies that support union membership and/or collective bargaining have better population health outcomes. These population-level policies are shaped by key forces that need ongoing attention. They include the power of markets and business, particularly globalised companies, unemployment, job security and financial pressures, with income inequities being experienced by many countries, families and communities (Raphael et al 2020). As health practitioners, we should have an

involvement with health and social policy decisions made by local and national government agencies, addressing health-promoting activities that acknowledge and take SDH into account. How we can advocate health-promoting policy formation is examined more closely in Chapter 2.

Primary, secondary and tertiary prevention

As one of the major elements of health promotion and health education, preventing ill health or injury is an instrumental goal of primary health care. Three levels of prevention, or preventative health, are widely accepted as encompassing the range of activities involved in preventing illness or injury. These levels, primary prevention, secondary prevention and tertiary prevention, distinguish between strategies aimed at maintaining health and wellbeing and preventing illness (primary), treating and limiting illness or injury (secondary), and rehabilitative or restorative actions (tertiary) (Guzys 2021a). The aim of primary prevention is to promote health by removing the precipitating causes and determinants of ill health or injury. These are also

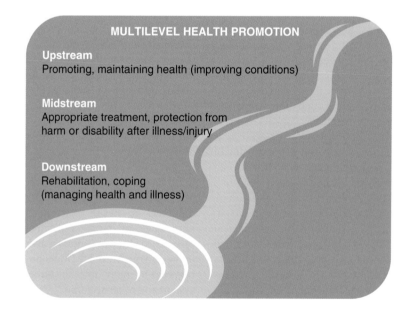

Figure 1.3 Primary, secondary and tertiary prevention

known as upstream strategies as they focus on healthy public policy and programs such as vaccination, tobacco control and promoting healthy lifestyles in areas such as nutrition, exercise and psychosocial environments. Secondary prevention includes screening for early detection and treatment of disease, often before symptoms are detected; for example, cervical and testicular cancer screening and treatment. Tertiary prevention is restorative, focusing on rehabilitation in a supportive community environment, such as cardiac and renal rehabilitation programs (Guzys 2021a, Parker & Baldwin 2019a).

Conceptualising health practitioners' activities across these three levels indicates a holistic, primary health care approach that can be applied across the lifespan. The metaphor of a waterfall illustrates this concept. Primary prevention activities at the community level are 'upstream' actions, such as developing educational materials to portray the benefits of nutrition or regular exercise to help individuals become health literate and make healthy choices. Besides offering encouragement for healthy individual choices, primary prevention includes lobbying the local council or government agencies to create the conditions that support these choices. This type of activity might include helping secure cost-effective foods or safe spaces for children to play. Secondary, or 'midstream', prevention includes such preventative activities as screening for skin cancer, conducting mammography clinics or establishing drop-in centres for adolescents or isolated older people. Tertiary prevention occurs 'downstream' and typically involves providing assistance or information to help people cope with a potentially disabling condition. This could involve the establishment of walking programs for those who have had a cardiac incident, support groups for family members coping with a loss or any measure that helps ensure continuity of care and health literacy, such as access to timely health advice (see Fig 1.3).

Nurses typically play an important role at all three levels of prevention. At the primary prevention level, it is common to see community health and practice nurses immunising children and public health or community health nurses working with a community to secure funding for a safe playground. At the secondary prevention level, a nurse practitioner may be seen running a youth drop-in centre (see,

for example, http://evolveyouth.org.nz/), while a practice nurse may be found undertaking tests to screen for cervical cancer. At the tertiary level, a specialist nurse may run a 'cardiac club' for people who have suffered a heart attack or a district nurse may do the same for people who have leg ulcers. These roles exemplify how health promotion is both a core skill and a theoretical underpinning of nursing practice.

Virtual health

Virtual or digital health refers to a range of technologies that can be used to assist clients in managing their health and wellbeing, including electronic health records, telehealth, wearable devices such as fitness trackers and the field of emerging artificial intelligence. These technologies have the potential for individuals, families and communities to have real time access to health and social services by overcoming barriers such as distance and lack of physical access. Health services are also able to monitor health system performance more accurately. However, digital technologies enhancing virtual health have limitations without privacy provisions, and if clients do not have the ability to access or understand information that is meaningful and relevant for their needs (AIHW 2020b). Health communication and health literacy are two major issues relating to these services.

The impact of the COVID-19 pandemic has highlighted the need for digital technologies, particularly for families requiring parent support. Recent research has highlighted how early parenting services have needed to modify their service provision to assist parents in virtual communities. Benefits have included a wider accessibility and reach of services and client receptiveness. Health practitioners have noted the need for client safety and confidentiality when delivering digital services, requirements for additional time to build online client relationships, technology disruptions and the need for staff development for this new approach (Bennett et al 2020). There are many examples of the use of digital health services for prevention and maintenance of health. It is vital that clients are able to work in partnership with community health professionals to develop meaningful online primary health care approaches.

Conclusion

Health and wellness are understood in different ways by different people and influenced by a multitude of environmental, contextual, ecological and social factors. In order to achieve good health and wellness we must base our practice on the principles of primary health care as a means of addressing the SDH, achieving equity, equality and inclusion, and promoting sustainable good health. It can be challenging for community health nurses to ensure they have the appropriate knowledge and skills to respond to the range of complex, socially determined issues. However, addressing health inequities through strengthening people's capacity to enhance their own health and wellbeing is a worthwhile and effective practice strategy. In the following chapter we will explore the impact of policy on practice, and the way in which policy contributes to creating the context within which we are able to bring a primary health care approach to our practice. But first, we will reflect on the big issues in this chapter and then introduce you to the Smiths and the Masons, two families who will join you on your journey through this book.

Reflecting on the Big Issues

This chapter outlined several 'big issues' including the following.

- Health is a state of balance between individual, social and environmental factors: the SDH.
- Being healthy includes wellbeing and happiness.
- Being healthy in any community means having equitable access to resources, empowerment, cultural inclusiveness, healthy environments and participation in decision-making.
- SDH have a significant role in determining the health status of people. These include biology/genetics, healthy child development, social supports, education/literacy, employment/working conditions, social environments, physical environments, health practices/coping skills, health services/resources and gender/culture.
- Healthy communities are the *synthesis* or product of people interacting with their environments when they work collaboratively to shape and develop the community in a way that will help them achieve positive health outcomes and capacities.

- Primary health care is a philosophy aimed at promoting social justice through the principles of accessible healthcare, appropriate technology, health promotion, cultural sensitivity and cultural safety, intersectoral collaboration and public participation.
- Primary health care principles focus on capacity building and empowerment of communities and those who reside in them.
- Social capital is created when people feel connected with others, developing mutuality and trust.
- Health literacy is empowering and a vital element of achieving equity in community health.
- Health practitioners undertake primary, secondary and tertiary prevention, using health promotion, appropriate technology and intersectoral collaboration.
- Health promotion is a combination of health education and helping people arrange the social, cultural and structural circumstances of their lives to maintain health.
- A range of charters and frameworks provide guidelines for health promotion across all communities.

Introducing the Smiths and the Masons

Australian family: The Masons

The Mason family lives in Maddington, a suburb of Perth, Western Australia (population 9136). The family consists of Colin (husband, age 44 years), Rebecca (wife, age 41), Emily (age 6), Caleb (age 4), Joe and Gemma (18-month-old twins). Emily goes to Maddington Public School, Caleb is about to start pre-primary, and Joe and Gemma go to day care two mornings a week. Rebecca attends a mothers' group organised through the twins' day care centre. They live in one of the older neighbourhoods, but on a street with several migrant families. Rebecca's mother lives in the wheatbelt, 3 hours' drive from Perth. Colin, who was previously a bricklayer, flies to a Pilbara mining site every 6 weeks for 4 weeks, works 12-hour shifts while he is in the mine, then returns home for 2 weeks. A downturn in the resource economy means Colin's work future is uncertain. He is facing redundancy and finds himself in a precarious work situation. Rebecca has struggled with her weight since giving birth to the twins and the child health nurse referred her to the GP, where she was diagnosed with metabolic syndrome. She is working with the practice nurse on a program of dietary management and activity. She goes to the gym two mornings a week while the twins are in day care and the rest of the time manages the home and family. Colin is relatively healthy but suffers from poor sleep habits related to his work and lifestyle. He enjoys a drink with his friends. Emily and Caleb are healthy, but Emily is having some difficulties coping with her first year of school. The twins are active but Gemma has eczema, which requires intermittent specialist treatment. Rising day care costs are making it difficult to keep the children in day care, which may impact on Rebecca's ability to get to the gym.

New Zealand family: The Smiths

The Smiths live in Papakura, South Auckland. The family consists of Jason (husband, age 34 years), Huia (wife, age 31), John (age 12), Aroha (age 8) and Jake (age 4). Jason works in the city as a senior adviser for a small Māori Land Trust. Huia works full-time as a Māori liaison teacher. John attends the local Kura Kaupapa Māori (Māori-language primary school) where he enjoys kapa haka (Māori dance). John has recently been diagnosed with a learning disability. Aroha also attends Kura Kaupapa. John and Aroha catch the bus to Kura most days but Huia drops them off when she can. Jake is 4 years old and attends a local Kōhanga Reo (Māori-language preschool). He is eligible for 20 hours of free preschool education available to all children aged 3 and 4 years in New Zealand. Jake also has asthma for which he has been hospitalised several times. Huia spends a lot of her free time at the local marae where she helps run a fitness program for elders. Jason struggles with his weight and has high blood pressure.

CASE
STUDY
1b

Promoting health for the Smiths and Masons

Strategies for promoting health in the three communities of the Smiths and the Masons are planned around the Ottawa Charter; that is, promoting healthy public policies, creating supportive environments, strengthening community action, developing personal skills and reorienting health services. For example, in the mining community we may want to debate the creation of wealth from the mining companies that provide employment versus the distribution of resources and services that may disadvantage some members of the community. The mining camp has a dearth of supportive services for Colin's health and wellbeing, especially as he suffers from isolation and a lack of work–life balance. Colin is also not included in the local community, and in some cases when he goes to town he is made to feel the resentment of the locals. Colin needs support for healthy ways of coping while he is up at the site, which involves some personal skill development and support from the mine site health service.

Maddington has assets and resources to support families, and several social networks for miners' wives. However, there is considerable stress on family life, with Rebecca having to get the children to child care, school and the child health nurse. Rebecca enjoys the social support of a group of wives of fly-in fly-out (FIFO) workers.

Like Maddington, Papakura has a range of services available for families but not all are considered culturally appropriate. The family struggles with finding appropriate child care and before and after school care to match their needs with both Jason and Huia working full-time. Jason has trouble accessing primary health care services due to the long hours he works and there is no workplace health program due to the small size of the trust he works for.

Reflective questions: How would I use this knowledge in practice?

1 Explain the link between climate change, social disadvantage and sustainable communities.

2 What is the difference between bonding and bridging social capital?

3 Create a brief map with an overview of the SDH that affect the health and wellbeing of the Smith and Mason families.

4 Identify one research question that would help inform your work with either the Mason or the Smith family.

5 How would you deal with the tensions in the mining town in such a way that would promote the health of both the townspeople and the mining employees?

6 What do you see as your role in building healthy public policy, creating supportive environments, strengthening community action, developing personal skills and reorienting health services in each of these communities?

7 Do you think the five strategies of the Ottawa Charter can yield health improvements for the host communities of Papakura and Maddington?

8 What level of advocacy could you engage in to make visible the need for community resources in the mining community?

9 How will you know if your strategies for health promotion are helpful?

References

Atanasova, S., Petric, G., 2019. Collective empowerment on online health communities: Scale development and empirical validation. J. Med. Internet. Res., 21 (11), e14392. Online. Available: https://doi.org/10.2196/14392.

Australian Bureau of Statistics (ABS). National Health Survey: Health literacy. ABS, Canberra.

Australian Institute of Health and Welfare (AIHW), 2018. Australia's health 2018. Australia's health series no. 16. AUS 221. AIHW, Canberra.

Australian Institute of Health and Welfare (AIHW), 2020a. Australia's health 2020. AIHW, Canberra.

Australian Institute of Health and Welfare (AIHW), 2020b. Digital health. AIHW, Canberra.

Baldwin, L., Fleming, M.L., 2019. Communities and organisational strategies. In: Fleming, M.L., Parker, E., Correa-Velez, I., (Eds), Introduction to public health, fourth ed. Elsevier, Sydney, pp. 143–153.

Bastable, S., 2014. Nurse as educator: Principles of teaching and learning for nursing practice, fourth ed. Jones & Bartlett Learning, MA.

Baum, F., 2003. Primary health care: Can the dream be revived? Dev. Pract., 13 (5), 515–519.

Becker, M.H. (Ed.), 1974. The health belief model and personal health behavior. Charles B. Slack, New Jersey.

Bennett, E., Simpson, W., Fowler, C., et al, 2020. Enhancing access to parenting services using digital technology supported practices. Child and Family Health Nursing, 17 (1), 4–11.

Center for Advanced Research on Language Acquisition. 2019. What is culture? University of Minnesota, Minneapolis, MN. Online. Available: https://carla.umn.edu/culture/definitions.html

Centers for Disease Control and Prevention (CDC). 2019. Culture and health literacy. Online. Available: www.cdc.gov/healthliteracy/culture.html.

Centers for Disease Control and Prevention (CDC). 2021. About social determinants of health. Online. Available: www.cdc.gov/socialdeterminants/about.html.

Curtis, E., Jones, R., Tipene-Leach, D., et al, 2019. Why cultural safety rather than cultural competency is required to achieve health equity: A literature review and recommended definition. Int. J. Equity Health, 18 (174), 1–17.

Durie, M., 1999. Whaiora: Māori health development, second ed, Oxford University Press, Auckland.

Economic Policy Institute (EPI), 2021. Unions help reduce disparities and strengthen our democracy. EPI, Washington, DC. Online. Available: https://files.epi.org/uploads/226030.pdf.

Ehrlich, K.B., 2020. How does the social world shape health across the lifespan? Insights and new directions. Am. Psychol., 75 (9), 1231–1241. Online. Available: https://doi.org/10.1037/amp0000757.

Fleming, M.L., 2019. Defining health and public health. In Fleming, M.L., Parker, E., Correa-Velez, I., (Eds), Introduction to public health, fourth ed, Elsevier, Sydney, pp. 3–15.

Fleming, M.L., Parker, E., Correa-Velez, 2019. Introduction to public health, fourth ed. Elsevier, Sydney.

Gostin L.O., Monahan J.T., Kaldor, J., et al, 2019. The legal determinants of health: Harnessing the power of law for global health and sustainable development. The Lancet, 393, 1857–1910. Online. Available: http://dx.doi.org/10.1016/S0140-6736(19)30233-8.

Green, J., Cross, R., Woodall, J., et al, 2019. Health promotion. Planning and strategies, fourth ed, Sage, United Kingdom.

Green, L.W., Kreuter, M.W., 2005. Health program planning: An educational and ecological approach, fourth ed, McGraw-Hill Higher Education, New York.

Gugglberger, L., 2019. The multifaceted relationship between health promotion and health literacy. Health Promot. Int., 34, 887–891. Online. Available: https://doi.org/10.1093/heapro/daz093.

Guzys, D., 2021a. Community and primary health care. In: Guzys, D., Brown, R., Halcomb, E., Whitehead, D., (Eds), An introduction to community and primary health care, third ed, Cambridge, Port Melbourne, pp. 3–21.

Guzys, D., 2021b. Empowering individuals, groups and communities. In: Guzys, D., Brown, R., Halcomb, E., Whitehead, D., (Eds), An introduction to community and primary health care, third ed, Cambridge, Port Melbourne, pp. 22–40.

Holst, J., 2020. Global health-emergence, hegemonic trends and biomedical reductionism. Glob. Health, 16 (42), 2–11. Online. Available: https://doi.org/10.1186/s12992-020-00573-4.

Huber, M., Knottnerus, J.A., Green, L., et al, 2011. How should we define health? BMJ, 343, d4163. Online. Available: https://doi.org/10.1136/bmj.d4163.

Huber, M., van Vliet, M., Giezenberg, M., et al, 2016. Towards a 'patient-centred' operationalisation of the new dynamic concept of health: A mixed methods study. BMJ Open, 5, e010091. Online. Available: https://doi.org/10.1136/bmjopen-2015-010091.

Keleher, H., 2020a. Public health in Australia. In Willis, E., Reynolds, L., Rudge, T. (Eds), Understanding the Australian health care system, fourth ed. Elsevier, Sydney, pp. 71–84.

Keleher, H., 2020b. Primary health care in Australia. In Willis, E., Reynolds, L., Rudge, T. (Eds), Understanding the Australian health care system, fourth ed. Elsevier, Sydney, pp. 85–99.

Kendall, G., Nguyen, H., Ong, R., 2019. The association between income, wealth, economic security perception, and health: A longitudinal Australian study. Health Sociol. Rev., 28 (1), 20–38.

Kickbusch, I., 2012. Addressing the interface of the political and commercial determinants of health. Health Promot. Int., 27 (4), 427–428. Online. Available: https://doi.org/10.1093/heapro/das057.

Labonté, R., Ruckert, A., 2019. Health equity in a globalizing era: Past challenges, future prospects. Oxford University Press, United Kingdom.

Lalonde, M., 1974. A new perspective on the health of Canadians. Minister of Supply and Services Canada, Ottawa, Ontario. Online. Available: www.phac-aspc.gc.ca/ph-sp/pdf/perspect-eng.pdf

Leonardi, F., 2018. The definition of health: Towards new perspectives. Int. J. Health Serv., 48 (4), 735–748. Online. Available: https://doi.org/10.1177/0020731418782653.

Luquis, R.R., 2021. Integrating the concept of cultural intelligence into health education and health promotion. Health Educ. J., 1–11. Online. Available: https://doi.org/10.1177/00178969211021884.

Makridis, C.A., Wu, C., 2021. How social capital helps communities weather the COVID-19 pandemic. PLoS ONE, 16 (1), e0245135. Online. Available: https://doi.org/10.1371/journal.pone.0245135.

Marmot, M., 2019. The art of medicine. Punitive social policy: An upstream determinant of health. The Lancet, 394, 376–377.

Marmot, M., Allen, J., Boyce, T., et al, 2020. Health equity in England: The Marmot Review 10 years on. Institute of Health Equity, London.

Marston, G., 2019. Public health and social policy. In: Fleming, M.L., Parker, E., Correa-Velez, I., (Eds), Introduction to public health, fourth ed, Elsevier, Sydney, pp. 85–97.

McKillop, A., Munns, A., 2021. Working in primary and community health sectors. In: Crisp, J., Douglas, C., Rebeiro, G., Waters, D. (Eds), Potter and Perry's fundamentals of nursing, sixth ed. Elsevier, Sydney, pp. 1413–1445.

McNicholas, C., Rhinehart, L., Poydock, M., et al, 2020. Why unions are good for workers—especially in a crisis like COVID-19. Economic Policy Institute, Washington, DC. Online. Available: https://files.epi.org/pdf/204014.pdf.

Milken Institute School of Public Health, George Washington University, 2020. Equity vs equality: What's the difference? Online. Available: https://onlinepublichealth.gwu.edu/resources/equity-vs-equality/.

Munns, A., 2021. Community midwifery: A primary health care approach to care during pregnancy for Aboriginal and Torres Strait Islander women. Aust. J. Prim. Health, 27, 57–61. Online. Available: https://doi.org/10.1071/PY20105.

National Aboriginal Health Strategy Working Party, 1989. National Aboriginal Health Strategy. Commonwealth of Australia, Canberra.

National Wellness Institute, 2020. The six dimensions of wellness. Online. Available: https://nationalwellness.org/resources/six-dimensions-of-wellness/.

Nutbeam, D., 2019. Health education and health promotion revisited. Health Educ. J., 78 (6), 705–709.

Nutbeam, D., Lloyd, J.E., 2021. Understanding and responding to health literacy as a social determinant of health. Annu. Rev. Public Health, 42, 159–173. Online. Available: https://doi.org/10.1146/annurev-publhealth-090419-102529.

Office of Disease Prevention and Health Promotion (ODPHP), 2020a. Determinants of health. Washington, DC, US Department of Health and Human Services, Washington, DC. Online. Available: www.healthypeople.gov/2020/about/foundation-health-measures/Determinants-of-Health.

Office of Disease Prevention and Health Promotion (ODPHP), 2020b. Social determinants of health. Washington, DC, US Department of Health and Human Services, Washington, DC. Online. Available: www.healthypeople.gov/2020/topics-objectives/topic/social-determinants-of-health.

Parker, E., Baldwin, L., 2019a. Refocusing public health: Emphasising health promotion and protection. In: Fleming, M.L., Parker, E., Correa-Velez, I., (Eds), Introduction to public health, fourth ed. Elsevier, Sydney, pp. 172–183.

Parker, E., Baldwin, L., 2019b. Contemporary practice. In: Fleming, M.L., Parker, E., Correa-Velez, I., (Eds), Introduction to public health, fourth ed. Elsevier, Sydney, pp. 184–196.

Patient Safety Network and Agency for Healthcare Research and Quality (AHRQ), 2019. Health literacy. Patient Safety Network and AHRQ, Maryland.

Pender, N.J., Murdaugh, C.L., Parsons, M.A., 2015. Health promotion in nursing practice, seventh ed. Pearson, New Jersey.

Ramsden, I., 1993. Cultural safety in nursing education in Aotearoa. Nurs. Prax. N. Z., 8 (3), 4–10.

Raphael, D., Bryant, T., Mikkonen, J., et al, 2020. Social determinants of health: The Canadian facts. Ontario Tech University Faculty of Health Sciences and Toronto, York University School of Health Policy and Management, Oshawa.

Rifkin, S.B., 2018. Alma Ata after 40 years: Primary health care and health for all—from consensus to complexity. BMJ Glob. Health., 3:e001188. Online. Available: https://doi.org/10.1136/bmjgh-2018-001188.

Sykes, S., Wills, J., 2018. Challenges and opportunities in building critical health literacy. Glob. Health Promot., 25 (4), 48–56. Online. Available: https://doi.org/10.1177/1757975918789352.

Taylor, J., O'Hara, L., Talbot, L., et al, 2021. Promoting health. The primary health care approach, seventh ed., Elsevier, Sydney.

United Nations, 2021. Sustainable development goals. United Nations Development Programme, New York.

Wakerman, J., Humphreys, J., Russell, D., et al, 2019. Remote health workforce turnover and retention: What are the policy and practice priorities? Hum. Resour. Health, 17 (99), 1–8. Online. Available: https://doi.org/10.1186/s12960-019-0432-y.

Webb, D., Small, R., Gregor, E., 2019. Universal health coverage for sustainable development. United Nations HIV, Health and Development Group (HHD) of the UNDP Bureau for Policy and Programme Support (BPPS).

Whitehead, D., 2003. A stage planning process model for health promotion/health education practice. J. Clin. Nurs., 36, 417–425.

Whitehead, D., 2021. Health-related planning and evaluation. In: Guzys, D., Brown, R., Halcomb, E., Whitehead, D., (Eds), An introduction to community and primary health care, third ed. Cambridge, Port Melbourne, pp. 188–205.

Wilkinson, R., Marmot, M. (Eds), 2003. Social determinants of health: The solid facts, second ed. WHO, Geneva.

World Bank, 2021. Social inclusion. Online. Available: www.worldbank.org/en/topic/social-inclusion.

World Health Organization (WHO), 1978. Declaration of the Alma-Ata. WHO, Geneva. Online. Available: www.who.int/publications/almaata_decration_en.pdf

World Health Organization (WHO), 1981. Global strategy for health for all by the year 2000. Health For All Series No. 3. WHO, Geneva.

World Health Organization (WHO), 2009. Milestones in health promotion. Statements from global conferences. WHO, Geneva.

World Health Organization (WHO), 2014. Health in all policies: Helsinki statement. Framework for country action. WHO, Geneva.

World Health Organization (WHO), 2017. Promoting health in the SDGs. Report on the 9th global conference for health promotion: All for Health, Health for All, 21–24 November 2016. WHO, Geneva.

World Health Organization (WHO), 2020a. Basic documents. Forty-ninth edition 2020.WHO, Geneva. Online. Available: https://apps.who.int/gb/bd/pdf_files/BD_49th-en.pdf.

World Health Organization (WHO), 2020b. Children: improving survival and well-being. WHO, Geneva. Online. Available: www.who.int/news-room/fact-sheets/detail/children-reducing-mortality.

World Health Organization (WHO), 2021a. Urban health initiative—A model process for catalysing change. Online. Available: www.who.int/publications/i/item/WHO-HEP-ECH-AQH-2021-1.

World Health Organization (WHO), 2021b. Social determinants of health. WHO, Geneva. Online. Available: www.who.int/health-topics/social-determinants-of-health#tab=tab_1.

World Health Organization (WHO), 2021c. Poverty. WHO, Geneva and Regional Office for Africa.

World Health Organization (WHO), 2021d. Health promotion. WHO, Geneva. Online. Available: www.who.int/teams/health-promotion/enhanced-wellbeing/first-global-conference.

World Health Organization (WHO), 2021e. Health promotion. WHO, Geneva. Online. Available: www.who.int/westernpacific/health-topics/health-promotion.

World Health Organization (WHO), 2021f. About health 2020. WHO, Geneva.

World Health Organization (WHO), 2021g. Nairobi call to action. WHO, Geneva.

World Health Organization (WHO), UNICEF, 1978. Primary health care. WHO, Geneva.

World Meteorological Organization (WMO), 2021. 2020 on track to be one of three warmest years on record. WMO, Geneva.

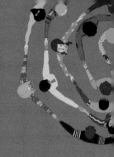

CHAPTER 2

Healthy policies for healthy communities

Introduction

Growing healthy communities does not occur in isolation from the political and economic drivers that influence our societies: local, national and global. This chapter outlines the Australian and New Zealand healthcare systems and the way in which policy is formed. This provides the basis from which we can situate primary health care within the current political context, enabling nurses and other health practitioners to engage in policy formation with their communities and understand how policy drivers influence practice.

The Australian and New Zealand healthcare systems both exist as part of a wider system of government. These wider systems comprise representative democracies whereby elected officials represent a group of people and make decisions on their behalf. The types of policies that drive both Australian and New Zealand health systems often depend on the elected government. An elected government that has a stronger neoliberal approach (e.g. advocates policies that revolve around privatisation, free trade, deregulation and tax cuts) may prefer a different approach to health policy than a government that has a more social democratic approach (e.g. prefers policies that support economic and social intervention to achieve social equity). Australian and New Zealand health policies often sit somewhere in the middle of this spectrum. Further detail on policymaking is found later in the chapter, but it is important to understand the approach of the government currently in power as this gives us greater

OBJECTIVES

By the end of this chapter you will be able to:

1 describe the Australian and New Zealand health systems

2 explain the impact of policy on primary health care practice

3 describe the features of a primary health care system that contribute to better health and wellbeing

4 analyse the successes, failures and policy gaps that have occurred in your national health policies

5 discuss the role of the nurse and other health practitioners in policy planning and implementation.

understanding of what health policies may be more likely and what approaches may be more effective when advocating change. As a matter of course, nurses and other health practitioners working in primary health care should have a good understanding of who the government of the day is, what impact their policies may have on practice and how they can influence these policies. In order to do this, it is important to understand how a health system works.

The Australian healthcare system

The system of healthcare in Australia is built on the principle of universal care for all citizens paid for by their taxes. Australia has a total annual expenditure on health of 10% of Australia's gross domestic product (GDP) (Australian Institute of Health and Welfare 2020). Health services are funded through Medicare, the national insurance scheme that provides each member of society with the ability to attend any one of a number of services at no cost, or, in the case of private providers such as general practitioners, by paying an additional surcharge or co-payment. Many people also have private health insurance, which covers them and their family for a wider range of services than are paid for by Medicare, including dental healthcare, massage, optometry and other services. Private health cover is subsidised through the private health insurance rebate and can be used for care in a public or private hospital. Because insurance costs are high, especially for families, having additional coverage advantages the most affluent, leaving the poor further disadvantaged. Means testing for private insurance subsidies were introduced in 2013 but inequities persist (Collyer et al 2020).

KEY POINT

Medicare is Australia's publicly funded universal healthcare system that provides all Australians with the ability to attend many healthcare services at no cost or at an affordable cost.

BOX 2.1

....

AUSTRALIAN STATUTORY AGENCIES

....

This box provides links to some of Australia's statutory bodies. A full list can be found at: www.health.gov.au/about-us/who-we-are/our-portfolio

- Australian Commission on Safety and Quality in Health Care (ACSQHC) (www.safetyandquality.gov.au)
- Australian Aged Care Quality and Safety Commission (www.agedcarequality.gov.au)
- Australian Institute of Health and Welfare (AIHW) (www.aihw.gov.au)
- Australian Digital Health Agency (www.digitalhealth.gov.au)
- Cancer Australia (www.canceraustralia.gov.au)
- National Health and Medical Research Council (NHMRC) (www.nhmrc.gov.au)

The Australian Government Department of Health (www.health.gov.au) has overall responsibility for healthcare in Australia, working through 19 statutory agencies and commissions. Box 2.1 describes some examples of these agencies. The Department of Health is responsible for national health policy, subsidisation of public hospitals, the Medicare Benefits Schedule, the Pharmaceutical Benefits Scheme and the Therapeutic Goods Administration, which monitors and regulates medicines, blood and tissue (Willis et al 2020). The Department also oversees a range of national health programs including those in ageing and aged care, mental health, Aboriginal and Torres Strait Islander health, primary and ambulatory care and health protection. Health protection includes public health surveillance, emergency preparedness and responses, food policy, chronic and communicable disease control, health promotion and harm reduction related to substance abuse (Willis et al 2020). Figure 2.1 shows the complex nature of the Australian health system, illustrating the differing tiers within the system and how each is required to create a comprehensive approach to health.

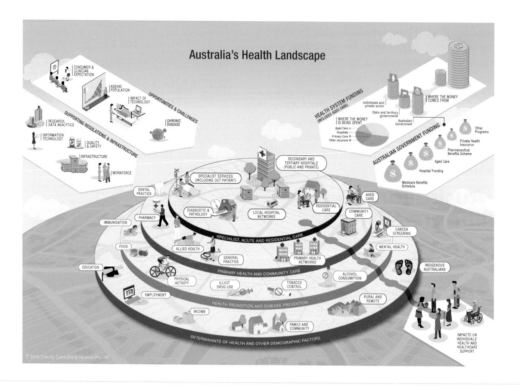

Figure 2.1 The Australian Health System

Source: www.health.gov.au/sites/default/files/australia-s-health-landscape_1.jpg. With permission from Gravity Consulting Services Pty Ltd.

The Australian health system is monitored through the Australian Health Performance Framework (AHPF) which measures health status, determinants of health and health system performance. Each category includes a range of indicators that can be broken down and analysed for specific population groups, providing a comprehensive overview of the performance of the system. The AHPF includes primary, secondary and tertiary measures.

Restructuring of health services is a regular occurrence in many state-based health and hospital services. Various administrative bodies take responsibility for individual hospitals, or district-level services. In most cases, a health service district will include both general and specialist hospitals, some specialising in certain populations (women and children) and others specialising in certain types of treatment (cancer care, various surgical specialties).

Where to find out more on …

Information on Australia's overall health performance:

- www.aihw.gov.au/reports-data/australias-health-performance/australias-health-performance-framework

Information on Australia's primary care performance:

- www.aihw.gov.au/reports-data/health-welfare-services/primary-health-care/data-sources

Information on Australia's hospital performance:

- www.aihw.gov.au/myhospitals

Certain hospitals are designated as state trauma centres, able to accommodate a wide range of emergencies, while others have the capacity for only minor emergency treatments, and are usually bypassed in emergencies of any substance. In addition to hospital services, patients in most health service districts have access to specialised drug and alcohol treatment services, state-based ambulance services, aged care, mental health hostels, the Australian Red Cross Lifeblood and the Royal Flying Doctor Service, which provides air transportation for health practitioners to attend to people in remote areas and for patient access to tertiary care. Although comparisons between different health systems are difficult because of variable reporting, among OECD countries, Australia compares well on such indicators as tobacco smoking, life expectancy and mortality from cardiovascular disease. Where we compare less favourably is on national indicators of infant mortality, obesity and alcohol consumption (OECD/WHO 2020). Most of these less favourable indicators are improving, but there remains a need to continue addressing inequities between different population groups to improve the overall health indicators. In the areas of alcohol consumption and obesity, the country is among the worst third of OECD countries (OECD/WHO 2020).

The Australian Government has developed a long-term national health plan comprising four pillars: 1. primary care; 2. supporting public and private hospitals; 3. mental health and preventive health; and 4. health research. Each pillar has a set of priority areas for action (Australian Government Department of Health 2019). Box 2.2 shows the priorities for primary care.

Although priorities can change according to a particular political agenda as noted earlier, the priorities for population health are generally non-partisan, and based on strong research evidence. In recent years, the government has also been working towards equitable distribution of digitally mediated communication and information. Access to digital technologies is an important equity issue, with those living in disadvantaged circumstances having the least access to health information. The National Digital Health Strategy is intended to help people become empowered partners in care, and to assist health practitioners interact with them and with one another (Australian Digital Health Agency 2019). A personalised health record, access to telehealth and

---

BOX 2.2

....

AUSTRALIAN GOVERNMENT DEPARTMENT OF HEALTH PRIORITIES FOR PRIMARY CARE 2019

....

- To put into operation the Commonwealth Government's 10-year primary healthcare plan, incorporating contemporary strategies such as genomics testing and telehealth
- Strengthen the responsibilities and scopes of practice of nurses and pharmacists in the development and delivery of primary healthcare
- Enhance access to novel drugs and therapies, noting recent multi-tumour treatments
- Recruit and provide an additional 3,000 doctors and nursing professionals to country areas
- Through primary healthcare strategies, preventable blindness in Indigenous communities will be brought to an end by 2025
- Through primary healthcare strategies, preventable deafness in Indigenous communities will be brought to an end
- Through primary healthcare strategies, rheumatic heart disease will be eliminated by 2030
- To progress a National Rural Generalist training program for doctors

Source: Adapted from Australian Government Department of Health, 2019. Australia's long-term national health plan to build the world's best health system. In Australian Government Department of Health (August). https://www.health.gov.au/sites/default/files/australia-s-long-term-national-health-plan_0.pdf

---

electronic prescriptions are the current cornerstones of the strategy that aims to improve health outcomes for Australians through better use of technology (www.digitalhealth.gov.au).

One of the most challenging aspects of the Australian health system is that responsibility for health services is distributed through Commonwealth, state, territory and local jurisdictions. This can cause duplication of effort and a lack of clarity in reporting mechanisms as well as cost-shifting (Krassnitzer 2020). Competition between acute and community services adds another layer of complexity. Community nursing services such as district nursing services are funded directly through regional health services, through contracts with public hospitals to provide specified services or through state or territory health departments. For older people, after many years of joint Commonwealth and state and territory funding, the bulk of community aged care services are now funded and controlled by the Australian Government through the Commonwealth Home Support Programme (CHSP). Older people with complex needs have their care funded through the Home Care Packages (HCP) program which supports older people to remain at home (Hodgkin & Mahoney 2020). My Aged Care is the primary portal for information related to aged care in Australia, linking policy, practice, referrals and resources. Further information can be found at www.myagedcare.gov.au.

For Australians under 65 with disability, the National Disability Insurance Scheme (NDIS) provides support for them, their families and their carers. The NDIS helps people with disability to receive the support they need to meet their needs including access to mainstream services, access to community services and support, maintaining informal support arrangements and receiving reasonable and necessary funding and equipment. The NDIS takes a lifetime approach to support, investing early in lives to make a difference in the longer term. Further information can be found on the NDIS website at www.ndis.gov.au. Disability is discussed further in Chapter 5.

Community nurses and other health practitioners can be employed by any of these agencies, attached to Commonwealth programs such as: the CHSP program; state or territory public health or education departments; district community services such as Silver Chain Nursing, Blue Care and Bolton Clarke; or a range of agencies responsible for specific population groups or those with a unique focus, such as the not-for-profit centres to help victims of violence, or torture and trauma survivors. In any context, health practitioners' registration to practise is governed by the National Registration and Accreditation Scheme (NRAS), which has oversight for accreditation, regulation and monitoring of all health practitioners. Professions in the scheme include chiropractors, dental practitioners, medical practitioners, nurses and midwives, optometrists, osteopaths, pharmacists, physiotherapists, podiatrists, psychologists, Aboriginal and Torres Strait Islander

health practitioners, Chinese medicine practitioners and medical radiation practitioners, each with their own accrediting body, such as the Nursing and Midwifery Board of Australia. The Australian Health Practitioner Regulation Agency (AHPRA) administers NRAS and provides administrative support to the National Boards.

KEY POINT

Australian nurses are registered with the Nursing and Midwifery Board of Australia and regulated through the Australian Health Practitioners Registration Authority (AHPRA).

Most Australian medical practitioners are self-employed general practitioners (GPs), or consultants who practise on a contractual basis in public, and sometimes private, hospitals. Allied health practitioners and paramedics are typically employed by hospitals or health districts, and some can charge a fee-for-service, including acupuncturists, podiatrists and naturopaths. Paramedics may also be employed by not-for-profit organisations such as the St John Ambulance Service. St John provides an air ambulance and ground ambulance service, and there are subsidised helicopters for beach patrols and surf rescues. There are also volunteer ambulance officers in rural ambulances and in attendance at metropolitan and rural events. Nurses and midwives can be employed in hospitals or health agencies, with many being appointed to government agencies at the state, territory, regional or local level. Some nurse practitioners and other nurse entrepreneurs have established clinics, and there are also midwives who work privately or in group practices to provide birthing services, or other consultations. Based on their insights into both the 'business' of health and the many dimensions of achieving better health for the population, these nurses should play an expanding role in policy development (Rasheed et al 2020).

As people age, their health and social needs frequently become more complex. Multiple health and social practitioners may become involved in the care of a person and this can result in poor coordination of services. One way of addressing this has been the development of integrated care. Integrated care is a systems response to increasing numbers of people living with long-term conditions and is being implemented in many countries including Australia and New Zealand. Integrated care has a number of definitions, but for the purposes of this discussion we will use a process-based definition that describes integrated care as the '... connectivity, alignment and collaboration within and between the cure and care sectors ... [designed] to enhance quality of care and quality of life, consumer satisfaction and system efficiency for people by cutting across multiple services, providers and settings' (World Health Organization [WHO] 2016, p. 4).

> **KEY POINT**
> ....
> Integrated care is an approach to ensuring people's care is coordinated, accessible and appropriate.

New models of care built around the concept of organising, managing and integrating health services so that people get the care they need, when and where they need it, and in ways that meet their needs in the most appropriate and effective ways is a worthy goal. The Western Sydney Integrated Care Program (WSICP) and the Gold Coast Integrated Care (GCIC) program are two examples of multilevel programs designed to improve patient-centred care in a complex system. Both programs use risk stratification (identification of those people with multiple co-morbidities and/or at greatest risk of hospitalisation) to ensure people's care is well coordinated (Scuffham et al 2017, Trankle et al 2019). Care facilitators, holistic assessment of needs, pro-active management of people with chronic or complex conditions and development of shared care plans are features of both models (Cooper et al 2015, Scuffham et al 2017, Trankle et al 2019). Evaluation of these models is under way, with qualitative findings from the Western Sydney model showing care facilitators were successful in helping people access appropriate services but

access to shared care records and electronic communication across sectors remain problematic (Trankle et al 2019).

The New Zealand healthcare system

Health and disability services in New Zealand are delivered by a complex network of people and organisations. Overall responsibility for the delivery of health services lies with the Minister of Health. The holder of this post is elected through the democratic process to government, and subsequently appointed to the role of Minister. The Minister of Health then works with the Ministry of Health to provide overall leadership, direction and stewardship for the healthcare system. The New Zealand Health Strategy (Ministry of Health 2016), He Korowai Oranga Māori Health Strategy (New Zealand Ministry of Health 2001 [updated 2013/14]) and Whakamaua: Māori Health Action Plan 2020-2025 (Ministry of Health 2020b) provide the direction for the current system of healthcare in New Zealand. Box 2.3 provides links to these documents.

> **KEY POINT**
> ....
> The New Zealand health system is guided by three strategic documents: the New Zealand Health Strategy (2016), He Korowai Oranga Māori Health Strategy (2001 [updated 2013/14]) and Whakamaua: Māori Health Action Plan 2020-2025 (2020).

District Health Boards (DHBs) provide the majority of public health services to New Zealanders. There are currently 20 DHBs in New Zealand, each mandated to plan, manage, provide and purchase services for the population of their district. This includes funding for public health services, primary health care services (through primary health organisations, discussed later in the chapter), aged care, and services provided by other non-government health providers including Māori and Pacific providers (www.health.govt.nz/new-zealand-health-system/overview-health-system).

BOX 2.3

NEW ZEALAND HEALTH SYSTEM STRATEGIC DOCUMENTS

- New Zealand Health Strategy: www.health. govt.nz/publication/new-zealand-health-strategy-2016
- He Korowai Oranga Māori Health Strategy: www.health.govt.nz/our-work/populations/maori-health/he-korowai-oranga
- Whakamaua: Māori Health Action Plan 2020-2025: www.health.govt.nz/publication/whakamaua-maori-health-action-plan-2020-2025

strategic direction and actions to improve health outcomes for Pacific people in New Zealand who experience significant disparities in health compared with non-Māori and non-Pacific people. The Healthy Ageing Strategy (Associate Minister of Health 2016) with its updated priority actions for 2019 to 2022 (www.health.govt.nz/our-work/life-stages/health-older-people/healthy-ageing-strategy-update/priority-actions-2019-2022) and the New Zealand Disability Strategy 2016–2026 (Office for Disability Issues 2016) provide further specific guidance in the areas of ageing and disability.

POINT TO PONDER

What differences can you identify between the Australian and New Zealand health systems?

Māori and Pacific providers play a particularly important role in the provision of services to their own population groups, emphasising culturally appropriate services as significant in achieving improved outcomes.

In 2019 and 2020 a Health and Disability System Review was undertaken to provide direction for future health provision in New Zealand. The review proposed removing all DHBs and creating one entity called Health New Zealand (HNZ), establishing a Māori Health Authority as an independent departmental agency with responsibility for advising the Minister on all aspects of Māori health policy, changing the focus of the system to population health with a much stronger emphasis on health promotion and outreach, and developing and implementing a New Zealand health plan to implement the New Zealand Health Strategy (Health and Disability System Review 2020). At the time of writing, implementation of the recommendations from the review was under way. Further information on progress can be found at https://systemreview.health.govt.nz/.

In addition to the health strategies outlined above, 'Ala Mo'ui: Pathways to Pacific Health and Wellbeing (Ministry of Health 2014) and the subsequent Ola Manuia Pacific Health and Wellbeing Action Plan 2020-2025 (Ministry of Health 2020a) both provide

DHBs employ a range of health practitioners to provide services including medical doctors, nurses, nurse practitioners and allied health staff, such as physiotherapists and occupational therapists. However, long waiting lists to receive care from public health services have seen the development of a robust private healthcare sector in New Zealand, particularly for the provision of surgical care. Many individual New Zealanders who can afford it choose to purchase their own health insurance policies to ensure they have access to surgical care quickly if they need it. However, for those people who cannot afford health insurance, poor access to surgical care can mean prolonged suffering and disability that is easily preventable. Many medical specialists work in both private and public health systems, potentially increasing the risk of long public health waiting lists and the inequities this creates. Improving access to elective surgery was one of six government targets designed to improve efficiency and care across the health sector, although strategies designed to achieve this target are not addressing the discrepancies in private/public surgical provision. The other five targets were: shorter stays in emergency departments (6-hour target), faster cancer treatment, increased immunisation, better help for smokers to quit, and raising healthy kids (www.health.govt.nz/new-zealand-health-system/health-targets). In 2019, the New Zealand Government directed the Ministry of Health to develop a new set of performance measures to replace the health targets. The Ministry has been asked to consider the following criteria (Ministry of Health 2021):

- a mix of health system and population health improvement measures
- alignment with government priorities (e.g. child wellbeing and mental health)
- be quantified and timed
- availability of data to monitor progress
- sector engagement and support
- focus on health issues with alignment to socioeconomic determinants.

Work on developing these measures continues in 2022. In the meantime, the system level measures (SLMs) framework continues to develop with an emphasis on collaboration with health system partners across primary, secondary and tertiary services. Information on the SLM framework can be found at www.health.govt.nz/new-zealand-health-system/system-level-measures-framework.

New Zealand continues to have significant disparities in health within its population—in particular Māori, Pacific people (as noted earlier) and those on lower incomes (Ministry of Health and Minister of Health 2020). Although child poverty rates were trending downwards prior to March 2020 (Weir 2021), child poverty remains a significant concern in New Zealand with approximately 18 to 22% of children living in low-income households (Duncanson et al 2020, Weir 2021) and approximately 20% of 0 to 17 year olds having unmet needs for primary care (Duncanson et al 2020). The New Zealand Government has a specific focus on the reduction of child poverty. In 2018, the *Child Poverty Reduction Act 2018* was passed into law with the aim of achieving a significant and sustained reduction in child poverty. Progress prior to COVID-19 was steady. This, combined with a renewed focus on achieving equity outcomes through focusing efforts on Māori, Pacific and high-deprivation communities, will hopefully see health outcomes for these groups improve.

KEY POINT

Health New Zealand (HNZ) will become the organisation responsible for planning, managing, providing and purchasing health services for New Zealanders.

HNZ will also be responsible for funding primary health care in the new system. There are currently 30 primary health organisations (PHOs) throughout New Zealand funded on a population basis to primarily support the provision of general practice and some other primary health care services to an enrolled population. PHOs vary in size and structure, are not-for-profit and provide services either directly by employing staff or through provider members. Most general practices are members of PHOs and provide the bulk of primary care services in New Zealand.

General practices charge a fee-for-service on top of the funding they receive through the PHO. Most general practices are run as businesses, usually GP-owned, and employ staff such as nurses within the business. This business model creates difficulties for practice nurses seeking to extend their practice, due to power imbalances inherent in employee and employer relationships, and traditional models of practice. It was hoped that population-based funding and the advent of PHOs would go some way towards addressing this issue, but change has been relatively slow. Growing population demands and the retirement of older GPs from rural areas have seen nurses stepping up to offer nurse-led clinics and, in some cases, buying into or starting their own general practices. However, funding arrangements make general practice ownership for nurses challenging (Hines & Ruddle 2017) and it is hoped the Health and Disability System Review will provide some solutions to address the public private system currently in place (Gauld et al 2019). New models of care including Health Care Homes and Integrated Family Health Centres also have the potential to provide new opportunities for nurses and other health practitioners, but caution is required as the models remain largely GP-centric.

In 2016, legislative changes enabled registered nurses working in primary health and specialty teams with appropriate qualifications to prescribe medicines and for nurse practitioners to become authorised prescribers (full prescribing rights). Other changes amending the terminology used in numerous pieces of legislation from medical practitioner to health practitioner has also addressed a number of barriers to practice. For example, nurse practitioners can now sign medical certificates and certify death. These incremental changes in policy and legislation are slowly enabling nurses to practise to the full extent of their knowledge and skills, improving access to healthcare for many despite the persistence of the business model in primary care.

POINT TO PONDER

Nurse-led clinics and nurses buying into general practices as business owners are increasingly common. What barriers currently exist that still limit nurses working in these areas?

Aged and residential care in New Zealand is provided through a mix of privately and publicly funded services. Large business conglomerates have bought out many of the aged and residential care providers in New Zealand that were traditionally run by charitable trusts. The New Zealand Government funds providers to deliver services to those in need, yet standards of care in aged and residential care facilities can be poor, with aged and residential care facilities featuring prominently in complaints to the Health and Disability Commissioner about standards of care (McDowell 2020). Visit www.hdc.org.nz to review case notes on complaints regarding aged care in New Zealand. Given the significant levels of funding provided by the government, further work is required to improve standards of care across the sector.

A unique feature of the New Zealand health system is the Accident Compensation Corporation (ACC). The ACC was established in 1974 and is, in effect, an insurance scheme that provides personal injury cover for all New Zealanders and some visitors. The ACC is funded through a mixture of levies from people's earnings, businesses, petrol and vehicle licensing fees and government funding. This means that if a person has an accident in New Zealand, the majority of costs associated with this will be covered by the ACC at no cost to the person. In return for this injury cover, an individual is unable to sue another person or company for personal injury except for exemplary damages (ACC 2020). There are inequities associated with ACC funding. For example, if an accident results in a person becoming permanently disabled, the ACC will fund all the care and equipment that person requires on an ongoing basis. On the other hand, if a person is permanently disabled due to a congenital abnormality or a medical condition, all costs associated with the disability are borne by the individual with limited financial support.

A further unique element of the New Zealand health system is the Pharmaceutical Management Agency or PHARMAC. PHARMAC is an agency of the New Zealand Government that decides, on behalf of DHBs, which medicines and related products are subsidised for use in the community and public hospitals. PHARMAC was established in 1973 as an attempt to control the spiralling costs of medicines in New Zealand. Its role is to get better value and better health outcomes for New Zealanders for the money spent on medicines. In 2019/20 PHARMAC saved NZ$87.4 million for reinvestment in new medicines (Pharmaceutical Management Agency Te Pātaka Whaioranga 2020). Further information on PHARMAC and how it works can be found online at https://pharmac.govt.nz/about/what-we-do/how-pharmac-works.

Paramedic care is provided largely by St John New Zealand. Exceptions include the Wellington Free Ambulance service covering the greater Wellington area, and air ambulance and rescue helicopter services, which are provided privately through a mix of government, philanthropic funding and corporate sponsorship. St John New Zealand has a significant volunteer base with volunteers providing the majority of ambulance services in rural areas. This has both advantages and disadvantages. Volunteerism is known to increase social capital in a community; however, increasing demands on volunteer ambulance officers and limited funding to employ full-time officers is increasing health risks for rural populations.

Primary maternity care in New Zealand is provided by lead maternity carers (LMCs). A woman selects an LMC to provide her maternity care throughout the duration of the pregnancy, birth and first weeks following birth. An LMC may be a midwife, general practitioner with a diploma in obstetrics or an obstetrician. Midwifery as a profession in New Zealand has its own distinct body of knowledge, scope of practice, standards of practice and code of ethics.

The *Health Practitioners Competence Assurance Act (HPCA Act) 2003* provides the legal framework governing the competency of health practitioners to practise in New Zealand. The HPCA Act is designed to protect public safety. A number of titles are protected under the Act, and only health practitioners registered under the Act are entitled to use these. Regulated professions include nursing, midwifery, medicine, pharmacy, physiotherapy and a range of other allied health professions. Registration of health practitioners is undertaken by the respective profession's council or board. For example, the Nursing Council of New Zealand is the statutory body that governs the practice of nurses, monitors and sets standards for practice and maintains the register of nurses. The Health Practitioner Disciplinary Tribunal (a separate but linked entity under the Act) is responsible for hearing and determining disciplinary proceedings brought against registered health practitioners under the *HPCA Act*.

Despite a number of inequities in the system, at present all New Zealanders have access to universal healthcare. New Zealand spends approximately $18 billion on health every year, representing approximately 9.2% of GDP (Te Tai Ōhanga The Treasury 2019a, The World Bank 2021). The impact of COVID-19 on New Zealand and the level of borrowing the government has undertaken in order to sustain the economy is predicted to have a significant impact on the country for many years to come (PwC 2020). Expenditure of $30 billion with an extra $20 billion available to assist in New Zealand's economic recovery has been funded through a public borrowing scheme meaning Crown debt as a percentage of GDP is forecasted to increase from around 20% pre COVID-19 to more than 50% by 2023 (PwC 2020). With an approach traditionally focused on fiscal savings in health, what this level of debt will mean for overall expenditure on addressing the social determinants of health is unknown. What is known is that when governments focus on fiscal restraint, health outcomes worsen (Francis 2013, Matheson 2013, Mosquera et al 2017).

KEY POINT

A focus on fiscal savings in health systems may result in poor outcomes for those people who are at greatest risk, including those who live in low socioeconomic areas, come from ethnic minority populations or who have existing long-term conditions or disability.

Politics, policymaking and healthcare

Policymaking for community health is basically a political process in which those in positions of power make decisions on how best to allocate resources. As health practitioners, it is our responsibility to be aware of how these decisions are made, and to advocate for equity in allocations to the communities we assist. This can take us into unfamiliar territory, carefully examining the needs and priorities of the community, while, at the same time, understanding the constraints on services and resources. Without policies, decisions for resource allocation could be made based on the loudest voices, the highest population or the desires of those best able to articulate their requests.

To work towards equitable distribution of resources requires policies that are fair. Fairness means there is advocacy for those who are most in need, whose voices are often silent. Fairness also means that those born to privilege are not overlooked, but their needs are carefully considered alongside those of the wider population. Guided by the principles of primary health care, we consider how policies and systems of health service are able to balance needs and services on the basis of social justice at the global, national, regional and local levels.

KEY POINT

A policy is a statement of intent that is implemented within an organisation or system as a procedure or protocol. A primary health care policy should result in equitable resource allocation.

National health policies are usually informed by and responsive to global priorities and local conditions. Ideally, state or regional priorities would also be designed to follow or complement the directions of national policies. However, where political agendas differ, this may not always be the case. So, for example, it is possible that in one Australian state or territory, policymakers could place a high priority on environmental issues in its health planning, whereas another might see child health as its greatest priority. Both states would be governed by the goal of better health, but they may change the distribution of resources according to their respective priorities. In countries such as New Zealand, where there is a single health department, policymaking is more consistent across the country, even though there may be some differences in the way different localities implement policies. Yet, even in this environment, there is a need for constant vigilance to ensure that policymaking is inclusive and that it results in all members of the community having equity of access to what they need to maintain good health.

Because of the complexity of health policymaking, it is important to understand how decisions are made. Optimally, decisions would be bi-directional: bottom-up and top-down. Local citizens' groups, health practitioners, town councils and city planners would convey the needs of local communities upwards to the regional, state and national levels, where they would participate in informed debates about health and healthcare. Policymakers would hear their voices and preferences, and attempt to accommodate multiple perspectives in the way they allocate resources for health. In this context, debates and decisions would be approached on the basis of equal partnerships and expedient information systems, so that all policy decisions would also be evidence-based or informed by the latest research and demographic data. Once considerations were aired and consensus was achieved, the policymaking group would communicate with the wider community, gathering further data and/or responses, which would instigate further cycles of input for decision-making. As a result, the policy would achieve three main outcomes. First, it would have a significant effect on improving the health of the population. Second, it would be fair. Third, it would be administered through efficient governance structures, with transparent goals, expectations, financial accountability and evaluation strategies. Yet, impediments to achieving this type of system remain for reasons that are often political and financial. Too often, political positions dictate the terms or targets of health decisions, especially if there are vested interests involved.

KEY POINT

In an ideal world, policymaking would be bi-directional: bottom-up and top-down, with local groups and individuals having a say in how health systems are structured and services are provided.

The main goal of health policymaking should be to improve and enhance health. This requires a strong healthcare system and decisive leadership to guide the way policies are developed. The ideal healthcare system is: ethical, fair and strategic in its endeavour to meet the needs of current and future communities; transparent in communicating its goals and capabilities; oriented towards community empowerment for informed choices; and resourced to the extent that it can support those choices. But the health system alone cannot create or sustain health. This is why there has been an urgent call from global health policymakers to incorporate health in all their policies. Health in All Policies (HiAP) is an approach to public policymaking that systematically considers the implications of all public policy decisions on health, considers the determinants of health and health systems, identifies synergies across policy sectors and seeks to avoid the harmful health effects of poor policies (Browne & Rutherfurd 2017, van Eyk et al 2020). HiAP also aims to improve the accountability of policymakers for health impacts at all levels of policymaking, and is based on social justice and the fundamental health-related human rights of populations and on the obligations of governments to uphold those rights (WHO 2014). If health was included in all policies, our governments would ensure health and safety in education, transportation, media advertising, food services and the environment. Community planning would include health considerations in their plans for housing, infrastructure and public works. Health planners would participate in policies for safe neighbourhoods, community policing and disaster planning. There would be health considerations in decisions made by departments of immigration and multicultural affairs, and health plans for primary industry development and innovation, workplaces and industrial relations. Health issues are embedded in each of these aspects of daily life, and affect people at all stages of the life course from family planning, safe maternity care, child protection and care, illness and injury prevention and management at all ages, to healthy ageing and end-of-life care. A good example of a HiAP approach is in South Australia where a HiAP team worked with teachers to engage with parents to increase literacy among children. Ultimately they found impacts at the individual level, with teachers changing their approach to engaging parents, as well as at the policy level where team members were invited by the Education Department to advise on the development of a system-wide literacy and numeracy strategy that included health aspects (van Eyk et al 2020).

KEY POINT

The health system alone cannot create or sustain health. Health must be considered in *all* policy development activities.

As mentioned previously, the defining purpose of a healthcare system lies in the provision of accessible, appropriate, equitable healthcare that is responsive to people's expectations. When equity is achieved, the healthcare system, its policies and the policies of other government departments are inclusive, and aligned with the social determinants of health (SDH). The fact that we live in conditions of *in*equity indicates that equity continues to be elusive, yet it is a worthy goal for our actions. To some extent, this may be due to the complexity of policymaking and all the competing interests that influence the outcome. However, some inequities persist because of events in the global and/or local environment. When global markets decline, there is a profound impact on countries that depend on these markets to sustain their population. If trade declines, unemployment increases and there is a major effect on family health and wellbeing. When families are unable to purchase goods and services, domestic trade suffers and more people become unemployed. When unemployment is high, there is a dramatic drain on public resources, and supports for those most in need are unavailable. This is a classic 'butterfly effect' where we can see the inherently complex and ecological perspective of policymaking. COVID-19 has had a significant impact on countries worldwide. Australia and New Zealand chose to approach the pandemic through the implementation of health-oriented policies to manage and eliminate the virus, but many people's livelihoods were affected by ongoing lockdowns, lower incomes and unemployment. While the spread of the virus through the community was initially restricted, the long-term impacts of these other determinants of health may remain unknown in the short term.

Ambrose Bierce (1842–1914), a United States author and satirist, once described politics as a 'strife of interests masquerading as a contest of principles'. In health policymaking there has always been a strife of interests, between rich and poor, urban and rural, young and old, sick and well, and those with competing biomedical or health promotion needs. Healthcare decisions revolve around distributive justice: who gets what. Ethically, the poor and disadvantaged should receive the lion's share of resources, as this would bring them up to the same level of opportunity as the rest of the population. However, no country in the world has achieved equity in resource allocation, leaving many people living impoverished lives.

While locally, Australia and New Zealand have a growing focus on achieving equity, particularly for their indigenous populations, at the global level, the United Nation's World Social Report 2020 focused on four 'megatrends' or global forces that are affecting inequality: technological innovation, climate change, urbanisation and international migration (United Nations Department of Economic and Social Affairs 2020). Each of the four megatrends has the potential to impact either positively or negatively on inequality. For example, technological innovation can create economic growth but can also displace workers, create income inequality and exacerbate poverty. We have the potential to harness these megatrends to create a more sustainable and equitable world, but this relies on countries developing and implementing policies that manage both the gains and the risks in each area rather than focusing solely on the gains (United Nations Department of Economic and Social Affairs 2020). Countries can draw on the Sustainable Development Goals to guide policy development to address megatrends. Alleviating global poverty is the first of the 17 goals and 169 targets outlined in the United Nation's 2030 Agenda for Sustainable Development (United Nations 2015). The 17 Sustainable Development Goals (SDG) (discussed in detail in Chapter 3) provide a platform for the social, economic and environmental development of the planet. The SDGs include a focus on universal access to health and wellbeing, universal education and sustainable approaches to production and consumption (United Nations 2015). From this foundation, policymakers can then assess the impact of action and inaction on community health in terms of the principles of primary health care: accessible healthcare, appropriate technology, health promotion and health education, cultural sensitivity and cultural safety, intersectoral collaboration and community participation.

KEY POINT

Globally, all governments must increase their efforts to address inequality through inclusion and sustainability.

Policy action at the national level: think global, act local

As health practitioners, we can be conscious and concerned about global issues and the failure of the global community to create either equity or equality. For those who wish to become global advocates, there are many lobby groups that welcome our participation. For others, becoming involved at the global level may not be possible; however, acting at a local level can encourage community participation in the policy arena, and ensure that professional knowledge and skills are used to the community's advantage. Box 2.4 provides examples of how nurses and other health practitioners can become engaged with policy formation.

To prepare for this type of advocacy it is important to be aware of global policies. Human rights policies such as the UN Convention on the Rights of the Child, their Declarations on the Elimination of Violence Against Women and the Rights of Indigenous Peoples, and WHO policies on women's and men's health, workplace equity and health and environmental protection can translate to local actions. Each of these policies brings together the main issues surrounding equity, cultural inclusion and family life. These policy areas therefore rely heavily on input from nurses and other health practitioners who are present, visible and working with people where they live, work and play. By working towards connecting the global policy agenda vertically (at different levels) and horizontally (through different services) we can promote better care across the life course from pregnancy to the end of life, incorporating maternity care, early childhood education, adolescent and adult physical and mental health, care of the homeless and vulnerable, and healthy ageing. Unfortunately, nurses' engagement in policy advocacy and formation remains low, with most policy work by nurses associated with implementation of policy rather than development (Rasheed et al 2020). If nurses are to continue to have a key role in policy development globally, we must advocate for nurses to hold senior positions within all health settings, including government. Fortunately, both Australia and New Zealand

BOX 2.4

ENGAGING WITH THE POLITICAL SYSTEM AND POLICY FORMATION

Having a say in the political process and the formation of policy is an essential role for nurses and other health practitioners. The practice experience of nurses and other health practitioners can help inform the development of robust policy and there are many different levels and ways in which nurses and other health practitioners can be involved in the process. Some simple ways to engage in the policy process are as follows:

- comment on or contribute to the development of a guideline or publication written by your workplace or professional organisation
- contribute to or comment on a proposed policy in your workplace or community
- join a group that is working on new policies or practices
- write or contribute to a submission during a policy consultation process
- make an oral submission to a workplace committee or a parliamentary select committee
- sign a petition, participate in a campaign or go on strike as part of union action
- send an email or letter to a manager, policy analyst or member of parliament.

(Clendon, 2013:1)

Using examples from everyday practice that reflect the knowledge, skill and impact nurses have on patient care is a useful approach to take in writing or making a submission. These real-life examples are helpful in informing policymakers of the reality of clinical practice and the potential impact of a proposed policy change.

Source: Adapted from Clendon, J., 2013. The value of engaging with the political process, New Zealand Nurses Organisation, Wellington, New Zealand.

senior policy positions worldwide. The appointment of Elizabeth Iro from the Cook Islands to Chief Nursing Officer (CNO) at the WHO in 2018 was the first time a CNO has ever been appointed at the WHO and hopefully signals an ongoing commitment to have nurses at the policymaking table, bringing their clinical and health promotion expertise to policy development.

KEY POINT

Clinical input is necessary in all policy areas from consultation and development to evaluation.

Policymaking is an iterative process involving and impacting many stakeholders including nurses and other health practitioners (Janssen & Helbig 2018). The policy cycle (see Fig 2.2) describes the way in which policy is formed and can be used to identify areas where nurses and other health practitioners can be and are involved. For example, frontline health practitioners have intimate knowledge of the issues facing communities and can help bring visibility to those areas where policy change is needed. Once an issue or problem is identified, local or national government will undertake policy analysis to research and inform decision-making around the new policy. As part of policy development, consultation with stakeholders and discussion with lawmakers and others will help direct the final shape of the policy. Next, the policy is completed and implemented. Changes in laws, by-laws, regulations and practice may be required to ensure successful implementation. Where frontline practitioners coordinate the implementation of policies, their ability to send evaluative information and practitioner-informed evidence back to political decision-makers is invaluable. Finally, policy evaluation takes place to ensure the policy is appropriately and legally implemented and the impact or outcome is what was intended.

Policies governing adult health such as the anti-tobacco strategies, women's and men's health, family-friendly workplaces, climate change adaptation, food security, national chronic disease strategies, falls prevention, healthy ageing, rural

currently have nurses at senior executive levels within their respective departments of health; however, as a profession, we must be vigilant to ensure these roles continue and that nurses retain

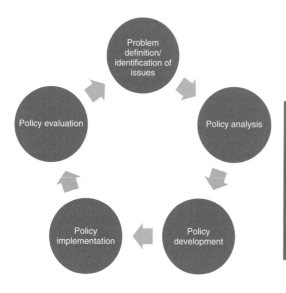

Figure 2.2 The policy cycle

health, social inclusion and mental health have been developed this way, with specific input; for example, from nurses in Australia and New Zealand. Where there are difficulties generating research evidence for change, health practitioners can provide informal information to policymakers in the context of community advocacy. The Healthy Ageing Strategy (Associate Minister of Health 2016) in New Zealand is an example of an important family policy initiative that relied heavily on input from nurses and other health practitioners prior to and during development. In these and other policy areas we are often seen as guardians of the community, ensuring health, protection from harm and cultural safety. Advocacy and involvement in policy is a competency requirement for nurse practitioners in Australia and New Zealand (Nursing and Midwifery Board of Australia 2021, Nursing Council of New Zealand 2012) and advocacy is a requirement of all registered nurses (Nursing and Midwifery Board of Australia 2016, Nursing Council of New Zealand 2016). Each of these policy areas continues to offer important opportunities to enact our social contract with society to promote health and social justice. Equally as important is the need for us to ensure that policies are framed within a caring discourse, especially those that have been developed with an emphasis on economics and the market. The central policy theme is equity, and the strategies for achieving equity must revolve around the SDH.

KEY POINT

Advocacy and involvement in policy is an important competency for nurse practitioners in Australia and New Zealand but all nurses, along with other health practitioners, have an important role to play as well.

Connecting policies with the social determinants of health

Poverty is pervasive and persistent in some countries of the world, but it is social injustice that kills people: unjust social structures, unfair distribution of society's benefits and responsibilities, poor policies, unfair economic arrangements and bad politics (Levy 2019). Social injustice occurs when an individual, community or society is denied fundamental human, economic, social, civil, political and/or cultural rights due to the inaccurate beliefs of those who hold power or influence (Levy 2019). People and communities affected by social injustice are more likely to experience poorer nutrition and have poor access to safe environments, less social support, less access to healthcare and poorer health outcomes; that is, they are more likely to be impacted by the SDH (Levy 2019). But equitable social policies that address these issues emanate from outside the healthcare system, in the economic environments of a nation or region (Rasanathan 2018). Unfortunately, progress on developing policies that address the SDH outside of the health system has been slow globally and there is still much work to be done to encourage countries to develop cross-sector policies that address the SDH (Rasanathan 2018). This holds true in both Australia and New Zealand. While both countries have made progress, inequities between population groups remain. Rasanathan (2018) encourages practitioners to look at different ways to frame the SDH so that the concept resonates with those outside of the health system and to prioritise actions towards health equity as a means to advocate for policy addressing SDH.

Another issue concerns the type of evidence that is acceptable by government decision-makers who may be unaware of the impact of local case studies that could provide exemplars for good and best policies elsewhere. Process evaluations, for example, provide evidence of what works well, where and why (Silies et al 2020), yet funding for this essential element of the policy process is frequently trimmed or diverted (Te Tai Ōhanga The Treasury 2019b). Evaluation of health policies themselves is also important—asking how well a policy worked and what the outcome was is an important feedback loop to inform future policy. New models of care are often developed in response to a range of pressures within a system. Issues such as the ageing population or workforce shortages may lead to new ways of working. However, new models of care must be evaluated carefully to ensure change is effective, cost-effective and has a positive impact where needed. A community nursing model developed in the Netherlands in the mid-2000s known as Buurtzorg (Neighbourhood Care) is underpinned by an ethos of autonomous practice and has proven exceptionally successful in retaining nursing staff and improving patient experience (RCN Policy and International Department 2016). However, just because a model is successful in one context (in this case the Netherlands) does not mean it is successful elsewhere (Chamanga et al 2020). A trial of the model in the United Kingdom (UK) found that although patient experience was good, regulatory and cultural differences between the two systems meant it was exceptionally difficult for the UK nurses to practise autonomously (Lalani et al 2019). This type of data is important to policymakers and underpins the importance of contextual, process-oriented evaluation in the community. To date, health service managers have been quick to adopt biomedical evidence, and, because political power frequently rests with the medical, technological and pharmaceutical industries, this is where the greatest level of funding is allocated. But equally important, if not more important, is ensuring funding is available for evidence-based, effective, preventive primary health care programs. Concentrating healthcare in urban, secondary-care environments deprives many segments of the population from access to appropriate care and prevention of illness and injury.

Policymaking and primary health care in rural areas

An inclusive approach to policy development resonates with a careful balance of comprehensive and selective primary health care. Equitable services can be provided from comprehensive primary health care systems that also accommodate selective care based on prioritised needs. Yet the logic of this type of policy environment has yet to be acknowledged by the 'strife of interests' among those competing for limited resources. Marginalised communities remain unable to control the key processes that control their lives and their health or to select what they need.

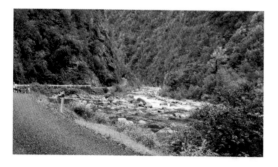

Figure 2.3 Rural and remote area health practitioners face a range of challenges that policymakers need frontline guidance to address. For example, geographical barriers can affect the delivery of health services in a timely manner.

They are subjected to inadequate services, and difficult living conditions that prevent them from being able to challenge power brokers or work towards building local capacity (Fig 2.3). A classic example is seen in the context of preventive interventions that benefit the affluent, subsequently widening disparities (Levy 2019). Another barrier to primary health care lies in policy decisions that see staff appointed to rural and remote areas for short periods of time, which are insufficient for community engagement and, ultimately, problem-solving. In some cases, they arrive in the community to find that they are expected to live in substandard, sometimes unsafe housing. The death of outback nurse Gayle Woodford in 2016 also highlighted the risks many nurses face when working in solo, remote positions. Despite policy changes requiring nurses in sole positions to be accompanied on home visits and after-hours call outs in the Northern Territory, South Australia (where Gayle was murdered) has so far failed to implement the full extent of requirements and there remains a push to roll 'Gayle's Law' out nationwide (ANMJ Staff 2021).

Nurses and other health practitioners in rural and remote positions have few opportunities for professional interaction or continuing education. In addition, with so many regional, state and national employers making decisions about their role in health and community development, there are mixed messages and variable expectations of their role. An example is seen in the policies governing the schedule of child health assessments in Australia, which can vary according to whether the child health nurse is employed by local, regional, state, national or Aboriginal services. These factors make it difficult to maintain the focus on primary health care. When communities and the people who care for them live in disadvantaged or unpredictable situations, their predominant focus is on day-to-day survival, which not only causes substandard health, but erodes social capital. Without political leadership that is committed to addressing the inequities of disadvantage, this situation will remain unchanged. The policy 'problem' is that, rather than try to mitigate the consequences of powerless groups, policymakers tend to shy away from restructuring healthcare, redefining labour relations or unemployment arrangements, or imposing regulations on environmental pollution, or taxes on alcohol or junk food that affect the poor disproportionately. Instead, spurred on by economic goals, social and health policies have continued to concentrate wealth in the hands of the powerful, which has left the poor and voiceless with a disproportionate amount of health-damaging experiences (Levy 2019, Rasanathan 2018).

KEY POINTS

Issues for policymakers

- Focusing on creating wealth rather than fair distribution of wealth
- Inadequate evidence for local policy implementation
- Dominance of biomedical rather than social evaluations
- Poor and disadvantaged are voiceless

Clearly, change is necessary, but it does not occur spontaneously. What is needed is an overt process of inviting community input, then an ongoing level of support. This would produce a combination of perspectives from the public, health practitioners, health planners and intersectoral policymakers to encourage multilevel, multidimensional approaches for better health. The key to success in accommodating such a breadth of opinions is authentic communication between all participants and particularly local stakeholders (Health in All Policies Team Community and Public Health 2018). But first, those in charge of healthcare have to extend the invitations, then practitioners need to become active and persistent advocates for communities, engaging with people to gain their support and input. In this era there is room for optimism, as the centrality of community engagement is being acknowledged in the contemporary policy environments of both Australia and New Zealand.

New Zealand's strong commitment to primary health care was reflected firstly in their Primary Health Care Strategy (King 2001), and latterly with the integration of primary health care into the New Zealand Health Strategy (Ministry of Health 2016) and Health and Disability System Review (Health and Disability System Review 2020). Australia has now begun to follow suit, at least in the rhetoric surrounding primary health care, committing the Commonwealth, states and territories through the 2011 National Health Reform Agreement (NHRA) to work together on preventive health strategies and system-wide policy and statewide planning for general practice and primary health care, and in 2013, developing a National Primary Health Care Strategic Framework. In 2015, 31 Primary Health Networks (PHNs) were established to coordinate primary health care delivery, address local healthcare priorities, support health practitioners and improve access to primary care (see www.healthdirect.gov.au/primary-health-networks-phns). The most recent NHRA signed in 2020 signalled the continuation of a commitment to primary health care and ongoing support for PHNs (see www.health.gov.au/initiatives-and-programs/2020-25-national-health-reform-agreement-nhra for more details).

PHNs have two key objectives: (1) to increase the efficiency and effectiveness of medical services for patients, particularly those at risk of poor health outcomes; and (2) improve coordination of care to ensure patients receive the right care, in the right place, at the right time (Ernst & Young 2018).

Evaluation of PHNs found that while they are largely achieving what they set out to do, they could expand their remit to focus on health services rather than just medical services and they need to engage more with their communities (Ernst & Young 2018). Focusing too closely on general practice risks siloing service provision and excluding NGO providers who often have close relationships with their communities.

In both Australia and New Zealand, attempts to devolve services traditionally provided in hospital settings to community settings have had mixed results. One of the primary issues has been the introduction of charges by some providers for services that were provided for free in hospitals. For example, the treatment of cellulitis (a common bacterial infection) usually requires intravenous antibiotics. In the past, a person was admitted to hospital for 2 to 3 days for treatment. Now, the person is treated in the community either at home or at their general practice. Although funding for the service has devolved to general practice, because general practice is run as a business, a consultation fee can be charged to the person in addition to the government funding. This can have major implications for low-income individuals and families and actually contribute to a delay in seeking treatment rather than improve access. It is essential that policy development in relation to devolution of services ensures equitable access to services is maintained.

Healthcare: building a better system

Three decades ago, few healthcare planners were concerned with the SDH. Yet gradually, as more evidence came to light, policymakers throughout the world came to realise that good health evolves from equity and the social aspects of people's lives, supported by an accessible healthcare system. Resources and good management practices play an important role, but there are other critical elements of a health system that contribute to the health of any given population. These are listed as health system features in Box 2.5. The outcome of good stewardship should be achieving the goals for a healthy society as listed in Box 2.6. Since the health communities of the world began to focus on the

BOX 2.5

....

HEALTH SYSTEM FEATURES

....

- Healthcare systems should be fair, not focused on privileging hospital care funding at the expense of prevention or community care.
- Universal care, along with universal systems of health insurance, can help reduce the disadvantage experienced by those already disadvantaged by socioeconomic status and health status.
- A health system should provide appropriate, adequate and culturally acceptable care for the most vulnerable.
- The majority of healthcare needs are in chronic disease and disability management and these must be met with continuity of care between the acute and the home and community settings.
- Service decisions should be made in partnership with health-literate end users of the system.
- Efficiencies in the system should carefully balance technological and biomedical care with community care.
- Health information systems are integral to efficient and effective services.
- Effective systems are person-oriented, so they deal with waiting lists and the patient journey through hospital to home and community from a client, rather than a service-provider perspective.
- A self-regulating system monitors and addresses threats to patient quality and safety.
- Adequate service provision relies on sufficient health practitioners, educated appropriately for their scope of practice and employed across all settings to practise at their level of competence.
- A robust healthcare system is based on research evidence as a basis for good and best practice.
- A healthcare system should include best practice in health promotion to strengthen capacity.

BOX 2.6

....

GOALS FOR HEALTHY SOCIETIES

....

1 Inclusivity and fairness—through a values-based commitment to equity, freedom, social inclusion and capacity development.
2 Equality—where people of all genders and members of minority groups are treated equally for common needs.
3 Cultural safety—through culturally competent management and clinical systems to ensure that all care processes acknowledge diversity, difference and ability, with an ultimate aim of empowerment.
4 Responsive health systems—with timely, affordable, safe and coordinated care.
5 Support for healthy behaviours—by arranging structural features of the environment to support people in achieving and maintaining health.
6 Sustainable ecosystems—through public awareness and action on preserving the environment.
7 Evidence-based, evidence-informed management of health and healthcare, where research, interventions and policy analysis are interlinked and translated into better health.
8 Democratic citizen participation—where all voices are heard.
9 Social capital is valued—human, spiritual, cultural and social capital is seen as equal to economic capital.
10 Adequate and appropriate resources—there is congruence between needs and resources.
11 Well managed for best processes and best practices—good stewardship and strong community leadership is rewarded and supported.
12. Development of goals and strategies—on the basis of multiple levels of influence by an appropriate, well-educated and satisfied workforce

SDH, we have had a closer global connection to those things that help and those that hinder our quest for health and wellness. Rapid communication brings into our consciousness the cold, hard reality of health inequalities. We are responding to a wider breadth of knowledge on the quality as well as the quantity of life, and as a backlash against the failures of the market to improve health in the population. Given the financial, demographic, environmental and epidemiological threats of modern society, it will take great leadership to nurture our communities and render our healthcare systems safe, effective and efficient. As health practitioners,

we must remain in our imperfect healthcare systems to improve, rather than abandon, our roles as purveyors of health. Every health practitioner has a certain sphere of influence, which can be used to build the capacity of a human community to shape its culture and its future (Burke 2016). This is leadership. It grows from a dialogue between people, between those of us in the healthcare professions and those who need us. We must use our leadership and our ability to generate evidence for practice to advance the goals of primary health care with a common language and the wisdom gleaned from community engagement.

Conclusion

In this chapter we have explored the way in which health systems and policy create the environment in which we work. Understanding how policies drive health practice enables us to be fully engaged with the policy formation process and contribute our frontline knowledge to policy development. In Chapter 3 we will continue our exploration of community and examine the notion of communities of place but before we do, we reflect on the big issues described in this chapter and we return to our case study to consider policies affecting the lives of the Smith and Mason families.

Reflecting on the Big Issues

- Policymaking is a political process of deciding how resources are allocated.
- Many local policies are linked to global and regional goals.
- All policies influence health, and most policies are linked with one another, which means there is a need for health to be considered in all policymaking.
- Community members should have a voice in policymaking.
- Nurses, midwives and other health practitioners should upskill themselves to engage in policymaking.
- Nurses, midwives and other health practitioners can help communities develop a level of health literacy

that would facilitate their participation in policy development.

- Healthcare systems continue to privilege hospital and high-tech care over community care.
- Despite policies designed to address inequities, these persist in access to care, with the most disadvantaged often excluded from the services they need.
- Primary health care can provide the fairest systems of health care.
- An ideal healthcare system is based on the social determinants of health.

Policy Implications for the Smith and Mason families

The occupational health nurses at the Pilbara mine where Colin is employed work within national occupational health and safety policies, which are meant to protect workers. There are few discrepancies in workplace practices given the high-risk environment of the mine.

Government policies that affect both families include those addressing financial matters, such as government spending on early childhood education, social service provision, women's health policy, men's health policy and children's policies such as healthy schools policies. Families in both countries are affected by global economic policies. The Mason family are particularly affected due to the need to generate wealth from the resources of Western Australia, but the uncertainty of the resources boom and the demise of the mining tax

may have an unexpected impact on Colin's employment. Further, the economic impacts of COVID-19 may impact families on both sides of the Tasman.

In New Zealand, Huia has taken up a new position as Māori teacher liaison officer. Even before she was employed, she had to undergo a safety check to ensure she is safe to work with children. This is a compulsory requirement of the *Vulnerable Children's Act 2014*. The Whānau Ora policy has enabled new wrap-around services to be offered in the Papakura community as well, and this appears to be making a difference for some families in the community. Aroha, who is 8, had been complaining of a sore throat and was able to get this checked out at the sore throat clinic offered by the school nurse, which is funded by the government to prevent rheumatic fever.

Reflective questions: How would I use this knowledge in practice?

1 Internationally, population health policies can vary according to factors such as culture, economics, political systems and the environment. Find and review the Australian and New Zealand population health policies available on the websites listed below and reflect on the enabling and challenging factors for population health approaches in each country: www.aihw.gov.au and www.health.govt.nz.

2 Identify the factors influencing policy development in your health service district or primary health organisation.

3 Explain why policy development is guided by the mantra 'think global, act local'.

4 What strategies would you use to ensure Rebecca Mason's level of health literacy is adequate for caring for her family?

5 How can a country's primary health care system promote access and equity in services?

6 What steps could you take to support ongoing development of an effective primary health care system in Australia or New Zealand?

7 Group exercise: Policymaking and nurses

Break into groups of two or three and consider the following questions.

a What is policy and why is it important for nurses to have a good understanding of this?

b What role do nurses have in the policymaking process?

Share your thoughts with the wider group.

8 Policy action exercise: Australian and New Zealand successes and gaps

Some consider policies in the following areas a success, others a work in progress and still others consider some of the policies a failure or even a complete gap. Search out these policy areas and reflect on how successful they are and why.

• Employment

• Food safety, security

• Tobacco legislation

• Affordable child care

• Mandatory seatbelts

Reflective questions: How would I use this knowledge in practice?—cont'd

- Healthy schools, workplaces
- Healthy ageing
- Disability insurance
- Drug and alcohol
- Social inclusion
- Distribution of health practitioners

- Migration
- Mental health
- Rural health
- Women's and men's health
- Indigenous health
- Climate change

References

Accident Compensation Corporation (ACC), 2020. What we do. Online. Available: www.acc.co.nz/about-us/who-we-are/what-we-do/.

ANMJ Staff, 2021. Scholarship in memory of Gayle Woodford makes lasting impact. Aust. Nurs. Midwifery J., 17 March. Online. Available: https://anmj.org.au/scholarship-in-memory-of-gayle-woodford-makes-lasting-impact/.

Associate Minister of Health, 2016. Healthy Ageing Strategy. Ministry of Health, the Netherlands. Online. Available: www.rug.nl/research/healthy-ageing/programme-healty-ageing?lang=en.

Australian Digital Health Agency, 2019. Digital Health Strategy 2018-2022. (February). https://ehealthresearch.no/files/documents/Undersider/WHO-Symposium-2019/1-3-Skovgaard-ENG.pdf.

Australian Government Department of Health, 2019. Australia's long-term national health plan to build the world's best health system. Australian Government Department of Health (August). Online. Available: www.health.gov.au/sites/default/files/australia-s-long-term-national-health-plan_0.pdf.

Australian Institute of Health and Welfare, 2020. Health expenditure Australia 2018–19. AIHW (Ed.). AIHW, Canberra. Online. Available: www.aihw.gov.au/getmedia/a5cfb53c-a22f-407b-8c6f-3820544cb900/aihw-hwe-80.pdf.aspx?inline=true.

Browne, G.R., Rutherfurd, I.D., 2017. The case for 'environment in all policies': Lessons from the 'Health in All Policies' approach in public health. Environ. Health Perspect., 125 (2), 149–154. Online. Available: https://doi.org/10.1289/EHP294.

Burke, S.A., 2016. Influence through policy: Nurses have a unique role. Reflect. Nurs. Leadersh., 42 (2), 1–3. Online. Available: https://nursingcentered.sigmanursing.org/commentary/more-commentary/Vol42_2_nurses-have-a-unique-role.

Chamanga, E., Dyson, J., Loke, J., et al, 2020. Factors influencing the recruitment and retention of registered nurses in adult community nursing services: an integrative literature review. Prim. Health. Care. Res. Dev., 21, e31–e31. Online. Available: https://doi.org/10.1017/S1463423620000353.

Clendon, J., 2013. The value of engaging with the political process. New Zealand Nurses Organisation.

Collyer, F., Willis, K., Keleher, H., 2020. The private sector and private health insurance. In: Willis, E., Reynolds, L., Rudge, T. (Eds), Understanding the Australian health care system, fourth ed. Elsevier, Sydney, pp. 37–52.

Cooper, H., McMurray, A., Ward, L., et al, 2015. Implementing patient-centred care in the context of an integrated care program. Int. J. Care Coord., 8 (4), 72–77.

Duncanson, M., Richardson, G., Oben, G., et al, 2020. Child poverty monitor 2020: Technical report. Online. Available: https://ourarchive.otago.ac.nz/bitstream/handle/10523/10585/CPM_2020_TECHNICAL REPORT.pdf?sequence=6&isAllowed=y.

Ernst & Young, 2018. Evaluation of the Primary Health Networks Program: Final report. Online. Available: www.health.gov.au/sites/default/files/documents/2021/06/evaluation-of-the-primary-health-networks-program.pdf.

Francis, R., 2013. Report of the Mid Staffordshire NHS Foundation Trust Public Inquiry: Executive summary. Online. Available: https://www.gov.uk/government/publications/report-of-the-mid-staffordshire-nhs-foundation-trust-public-inquiry.

Gauld, R., Atmore, C., Baxter, J., et al, 2019. The 'elephants in the room' for New Zealand's health system in its 80th anniversary year: General practice charges and ownership models. N. Z. Med. J., 132 (1489), 8–14. Online. Available: www.nzma.org.nz/journal-articles/the-elephants-in-the-room-for-new-zealand-s-health-system-in-its-80th-anniversary-year-general-practice-charges-and-ownership-models.

Health and Disability System Review, 2020. Health and Disability System Review: Final report / Pūrongo Whakamutunga. Health and Disability System Review. Online. Available: https://systemreview.health.govt.nz/assets/Uploads/hdsr/health-disability-system-review-final-report.pdf.

Health in All Policies Team Community and Public Health, 2018. Tools to support a health in all policies approach: A guide for moving from theory to practice. In: Tools to support a HiAP approach. Canterbury District Health Board.

Hines, K., Ruddle, R., 2017. Through the looking glass: the perspective of a nurse and practice manager-owned general practice. J. Prim. Health Care, 9 (3), 191–192. Online. Available: https://doi.org/10.1071/HC17035.

Hodgkin, S., Mahoney, A., 2020. The aged care sector: Residential and community care. In: Willis, E., Reynolds, L., Rudge, T. (Eds), Understanding the Australian health care system, fourth ed. Elsevier, Sydney, pp. 121–135.

Janssen, M., Helbig, N., 2018. Innovating and changing the policy-cycle: Policy-makers be prepared. Government Information Quarterly, 35 (4), S99–S105. Online. Available: https://doi.org/10.1016/j.giq.2015.11.009.

King, A., 2001. Primary health care strategy. Ministry of Health, Wellington.

Krassnitzer, L., 2020. The public health sector and Medicare. In: Willis, E., Reynolds, L., Rudge, T. (Eds), Understanding the Australian health care system, fourth ed. Elsevier, Sydney, pp. 18–36.

Lalani, M., Fernandes, J., Fradgley, R., et al, 2019. Transforming community nursing services in the UK; lessons from a participatory evaluation of the implementation of a new community nursing model in East London based on the principles of the Dutch Buurtzorg model. BMC Health Serv. Res., 19 (1), 945. Online. Available: https://doi.org/10.1186/s12913-019-4804-8.

Levy, B.S., 2019. The impact of social injustice on public health: Introduction. In: Levy, B.S. (Ed.), Social injustice and public health, third ed. Oxford University Press, pp. 3–20. Online. Available: https://doi.org/10.1093/oso/9780190914653.003.0001.

Matheson, D., 2013. From great to good: How a leading New Zealand DHB lost its ability to focus on equity during a period of economic constraint. Online. Available: http://publichealth.massey.ac.nz/assets/Uploads/From-Great-to-Good-Final.pdf.

McDowell, M., 2020. Health and Disability Commissioner annual report for the year ended 30 June 2020 (June). Online. Available: www.hdc.org.nz/media/5696/hdc-annual-report-2020.pdf.

Ministry of Health, 2001. He Korowai Oranga: Māori health strategy. Wellington.

Ministry of Health, 2014. 'Ala Mo'ui: Pathways to Pacific health and wellbeing 2014–2018. Ministry of Health, Wellington.

Online. Available: www.health.govt.nz/system/files/documents/publications/ala-moui-pathways-to-pacific-health-and-wellbeing-2014-2018-jun14-v2.pdf.

Ministry of Health, 2016. New Zealand health strategy: Future direction (April). Ministry of Health, Wellington. Online. Available: www.health.govt.nz/system/files/documents/publications/new-zealand-health-strategy-futuredirection-2016-apr16.pdf.

Ministry of Health, 2020a. Ola Manuia: Pacific health and wellbeing action plan 2020–2025. Ministry of Health, Wellington. Online. Available: www.health.govt.nz/system/files/documents/publications/ola_manuia-phwap-22june.pdf.

Ministry of Health, 2020b. Whakamaua Māori health action plan, July. Ministry of Health, Wellington. Online. Available: www.health.govt.nz/system/files/documents/publications/whakamaua-maori-health-action-plan-2020-2025-2.pdf.

Ministry of Health, 2021. Health targets. 19 February. www.health.govt.nz/new-zealand-health-system/health-targets.

Ministry of Health and Minister of Health, 2020. Health and independence report 2019. Ministry of Health, Wellington.

Mosquera, I., González-Rábago, Y., Bacigalupe, A., et al, 2017. The impact of fiscal policies on the socioeconomic determinants of health. Int. J. Health Serv., 47 (2), 189–206. Online. Available: https://doi.org/10.1177/0020731416681230.

Nursing and Midwifery Board of Australia, 2016. Registered nurse standards for practice. Online. Available: www.nursingmidwiferyboard.gov.au/Codes-Guidelines-Statements/Professional-standards.aspx.

Nursing and Midwifery Board of Australia, 2021. Nurse practitioner standards for practice. Online. Available: www.nursingmidwiferyboard.gov.au/Codes-Guidelines-Statements/Professional-standards.aspx.

Nursing Council of New Zealand, 2012. Code of conduct for nurses. Nursing Council of New Zealand, Wellington.

Nursing Council of New Zealand, 2016. Competencies for registered nurses. Nursing Council of New Zealand, Wellington.

OECD/WHO, 2020. Health at a glance. In: Health at a Glance: Asia/Pacific 2020: Measuring progress towards universal health coverage. OECD Publishing. Online. Available: www.oecd-ilibrary.org/docserver/26b007cd-en.pdf?expires=1614328467&id=id&accname=guest&checksum=6595894C92A462BFCE9E49232F1524B0.

Office for Disability Issues, 2016. New Zealand disability strategy 2016–2026. Ministry of Social Development, Wellington. Online. Available: www.odi.govt.nz/assets/New-Zealand-Disability-Strategy-files/pdf-nz-disability-strategy-2016.pdf.

Pharmaceutical Management Agency Te Pātaka Whaioranga, 2020. The 2020 year in review. Online. Available: https://pharmac.govt.nz/assets/Uploads/2020-Year-in-Review.pdf.

PwC, 2020. Rebuild New Zealand. June, PricewaterhouseCoopers New Zealand. Online. Available: www.pwc.co.nz/pdfs/2020pdfs/PwC_Rebuild_NZ_2020_report.pdf.

Rasanathan, K., 2018. 10 years after the Commission on Social Determinants of Health: social injustice is still killing on a grand scale. The Lancet (British Edition), 392 (10154), 1176–1177. Online. Available: https://doi.org/10.1016/S0140-6736(18)32069-5.

Rasheed, S.P., Younas, A., Mehdi, F., 2020. Challenges, extent of involvement, and the impact of nurses' involvement in politics and policy making in the last two decades: an integrative review. J. Nurs. Scholarsh., 52 (4), 446–455. Online. Available: https://doi.org/10.1111/jnu.12567.

RCN Policy and International Department, 2016. Model, policy briefing the buurtzorg Nederland (home care provider). Online. Available: www.rcn.org.uk.

Scuffham, P.A., Mihala, G., Ward, L., et al, 2017. Evaluation of the Gold Coast Integrated Care for patients with chronic disease or high risk of hospitalisation through a non-randomised controlled clinical trial: A pilot study protocol. BMJ Open, 7 (6). Online. Available: https://doi.org/10.1136/bmjopen-2017-016776.

Silies, K., Schnakenberg, R., Berg, A., et al, 2020. Process evaluation of a complex intervention to promote advance care planning in community-dwelling older persons (the STADPLAN study)—study protocol. Trials, 21(1), 653. Online. Available: https://doi.org/10.1186/s13063-020-04529-2.

Te Tai Ōhanga The Treasury, 2019a. Revenue and expenditure. Online. Available: www.treasury.govt.nz/information-and-services/financial-management-and-advice/revenue-and-expenditure.

Te Tai Ōhanga The Treasury, 2019b. Guidance note: Best practice, monitoring, evaluation and review. Online. Available: www.treasury.govt.nz/publications/guide/guidance-note-best-practice-monitoring-evaluation-and-review.

The World Bank, 2021. Current health expenditure (% of GDP)—New Zealand. Online. Available: https://data.worldbank.org/indicator/SH.XPD.CHEX.GD.ZS?end=2018&locations=NZ&start=2007.

Trankle, S.A., Usherwood, T., Abbott, P., et al, 2019. Integrating health care in Australia: A qualitative evaluation. BMC Health Serv. Res., 19 (1), 954. Online. Available: www.ncbi.nlm.nih.gov/pmc/articles/PMC6907151/pdf/12913_2019_Article_4780.pdf.

United Nations, 2015. Transforming our world: The 2030 agenda for sustainable development.

United Nations Department of Economic and Social Affairs, 2020. World social report 2020: Inequality in a rapidly changing world. In: World Social Report 2020. United Nations. Online. Available: https://doi.org/10.18356/7f5d0efc-en.

van Eyk, H., Delany-Crowe, T., Lawless, A., et al, 2020. Improving child literacy using South Australia's Health in All Policies approach. Health Promotion International, 35 (5), 958–972. Online. Available: http://dx.doi.org/10.1093/heapro/daz013.

Weir, J., 2021. Latest release of child poverty statistics. Stats NZ. Online. Available: www.stats.govt.nz/tereo/news/latest-release-of-child-poverty-statistics.

Willis, E., Reynolds, L., Rudge, T. (Eds), 2020. Understanding the Australian health care system, fourth ed. Elsevier, Sydney.

World Health Organization (WHO), 2014. Health in all policies (HiAP): framework for country action. In: Health promotion international, 29, January. Online. Available: https://doi.org/10.1093/heapro/dau035.

World Health Organization (WHO), 2016. Integrated care models: An overview. Online. Available: www.euro.who.int/__data/assets/pdf_file/0005/322475/Integrated-care-models-overview.pdf.

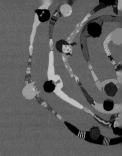

CHAPTER 3
Communities of place

Introduction

The notion of reciprocal determinism, whereby people affect and are affected by their environments, epitomises the relationship between health and place. Place is not just a location but refers to spaces that are meaningful for human interactions for individuals, families and communities. This may include physical, geographical and virtual communities as well as communities of affiliation. It is important to recognise that place can affect physical, social and emotional aspects of health and wellbeing and can be affected by the social determinants of health (SDH). In today's world, where there is an increasing concern about our global and local places, there is a need to look more closely at the intersection of health, place and our personal geographies and how we transit through multiple contexts along the pathways to good health. It is important for health practitioners to understand how micro- and macro-level influences can affect people's ability to develop enabling pathways and resilience or can further exacerbate issues. Micro level relates to factors affecting families at home and at community-level practice while macro-level considerations result from wider economic, regulatory, social and political government and non-government institutions (Smith et al 2019).

A primary health care lens highlights how communities within places, or communities of place, can promote health and wellbeing through ongoing interactions with their environments. In so doing, place has the potential to be adapted through community knowledge and action, expanding the

---

OBJECTIVES

By the end of this chapter you will be able to:

1 explain how knowledge of health and place can be used to promote health across a range of community settings

2 explore the impacts of COVID-19 on families and communities

3 discuss how local, national and global factors/ social determinants influence primary health care practice

4 explain how the health of people is influenced by virtual communities

5 identify strengths and challenges to sustaining health and wellness in urban, rural and remote communities

6 describe the importance of the Sustainable Development Goals (SDGs) on primary health care practice in Australian and New Zealand communities.

concept and management of health and wellbeing towards development of social capital, social cohesion and community identity (Iroz-Elardo et al 2020).

In this chapter, we expand on our analysis of community and explore how place impacts on health disparities between different groups within our communities and how these groups are able to enable and sustain their health and wellbeing. We start by looking more closely at local communities and build through to national and global communities. We also consider the Sustainable Development Goals and the relationship between these and interdisciplinary primary health care practice, virtual communities and their growing importance in a digital world and a range of existing unique communities including rural/remote, fly-in fly-out, refugee, Indigenous and migrant communities. We finish the chapter with an exploration of promoting health in communities of place.

The global community

As part of the global community, we need to be mindful that what occurs in one country affects all others. We depend on our natural ecosystems to provide life support throughout the world, and this affects our physical and psychosocial health and that of our communities. This emphasises the need to continually assess risks of issues such as climate change with associated impacts on communities, including food security, infectious diseases and housing (Victoria State Government 2020). The macro factors affecting the global community have a profound impact on our social world, particularly in terms of economic capabilities and our ability to access the social and cultural supports that help conserve our communities (Smith et al 2019). Globalisation is therefore relevant to family life across the age continuum and across generations, from birth and child care to education, employment, recreation and a comfortable retirement. Our globalised world has brought significant changes to community life, with significant changes to our culture and beliefs being influenced by areas such as social media, political groups and educational organisations (Correa-Velez 2019). Global technology has enhanced knowledge for many people, providing instant electronic access to a wealth of information, including health information and research data; however, it has also created inequities.

The term 'globalisation' refers to the interconnectedness of people and countries, with the opening of borders to enhance the flow of goods, services, finance, people and ideas, in addition to the changes in policies and practices facilitating these movements (World Health Organization [WHO] 2021a). Integration of economic capabilities means that economic decisions affecting people in all corners of the world are influenced by global conditions. Initially, a globalised world held the promise of increased markets for goods, borders through which people could pass freely, greater sharing of cultures, and economies of scale where goods might become cheaper because they could be bought and sold efficiently by large business concerns. Economic arrangements since globalisation have added wealth to various nations, reducing *absolute poverty*, which is a multidimensional phenomenon. It is a term that not only measures deprivation in relation to the amount of money needed to address basic needs of daily living but is also a human rights issue. People, families and communities are deprived of access to health services, education and adequate nutrition in addition to participation in political processes to protect their social and economic health and wellbeing (OHCHR 2021a). Inequities have become evident from the fact that global markets privilege those in control of trade relationships who have profited enormously from worldwide commercial endeavours at the expense of social, environmental and health concerns such as water and air quality (Emmanuel et al 2018).

Globalisation has also led to increased spread of infectious diseases and pandemics such as: the Ebola virus disease; HIV-AIDS; avian influenza subtypes A(H5N1), A(H7N9), A(H9N2) infections; and, in particular, the COVID-19 viral pandemic. The effects of COVID-19 have affected individuals and families, also influencing the ability of government and non-government community agencies to support populations across all age groups. Of note are the adverse physical and psychosocial impacts seen in disadvantaged communities, with SDH influencing the ability of people to manage safe COVID-19 environments while being able to maintain basic necessities such as employment, housing and food security (Callis et al 2020). Globally, extreme poverty has been rising due to social, health and civil disruptions caused by the COVID-19 pandemic, which have added to existing multifactorial conflicts and climate change. Significant and cohesive national and international policy actions are needed to ameliorate harmful human and economic consequences (World Bank 2021).

Chronic disease management has needed to take a global perspective. For example, international food supply and advertising along with tobacco production and distribution contribute significantly to chronic respiratory diseases and obesity, diabetes and renal disease. Further social health impacts are emerging in relation to unlawful income generation through human trafficking, adult and child forced labour and modern slavery, official corruption, child and adult prostitution and smuggling of migrants all targeting vulnerable people and communities (David et al 2019).

KEY POINT

Globalisation

Integration of the world economy through the movement of goods and services, capital, technology and labour.

In 2000, a global macro initiative coordinated by the United Nations developed the Millennium Development Goals (MDGs). A global partnership between participating countries agreed on eight targets to reduce extreme poverty and associated social issues by 2015. The goals were to: eradicate extreme poverty and hunger; achieve universal primary education; promote gender equality and empower women; reduce child mortality; improve maternal health; combat HIV/AIDS, malaria and other diseases; ensure environmental sustainability;

and develop a global partnership for development (WHO 2021b). The MDGs achieved many successes with their targets; however, they did not address the multidimensional nature of poverty, including conflicts, social inequality, vulnerability to natural disasters, public health challenges and environmental factors. In 2015, a further global development strategy was adopted by the United Nations. The Sustainable Development Goals (SDGs) were built on the successes of the MDGs with 17 goals addressing three broad dimensions of intersectoral sustainable economic, social and environmental development. With the aim of making positive changes by 2030, they reinforced and expanded targets from the MDGs, focusing on the origins of poverty and disparities for families and communities, along with investigating how social, economic and environmental determinants of health influence sustainable development. However, the current COVID-19 pandemic has slowed progress of the SDGs, worsening inequalities for vulnerable people and population groups. For example, globally, the pandemic has increased the burden of economic insecurity for women and children, in addition to limiting access to healthcare and food supplies. These have the potential to lead to malnutrition and death, particularly for those under 5 years of age and childbearing women (Bettelli 2021).

Nurses and other health practitioners have an important role to play in achieving these goals and addressing circumstances impacting on their effectiveness. The International Council of Nurses (ICN) highlights that nurses are key health professionals for the achievement of the SDGs, with primary health care being integral to the improvement of health and wellbeing (ICN 2021), but everyone has a role to play. The SDGs are not just about people in low-income countries, they affect everyone. Achieving the targets will improve the health of everyone, including ourselves.

Box 3.1 outlines the full list of SDGs.

Despite the global attention to poverty in developing countries, another effect of globalisation has been the loss of cultural identities, languages and the right to choice in securing the best level of health for the most number of people. The reality is that even as countries of the West celebrate new wealth, we are all aware that wealth is distributed unequally. So as the global community has continued to develop,

---

BOX 3.1

....

SUSTAINABLE DEVELOPMENT GOALS

....

Goal 1. End poverty in all its forms everywhere.

Goal 2. End hunger, achieve food security and improved nutrition and promote sustainable agriculture.

Goal 3. Ensure healthy lives and promote wellbeing for all at all ages.

Goal 4. Ensure inclusive and equitable quality education and promote lifelong learning opportunities for all.

Goal 5. Achieve gender equality and empower all women and girls.

Goal 6. Ensure availability and sustainable management of water and sanitation for all.

Goal 7. Ensure access to affordable, reliable, sustainable and modern energy for all.

Goal 8. Promote sustained, inclusive and sustainable economic growth, full and productive employment and decent work for all.

Goal 9. Build resilient infrastructure, promote inclusive and sustainable industrialisation and foster innovation.

Goal 10. Reduce inequality within and among countries.

Goal 11. Make cities and human settlements inclusive, safe, resilient and sustainable.

Goal 12. Ensure sustainable consumption and production patterns.

Goal 13. Take urgent action to combat climate change and its impacts.*

Goal 14. Conserve and sustainably use the oceans, seas and marine resources for sustainable development.

Goal 15. Protect, restore and promote sustainable use of terrestrial ecosystems, sustainably manage forests, combat desertification and halt and reverse land degradation and halt biodiversity loss.

Goal 16. Promote peaceful and inclusive societies for sustainable development, provide access to justice for all and build effective, accountable and inclusive institutions at all levels.

Goal 17. Strengthen the means of implementation and revitalise the Global Partnership for Sustainable Development.

*Acknowledging that the United Nations Framework Convention on Climate Change is the primary international, intergovernmental forum for negotiating the global response to climate change.

Source: Reprinted from World Health Organization (WHO), 2015. Health in 2015: from Millennium Development Goals to SDGs, Sustainable Development Goals. WHO, Geneva.

---

there have been greater disparities between rich and poor countries, and between the rich and poor within most countries. Clearly, globalisation has wreaked havoc with the SDH. The effects of decisions cascade throughout society, affecting the poor and vulnerable, including women workers, migrants, different cultural groups, rural and urban dwellers and families.

FAMILIES

Positive family environments are integral to the development of children's lifelong physical and psychosocial development. Family structure and function underpin each member's ability to maintain their health and wellbeing. However, families frequently experience health and psychosocial challenges which are optimally addressed through holistic, place-based approaches.

Health inequalities are underpinned by a complexity of psychosocial, environmental and cultural issues that impact on populations and communities as a whole. Place-based approaches recognise the necessity of addressing these determinants with a community-level bio-ecological and resources focus. This enables larger differences in health and wellbeing to be made at the level of population health, thereby enhancing supportive environments for families (Public Health England 2021).

As health practitioners, we work in partnership with families, advocating through a respectful and culturally sensitive approach, helping them to engage with their chosen community and develop sustainable outcomes in the face of social adversities such as poverty, homelessness, lack of transport and economic and social marginalisation. Chapter 7 explores the concept of family in greater detail.

URBAN COMMUNITIES

Globally, there is a greater proportion of people living in urban areas compared with those in rural areas. Urban communities, consisting of towns and cities, are accounting for over 50% of the world's population. This is anticipated to rise to 5 billion people by 2030, accompanied by vast social, economic and environmental changes. These provide opportunities for enhanced health and wellbeing with a greater range of resources. However, urban expansion and informal settlements can result in a rise in inequity, leading to poor living conditions, lack of access to essential services, poverty and food insecurity (United Nations Population Fund 2020). Forms of pollution, such as noise, water and soil contamination, combined with lack of green spaces and opportunities for physical activities, also contribute towards contemporary health burdens. These include risks of infectious diseases such as influenza, COVID-19 and tuberculosis, and accompanying non-communicable diseases including respiratory conditions, cancers and cardiac diseases. Additionally, psychosocial adversity and poor living conditions increase possibilities for anxiety and depression, and injuries due to violence (WHO 2021c). Furthermore, there have been very significant global adverse impacts on

natural environments, biodiversity and ecosystems which have subsequently reduced capabilities of families and communities to maintain their wellbeing (WHO Regional Office for Europe 2021).

Recent Australian research has highlighted the impacts of living in urban high-rise apartment buildings, which have influenced the mental health of adults and children. Poor psychosocial outcomes and feelings of wellbeing have been noted, especially for those in economically and socially disadvantaged neighbourhoods (Larcombe et al 2019). The consequences of COVID-19 management in Melbourne, Victoria, was felt during July 2020 when approximately 3000 residents from nine inner-city public housing towers, including a high number of multicultural families, were placed in immediate lockdown to reduce widespread infection of the disease. They were not able to leave their units for between 5 and 14 days. The strategy did stop the spread of COVID-19 cases within these communities; however, there was considerable stress experienced by residents who required interpreters and information in non-English formats due to delays in accessing these resources. These experiences were further compounded by a lack of culturally specific mental health support (Victorian Ombudsman 2020), demonstrating a need for health practitioners to participate in ongoing community assessments. This includes having up-to-date data on their communities to help facilitate timely and culturally appropriate responses to urgent community and public health situations.

The need for resources and infrastructure to combat issues such as crowded housing, food and water security, air pollution and inadequate social services, particularly in times of crisis such as the COVID-19 pandemic, places pressure on countries at both national and community levels to manage sustainable and socially inclusive environments for individuals, families and communities. Interdisciplinary, coordinated efforts across government and non-government agencies are needed to address these challenges (Organisation for Economic Co-operation and Development [OECD] 2020).

Homelessness, as an ultimate marker of disadvantage and inequality in society, is a particular concern, especially as a human rights issue. The ability of individuals and families to maintain their health and wellbeing when homeless is severely impaired, with preventable death a notable concern. Lack of appropriate housing is frequently associated with violence, which does not provide safe, stable physical and psychosocial environments for children and their families, including development of low self-esteem. Having no fixed address lessens opportunities to engage with social support services and gain employment, thereby exacerbating poverty and disadvantage (OHCHR 2021b).

KEY POINTS
....

Up side, down side to the city

• More services, more jobs, more people

• Higher costs, poverty

• Inequities

• Substandard housing, crowding

• Fewer family supports

• Crime, pollution

Cities can also be seen as a community of place, supporting health environments where people have choices that can help them reach their maximum potential. The Healthy Cities initiative is a strategy supported by the WHO, with an intersectoral approach involving people such as health practitioners, and representatives of recreation, police, social services, voluntary organisations and community members of all ages. The model of Healthy Cities is to create awareness of the importance of place in achieving and maintaining health, with community participation being a high priority. Healthy Cities initiatives have instigated actions to take a human approach to development, increase recreational spaces based on the needs in communities and promote connectedness between people for health, education and quality of life. Notably, city government and non-government organisations have been central to developing COVID-19 pandemic policies and responses, thereby reducing long-term economic and social disadvantages (WHO 2021d).

A Healthy City initiative is seen in the interdisciplinary approach undertaken by the Queensland City of Logan, where there are over 20 community hubs, community and family centres facilitating equity for children and families. Universal and targeted prevention and social inclusion activities are available through community health nurses, allied health professionals and peer support (Logan Together 2018).

An extension of the Healthy Cities movement is the WHO Age-Friendly City concept, designed to provide optimal opportunities for health, participation, security and quality of life for older citizens. Eight initiatives to support city and community structures and services that optimally address the needs of older people have been identified: the built environment, transport, housing, social participation, respect and social inclusion, civic participation and employment, communication, and community support and health services (WHO 2021e). Each of these initiatives will need to be developed on a local or regional basis to ensure they are responsive to the specific needs and resources of various geographical areas.

The Healthy Cities program and WHO Age-Friendly City concepts promote micro-level equity for families and communities, but rely on macro-level political commitment and support. Government policies in Australia and New Zealand seek to facilitate universal publicly funded healthcare systems for hospitals and primary health care in addition to social support systems that assist in enabling SDH (The Commonwealth Fund 2021 a,b). Both governments also liaise with non-government organisations to diversify the planning and delivery of health and social services. These policies extend from urban communities to rural communities.

RURAL COMMUNITIES

Rural communities have a number of unique challenges that have left many more people disadvantaged by poorer health than city dwellers. The most glaring challenge is difficulties in accessing both primary health care services and specialist health professionals, which is the case in both Australia and New Zealand. A complex array of factors contribute to poorer health outcomes in rural and remote areas, with remoteness differing from rurality according to population size and increasing distance from services (Australian Government Department of Health 2021). (See Box 3.2.) SDH such as geographical isolation impact on education and employment opportunities, and there are increased injury risks related to occupations (Australian Institute of Health and Welfare [AIHW] 2019). As we discuss later in the chapter, globalisation has meant that much health service planning is no longer undertaken on the basis of need alone, and there is a need for government policies and resources that are designed specifically for rural and remote healthcare needs, reflecting the uniqueness of inequalities for individuals, families and population groups living outside urban areas (Australian Medical Association [AMA] 2019).

KEY POINTS

....

Up side, down side to rural life

- Strong sense of community
- Stable family home
- Few health, social services
- Social, cultural isolation
- Family burden of caring
- Few education, employment, recreational opportunities
- Declining economy

The issue of access to care in rural and remote areas has been addressed through a number of innovations, in Australia these have primarily been aimed at flying in health practitioners who conduct clinics or community assessments, but are then not able to provide the long-term attention the community needs. As a result, many rural people have less preventative care, such as screening, than urban residents, and ongoing poorer health outcomes. They may need lengthy and disruptive trips to urban tertiary health centres and may not be able to undertake effective self-management of chronic conditions. Lack of access to continuing health professional services has the potential to impact on

health recovery trajectories (National Rural Health Alliance [NRHA] n.d.). Of note is the urgent need for mental health assistance across Australia and New Zealand. People are experiencing a unique range of economic and health stressors, and rates of suicide and self-inflicted injuries increase with remoteness. Indigenous peoples experience unique psychosocial and mental health needs, with suicide rates, for example, for Aboriginal and Torres Strait Islander people in Australia being substantially higher than non-Indigenous Australians (AIHW 2020a, NRHA 2021).

Rural communities also have high levels of disadvantage because of restricted access to the range of goods and services that their urban counterparts enjoy. With shrinking economic resources, many services such as banks and commercial outlets have closed down, and this has led to a decline in the infrastructure for those who remain. Other problems include the lack of educational, employment and recreational opportunities that would enhance health literacy and social interaction. These factors all contribute to higher morbidity and mortality rates for rural people, compared with those who live in cities, which is evident in the significant and unacceptable gradient in health and wellbeing that worsens with distance from capital cities (AIHW 2020b). Population ageing has affected a growing number of rural residents, and many of these people have chronic diseases. There is a need for a strengths-based, culturally safe approach to health and wellbeing for older Indigenous people, with culturally proficient staff and culturally safe venues recommended to help facilitate positive health behaviours (Wettasinghe et al 2020). Similarly, those needing mental health services and guidance often have difficulty accessing services and may profit from a range of interdisciplinary, collaborative and integrated strategies. However, the mental health workforce tends to reduce in rural and remote locations, resulting in inconsistency with increasing requirements for support (NRHA 2021).

Sustainable health outcomes in rural communities are not achievable without a primary health care approach. Issues such as affordable and accessible housing, fuel, healthy food, education, health literacy and culturally secure health and social services underpin healthcare provision for rural individuals, families and communities (Rural Health Information

BOX 3.2

PRACTICE PROFILE: FLIGHT NURSE

Hi. My name is Kate and I am a flight nurse.

What the role entails:

Flight nurses (FNs) have specialised training in critical care nursing and midwifery. They deliver all-encompassing critical, emergency and pre-hospital care for patients of all kinds aboard an aircraft. They also provide community-based healthcare such as child health services and diabetes clinics.

Perhaps the most visible part of the FN's job is the primary retrievals that treat trauma victims. These patients have usually been injured in a remote location and standard ground transportation may not be accessible or it might take considerable time to reach the patient. FNs stabilise these patients, administering emergency care and preparing the patient for treatment at a tertiary facility. Duties range from basic first aid to starting IVs, administering medication or performing advanced resuscitation techniques.

Another common scenario involves inter-hospital patient transfers. Patients might need to be transferred to a tertiary centre to obtain lifesaving treatment that is unavailable at the original facility, such as an angioplasty. Secondary to patient comfort and safety during the flight, an FN's role is to liaise with medical practitioners at the transferring and receiving facilities, ensuring that all pertinent information, patient files and belongings are received and delivered into the right hands.

How I came to be in the role:

I did my graduate year in rural Western Australia and got to work in the local hospital's emergency and high-dependency units. Many of these patients needed transfer to a tertiary hospital in Perth for further and ongoing treatment. The majority of these patients were flown to Perth with the Royal Flying Doctor Service (RFDS). I was fortunate to accompany patients in the ambulance from the hospital to the RFDS hangar for transfer to Perth. I got to meet some of the FNs transferring the patients and I admired their confidence, knowledge base and autonomy. One of the FNs noted my enthusiasm and took the time to show me around the aircraft, its equipment and inside the local base. She also gave me some advice on some courses that would help me get to my goal of being an FN. That experience, and that FN's kindness and patience, started me on the path to become a flight nurse.

What I find most interesting about the role:

There are so many interesting aspects of this role! The fact that you don't know what type of patients you are going to get each day—it could be a premature baby requiring ventilation, an elderly patient with a fractured hip needing surgery, a woman in preterm labour or being first on scene to a patient in a remote location involved in a motor vehicle crash. The excitement, variety and autonomy in the role, combined with the amazing views from your office window, makes it a fabulous experience.

Advice for anyone wanting to become a flight nurse:

Go for it! You need to hold a dual registration in nursing and midwifery, as well as previous critical care experience in emergency or the intensive care unit. Ideally, a postgraduate qualification in critical care will increase your chances of getting a job. While gaining clinical experience and consolidating your practice in these areas, there are a few courses to consider including: advanced life support, advanced life support obstetrics, advanced paediatric life support, pre-hospital life support and trauma nursing care course. It also pays to get rural and remote nursing experience.

Hub [RHIhub] 2021) and need to be integral to an intersectoral approach for care planning. Of note is the rise in telehealth interventions in rural and remote locations, within health centres and in people's homes. Digital technology provides significant opportunities for enhanced access to services; however, this depends on availability of digital hardware and technical skills (Bennett et al 2020). Factors in the global environment may also impact on policies to achieve sustainable health outcomes across rural and urban environments and within distinctive communities. We turn our attention to these now.

Where to find out more on …

Rural health

There are a wide range of health and social challenges for individuals, families and communities in rural areas of Australia and New Zealand. Fact sheets on a variety of these issues are available through the National Rural Health Alliance (http://ruralhealth.org.au/factsheets/thumbs) in addition to the Rural Health Alliance Aotearoa New Zealand's Rural Health Road Map 2019 (https://rhaanz.org.nz/wp-content/uploads/2019/11/Rural-Health-Road-Map-2019.pdf).

Contemporary issues within distinctive communities

Within global, national and local communities there are distinctive and special populations. In this next section of the chapter, we will explore some specific examples and circumstances, and review the impact of the SDH and primary health care approaches to the health and wellbeing of people within these communities.

VIRTUAL COMMUNITIES

A contemporary perspective of health and communities of interest sees internet networks as virtual communities, where relationships are created and maintained (Taylor et al 2021). This approach is appropriate to today's lifestyles where most of us influence and are influenced by multiple local, national and international places on the web through our virtual networks with others. These places can be described as 'relational', compared to the conventional view of 'place' as a specific geographical location. In our technological world, the various forms of internet networks that bind people together can also be considered communities, albeit as virtual places. From this perspective, people can enjoy membership in multiple communities that are settings for health promotion through social media tools such as Facebook, Twitter, blogs, smart phones, SMS messaging, telephone-assisted devices and self-tracking devices. Linking vulnerable people into online groups can help to reduce social isolation and enhance a sense of belonging (Taylor et al 2021). Electronic devices and social media that expedite communication are instrumental to health and wellness because they act as conduits for people to develop advocacy skills, exchange knowledge on health, become socially engaged with others and receive information from health practitioners or other sources when they need guidance or support. Social and electronic media therefore play an important role in enhancing health promotion and health education, and ultimately social capital for individuals, families and communities. Working with social and mass media requires a range of effective communication skills to increase knowledge, influence social norms and public opinion and enhance behaviour change, which necessitates working collaboratively with media professionals (Taylor et al 2021). Virtual networks can therefore be seen as enabling places for health. Examples of virtual communities include private Facebook groups for families of children with a rare disease, gaming communities or special interest communities such as people with an interest in mountain biking or needlework.

However, virtual spaces can also create risks to health in similar and novel ways to physical communities. Such risks may include cyber bullying and sexual predation. Other risks are related to eyesight damage from the constant connection to screens, and behavioural effects that see some people become socially isolated or depressed from interacting almost exclusively with online sites rather than individuals. These risks must be managed to ensure virtual networks remain safe environments for all those who choose to use them.

FLY-IN FLY-OUT COMMUNITIES

Fly-in fly-out (FIFO) or, in some cases, drive-in drive-out (DIDO) refers to the type of work arrangements that have become common in the mining and health professions throughout Australia and New Zealand. Workers usually work a scheduled roster in rural or remote geographical locations, where food, accommodation, health services and a range of recreational activities are provided. This is followed by a set number of days at home (Safe Work Australia 2020).

While they are away, employee working hours are long with minimal time off. There is increasing evidence that FIFO and DIDO workplaces can impact on the mental health and wellbeing of workers. Long working hours and continual shifts highlight the unique demands of such work, with workers reporting feelings of loneliness, isolation and bullying.

Multidisciplinary innovative strategies are needed to prevent psychosocial deterioration and promote mentally healthier employees. Partners and families of these workers may also have a high risk of psychological issues and could benefit from targeted family support initiatives (Parker et al 2018).

During the COVID-19 pandemic, mining rosters were continued in Australia under modified arrangements. However, emotional wellbeing was adversely impacted with workers feeling less happy and optimistic. A range of protective factors were promoted to enhance mental health and wellbeing during this time, including regular communication with family and home and COVID-19 testing, with interdisciplinary on-site teams placing a priority on mental and physical health, and developing innovative activities to maintain social connectivity (Gilbert et al 2020).

Where to find out more on ...

Mental health and wellbeing and support for families of FIFO and DIDO workers

There is a wide range of psychosocial challenges impacting on FIFO/DIDO, FIFO and DIDO workers and their families in Australia and New Zealand. Information on support services is available through the Department of Mines, Industry Regulation and Safety: www.dmp.wa.gov.au/Safety/Information-for-families-25133.aspx.

KEY POINTS

The potential effects of FIFO employment are:

- substantial wages
- compressed work schedules
- intermittent parenting
- low sense of community
- accommodation difficulties
- lifestyle risks for workers
- isolation of partners
- marital pressures
- stress
- fly-over effects on community
- low social capital
- inadequate community services
- destruction of Indigenous land
- pressure on infrastructure.

COMMUNITIES OF AFFILIATION

Some people are bound by occupation to communities such as FIFO families, and this can affect health and social behaviours. Other occupations connect people together by virtue of shared values and attitudes, and this is evident for many health practitioners who travel throughout the world. Our own experiences have shown that meeting another member of the profession often results in an instant connection based on a common commitment to health and wellbeing. Other occupations may have less of a community connection, and some people prefer to maintain their distance rather than develop a connected relationship with co-workers. So the ties that bind members of an occupational community fall along a continuum of connectedness from very little to very strong linkages.

On the other hand, members of religious or faith communities tend to have a strong sense of community that is based, again, on a common commitment. Cultural groups may also feel a strong sense of community, but this varies with the particular culture and subgroups within that culture. Community bonds may be based on such things as age, gender, family structure and whether or not people are bound together by social, occupational or religious affiliation. For example, a group of Pacific Island elders who live in a particular neighbourhood and attend a common church may share a close social bond, while another group of seniors from the same region may have a separate, distinctive sense of community outside the group. The children and grandchildren of both groups may not feel part of either community, and instead may create their social bonds in communities bound together by study, sports or recreational activities. These differences caution us against making generalisations about people and their community memberships on the basis of ethnicity, which is important to consider when working with migrant or refugee populations.

MIGRANT AND REFUGEE COMMUNITIES

International migration is a feature of globalisation, with economic, political and social inequities and conflict underlying short- and long-term movements of people between countries. The term *migrant* can be politically defined and redefined and is a current topic of interest worldwide. For example, the designations of migrant and refugee can be used interchangeably but it is important to acknowledge their differences. Migrants move voluntarily for economic, lifestyle and family reasons as compared to refugees who involuntarily leave their home countries due to physical, social and religious conflict and persecution. In contrast, asylum seekers are requesting another country's protection from oppression and discrimination, and are waiting on legal recognition of their refugee status (Amnesty International 2021). This is supported by the United Nations High Commissioner for Refugees (UNHCR 2010) which highlights the deadly consequences for people who are denied asylum when governments conflate the two terms, effectively removing legal protections for refugees (see Box 3.3). Of note are people from all these groups who are at risk of human trafficking or slavery. Unaccompanied minors are especially vulnerable to exploitation (WHO 2019).

Further categories include temporary workers who may have entered a country under specific employment and education programs, and undocumented persons, who have no status in their new country. There is deep inequality for these workers who are employed in insecure work conditions, with exclusion from social security benefits, and with increased risk of

---

BOX 3.3

THE CONVENTION RELATING TO THE STATUS OF REFUGEES

The Convention Relating to the Status of Refugees was adopted by the UNHCR in 1950–51. Information on the Convention and the updated 1967 Protocol Relating to the Status of Refugees can be located at: www.unhcr.org/3b66c2aa10.html.

The basic minimum standards for the treatment of refugees are highlighted.

Source: United Nations High Commissioner for Refugees (UNHCR), 2010. Convention and protocol relating to the status of refugees. UNHCR, Geneva.

underpayment, overwork, sexual harassment and dismissal after complaints to employers (Farbenblum & Berg 2020, Lees & Niner 2021). Of further concern is the complex issue of stateless persons and families who are not classified as citizens of any country. Loss of citizenship can occur when a country ceases to exist, or when a country implements discriminative statutes and cancels the nationality of certain population groups (UNHCR 2021).

Accessible, culturally appropriate primary health care is frequently lacking for many of these categories of families and workers, including strategies for addressing posttraumatic disorders. Adverse social and cultural determinants of health including language difficulties, prejudice and discrimination, poor housing and living conditions, unemployment and inadequate understanding of their rights severely impacts their ability to assimilate with their host countries and maintain basic standards of physical and psychosocial health and wellbeing (WHO 2019).

Current estimates are that 3.5% of the world's population or 244 million people are classified as international migrants. In recent years, the number of migrants moving to high-income countries has declined slightly while increasing elsewhere, particularly in upper middle-income countries. Internationally, the number of refugees in 2018 was 25.9 million, with 52% under the age of 18 years. Additionally, the global population of stateless people was 3.9 million (McAuliffe & Khadria 2019, pp. 3–4).

Migrants enrich communities through economic development and cultural diversity through their contributions to their host country's cultural, civic and economic environments. Migration can influence health risk due to factors associated with health engagement, but resettlement can also be correlated with improved health due to access and positive intention for health-seeking behaviours (McAuliffe & Khadria 2019). Refugees and migrants need transitory or ongoing support with their relocation, with an interdisciplinary primary health care approach by community health nurses and other practitioners needed to promote socially inclusive, accessible policies and strategies.

Research has demonstrated that significant adversity early in life can impair healthy development during childhood and adult life. Contributory causes include the social determinants of poverty, community violence and impacts of contaminated water and poor food security. Children and their families relocating to new countries, escaping violence and disasters, and living in substandard living situations in host nations, experience high risks of lifelong impairments in physical and psychosocial health (Shonkoff et al 2021). These issues highlight the need for community health practitioners to understand the impacts of adverse childhood experiences and develop partnerships with families, communities and other health professionals to develop culturally appropriate, family-centred care pathways.

Chapter 9 explores the refugee experience in the context of inclusive communities.

INDIGENOUS POPULATIONS

Australian Aboriginal and Torres Strait Islander and New Zealand Māori families and communities have a richness in their family lives and relationships to their communities. The original inhabitants of both countries enjoy strong family and cultural ties that positively influence their relationships and sense of wellbeing. However, historical and contemporary public social and health policies have had negative influences on their ability to maintain healthy families and communities (Gray et al 2020). Culturally reflexive healthcare provision is needed from nurses and other health practitioners, working in partnership with these vulnerable populations to investigate their self-perceived needs and pathways forward. This area of practice will be explored in greater detail in Chapter 9.

Promoting health in communities of place

People's most immediate environment is significant for maintaining their health and wellbeing. Planning for health promotion and health education activities needs to reflect a settings approach and communities of place, where interdisciplinary strategies aim to improve protective health and social factors and moderate risks for individual, family and community wellbeing across each specific setting. This approach recognises that health and health promotion are influenced by the various settings where people live, work and play (Taylor 2021, p. 248). Effective health promotion plans begin with knowledge of the local context, the SDH that either enhance or constrain health and wellbeing in that environment, and individual or family factors that may be influencing personal choices. As noted earlier in the chapter, place is where people share meanings and understanding of their daily lives, which influences the extent to which they can socialise and develop their sense of social wellbeing (Van Otten & Dutton 2020). Some places are more conducive to good health than others. For example, some communities enable and sustain health and wellbeing through community action to enable social connectedness and spaces for physical activity (Taylor et al 2021). Relative disadvantage may include disempowering settings where there is a lack of employment opportunities and the presence of victim blaming for poor social circumstances. Contemporary settings affecting health and behaviour include the internet and a range of social networking sites, including visual media which can demonstrate desired behaviour (Taylor et al 2021). Examples of settings approaches are explored in the following paragraphs; however, you may encounter more settings in your varied practice situations.

HEALTH PROMOTION IN THE CITY

As discussed earlier in the chapter, promoting the health of urban communities begins with the global commitment to healthy cities, where community participation and empowerment, intersectoral partnerships and participant equity are integral features of health in numerous cities throughout the world. Locally, many Healthy Cities initiatives begin at the neighbourhood level, recognising the determinants of health and the necessity to work in partnership across a range of government, non-government and voluntary organisations. The key to achieving target initiatives is the involvement of local people in decision-making, with the engagement, collaboration and capacity-building processes as important as the outcomes (WHO 2021f).

HEALTH PROMOTION IN HOSPITALS

Throughout the past two decades the Health Promoting Hospitals (HPH) concept has been used to encourage hospital staff to engage in health promotion and health education, in order to improve the health of patients and staff. This work was developed by the WHO, recognising hospitals as a setting for reorientation of health. Structures, cultures, decisions and processes are supported to include health promotion in hospitals and health services for patients, their families and staff (International Network of Health Promoting Hospitals and Health Services 2021). Nurses have reported more confidence in their employment, with enhanced work satisfaction, less illness, less staff turnover and, subsequently, decreases in patient morbidity and mortality. Of note are current HPH initiatives to reduce hospital emissions and waste through the Global Green and Healthy Hospitals framework (Taylor et al 2021).

RURAL HEALTH PROMOTION

Like health promotion in the city, promoting health in rural communities is dependent on understanding people and place factors. Rural culture can provide a structure for higher levels of social capital and cohesiveness; for example, higher rates of volunteering (AIHW 2019). This is not to imply a homogeneous culture in rural and regional areas, but there are shared cultural norms among rural people that need to be recognised for the development of effective health promotion activities. Health outcomes are poorer outside major cities, with common issues being diabetes, coronary heart disease and motor vehicle crashes. Multifactorial determinants of health impact on rural and remote populations that contribute to these outcomes, such as availability of fresh fruit and vegetables, differences in access to services and factors associated with driving (AIHW 2019).

POINT TO PONDER

People who live in rural or remote regions frequently have poorer access to health promotion programs. What specific role could you see a nurse or other health practitioner undertaking to improve access to health promotion for rural families?

In many rural and regional areas, there is often closer collaboration between primary care and primary health care services, both with an interest in integration of services. Health prevention activities, along with early and chronic disease management, are usually delivered in general practice primary care and community-based settings (AIHW 2019). As such, in some cases it is important to develop selective and comprehensive primary health care programs. In many rural areas one of the greatest needs for engaging local communities is in enabling mental health literacy and supports. With the decline of the rural economy, young people often feel isolated from their peers at a time when social connections are most important. Adolescents may be receptive to health education messages that encourage responsible alcohol consumption, or other healthy behaviours, but in rural areas even when programs or services are available, they may not access these because of the stigma of the entire community knowing their reasons for attending a clinic or service. Valuable sources of information for rural and regional communities are the Australian National Rural Health Alliance (www.ruralhealth.org.au) and the Rural Health Alliance Aotearoa New Zealand (https://rhaanz.org.nz/).

HEALTH PROMOTION IN SCHOOLS

Health Promoting Schools (HPS) are also place-based settings for health promotion, developed around a whole-of-school approach to engage students, their families and staff in promoting their health and that of their school. Nurses and other health practitioners in both Australia and New Zealand are actively engaged in promoting health in schools (Taylor et al 2021), with HPS recognised as focusing on non-communicable diseases (NCDs) by positively promoting healthy development and health-seeking behaviours through activities such as physical activity, appropriate nutrition and bullying prevention. A whole-of-school approach is necessary, with governance, intersectoral working and sustainability being features of successful implementation. Current challenges that require more evidence and action are the need to address equity and disparities between geographical regions that are impacted by a range of social and cultural determinants of health (WHO & UNESCO 2020).

Schools are regarded as important health promotion settings as prevention and promotion activities can help address the social gradient through capacity building for health. The WHO developed six key strategies that have been used internationally for development of policies, practice and research: healthy school policies, optimal physical environment, positive social environment, capacity-building approaches to individual health skills, and availability of community links and health services (Dadaczynski & Hering 2021, WHO/WPRO 1996).

Promoting awareness of mental health issues, particularly for adolescent mental health and bullying in primary and secondary schools, is an essential component of primary health care practice in schools. Nurses and other practitioners working in schools need an awareness of the social dynamics and power imbalances that exist in schools as a great deal of their practice is spent helping students and their families with mental health, physical and online bullying and a range of psychosocial issues. This includes the safe use of technology, as online support and care plays a significant role in management of mental health and wellbeing (Moyes 2019, Nelson et al 2019).

Assisting school-aged children to address negative peer influences and develop a general sense of belonging and empowerment helps community health practitioners working in schools to target negative body image in both male and female students. If left unaddressed, this has the potential to develop into poor adult psychosocial health (Gattario & Frisén 2019). These practitioners are also instrumental in facilitating safe environments for sexual health services and health promotion to students, their families and whole school communities. There is a diverse range of health concerns in this area which requires sensitive, non-judgmental communication and liaison skills with the practitioner's ability to be inclusive of the sexual health needs of diverse cultural and sexual identity students being paramount (Guys 2021).

HEALTH PROMOTION THROUGH VIRTUAL TECHNOLOGIES

The internet is increasingly becoming a valid tool for health promotion with a wide variety of approaches that can be used by health practitioners and community members for information, mass communication, peer interaction and community engagement (Taylor et al 2021). However, access to computers can be a problem for people experiencing disadvantage which creates barriers to participation. Digital exclusion is related to economic and social factors. People impacted by adverse SDH such as poverty, lower educational attainment, unemployment and underemployment are significantly less digitally included. Geography also plays a critical role, with access to the internet being greater in urban areas than rural and remote regions. Indigenous Australians in both urban and regional areas are relatively less able to engage with digital technology. This is exacerbated by increasing remoteness which impacts particularly on access and affordability (Thomas et al 2020).

Digital exclusion is especially prevalent in periods of social disruption and community lockdowns such as during the COVID-19 pandemic. Families without adequate internet access, senior citizens and people experiencing stress across a range of physical and psychosocial domains were, and continue to be, particularly vulnerable to social isolation and lack of reliable information during the pandemic (Drane et al 2020, Thomas et al 2020).

There is also a caution for practitioners in using the internet for health education. Information placed on the internet is publicly accessible in perpetuity, and is discoverable by a court of law even when deleted. While the internet can provide valuable information to healthcare consumers, practitioners must be careful that any postings maintain client confidentiality, and that they are accurate and represent best available knowledge at the time they are disseminated (National Council of State Boards of Nursing, Inc. [NCSBN] 2018).

KEY POINTS

Trends in health promotion and health education include:

- social media for health information
- smart phones
- addressing the digital divide
- online peer support.

One of the challenges of health promotion and education is to help maintain integrity in the type, level and appropriateness of information people are accessing from the internet. As health practitioners, we can fulfil an enabling role by providing access to expertise, research evidence and contextual information that will assist people in making healthy choices and finding the resources they need, along with providing guidance on accessing credible and reliable information.

Conclusion

The implications of these discussions on communities of place are twofold. First, they indicate that place is very important to health. Second, as professional advocates, we have an obligation to stay abreast of new evidence-based knowledge and strategies that will help us maintain professional competence to work in partnership with virtual and geographical communities, whether they are located locally, nationally or globally. These activities are developmental, in that by working collaboratively the knowledge, skills and self-confidence of individuals, families and communities are developed, ultimately empowering them in their lifelong health and wellbeing. Facilitating and enabling community empowerment also helps develop the skills of health practitioners. Every opportunity to work with a community is unique and yields new information that community health practitioners working in partnership with individuals, families and communities can use to consolidate and refine health promotion skills. In this respect, advocacy is a deliberate two-way process of mutual development. In the next chapter we focus on the role of the practitioner and the differing ways they work with communities and other health practitioners.

Conclusion—cont'd

Please reflect on the big issues below before reading the case study involving the Smith and Mason families. Consider how you can use your new-found knowledge from this chapter to work in partnership with families to identify their strengths and challenges, and guide ways forward.

Reflecting on the Big Issues

- Being healthy in any community means having equitable access to resources, empowerment, cultural inclusiveness, healthy environments and participation in decision-making.
- Global factors have an impact on all types of communities.
- Place is important to health because it constitutes as well as contains social relations.
- The reciprocal relationship between health and place means that some places can enhance health potential, while others may create risks to health.

- A relational view of health sees health as dynamic, and created through either virtual or visible networks.
- Social capital means that communities can accumulate social assets.
- Distinctive and special populations within our communities need supportive primary health care approaches to enhance their capacity to maintain their health and wellbeing.
- The relationship between health and place is a major consideration in promoting health and advocating for the community.

CASE STUDY | The Smith and Mason families' communities

Papakura is a working-class suburb of South Auckland with large Māori and Pacific populations. Jason and Huia have recently built a new home on the outskirts of Papakura, approximately 5 minutes' drive to the local shopping centre and a 40-minute drive to central Auckland where Jason works. Huia's family lives in the Papakura area and, although Jason and Huia could afford to move to more affluent suburbs, she wants to stay close to her extended family.

Maddington is a leafy, older suburb of Perth, with large, comfortable homes and a growing multicultural population. The suburb contains major residential, retail and industrial sections as well as some semi-rural areas. Unusual for a large city suburb, Maddington has several vineyards and orchards from a previous era when it was primarily agricultural. The community has a railway station and is engaged in transit-oriented development planning. The area also has a large shopping centre and a technical college, and it is within 10 kilometres of a major university. The Masons live in a three-bedroom home close to a park and within a short drive to most of the local schools and services. They are only 10 minutes away from the freeway which helps Colin's commute to the airport.

The mining site where Colin is employed is in the Pilbara region of Western Australia. The mine operates 24 hours a day, 365 days a year. It is close to several small communities where some of the mine's service personnel live. The men live in single men's quarters in the mining camp where they have some access to amenities such as a gym, recreation hall and some internet access on most days.

Reflective questions: How would I use this knowledge in practice?

1 Identify the primary, secondary and tertiary steps that can be taken to promote health in a relational community, such as one connected by social media.

2 Intersectoral collaboration is essential for addressing the SDGs. Consider the health professional skill mixes needed in different global communities to address community health challenges.

3 Consider how globalisation may affect your practice. How will globalisation affect job opportunities for new graduates, and the drive for efficiencies and cost savings within health services?

4 Can you identify any influences on the Mason and Smith families from global factors?

5 Which of these factors are evident in Colin's (mining) workplace community?

6 How could the Smith and Mason families potentially use social media for their adult and children's health

needs and to maintain their wellbeing? Consider their urban and rural locations.

7 Conduct a web search of the two communities of Maddington, Western Australia and Papakura, New Zealand. From the online information describe the relationship between health and place in each community.

8 What would constitute social capital in each of these communities?

9 What are the most important assets available to those who live in large cities?

10 Describe a relational community in which you are a member.

11 What are the barriers to empowerment for rural communities?

References

Amnesty International, 2021. Refugees, asylum seekers and migrants. Online. Available: www.amnesty.org/en/what-we-do/refugees-asylum-seekers-and-migrants/.

Australian Government Department of Health, 2021. Australian statistical geography standard—Remoteness area. Department of Health, Canberra.

Australian Institute of Health and Welfare (AIHW), 2019. Rural and remote health. Cat. No. PHE 255. AIHW, Canberra.

Australian Institute of Health and Welfare (AIHW), 2020a. Suicide and self-harm monitoring. AIHW, Canberra.

Australian Institute of Health and Welfare (AIHW), 2020b. Australia's health 2020. AIHW, Canberra.

Australian Medical Association (AMA), 2019. 2019 AMA rural health issues survey. Improving care for rural Australia. AMA, Canberra.

Bennett, E., Simpson, W., Fowler, C., et al, 2020. Enhancing access to parenting services using digital technology supported practices. Australian Journal of Child and Family Health Nursing, 17 (1), 4–11. Maternal, Child & Family Health Nurses Australia.

Bettelli, P., 2021. What the world learned setting development goals. International Institute for Sustainable Development (IISD), Canada. Online. Available: www.iisd.org/system/files/2021-01/still-one-earth-MDG-SDG.pdf.

Callis, Z., Seivwright, A., Orr, C., et al, 2020. The impact of COVID-19 on families in hardship in Western Australia. The 100 Families WA project (Anglicare, Centrecare, Jacaranda Community Centre, Mercycare, Ruah Community Services, Uniting WA, Wanslea, WACOSS, The University of Western Australia [Centre for Social Impact and the School of Population and Global Health]), Perth. Online. Available: https://doi.org/10.25916/5f3b2a5e4bb42.

Correa-Velez, I., 2019. Global health. In: Fleming, M.L., Parker, E., Correa-Velez, I., (Eds), Introduction to public health, fourth ed. Elsevier, Sydney, pp. 197–212.

Dadaczynski, K., Hering, T., 2021. Health promoting schools in Germany. Mapping the implementation of holistic strategies to tackle NCDs and promote health. Int. J. Environ. Res. Public Health, 18, 2623. Online. Available: https://doi.org/10.3390/ijerph18052623.

David, F., Bryan, K., Larsen, J.J., 2019. Migrants and their vulnerability to human trafficking, modern slavery and forced labour. International Organization for Migration, Switzerland.

Department of Mines, Industry Regulation and Safety, 2021. Information for families. Government of Western Australia, Perth.

Drane, C.F., Vernon, L., O'Shea, S., 2020. Vulnerable learners in the age of COVID-19: A scoping review. Aust. Educ. Res. Online. Available: https://doi.org/10.1007/s13384-020-00409-5.

Emmanuel, A.W., Jerry, C.S., Dzigbodi, D.A., 2018. Review of environmental and health impacts of mining in Ghana. J. Health Pollut., 17, 43–52.

Farbenblum, B., Berg, L., 2020. International students and wage theft in Australia. Migrant Worker Justice Initiative, University of New South Wales and University of Technology Sydney, Sydney.

Gattario, K.H., Frisén, A., 2019. From negative to positive body image: Men's and women's journeys from early adolescence to emerging adulthood. Body Image, 28, 53–65. Online. Available: https://doi.org/10.1016/j.bodyim.2018.12.002.

Gilbert, J., Fruhen, L., Parker, S.K., 2020. Summary of findings. FIFO worker mental health and wellbeing: The impact of Covid-19. Centre for Transformative Work Design, Perth.

Gray, S., Biles, B., Biles, J., 2020. Exploration of history, culture, cultural bias, race and racism. In: Biles, B., Biles, J. (Eds), Aboriginal and Torres Strait Islander Peoples' health and wellbeing. Oxford University Press, Docklands, pp. 27–46.

Guys, D., 2021. School and youth health nursing. In: Guys, D., Brown, R., Halcomb, E., Whitehead, D., (Eds), An introduction to community and primary health care, third ed. Cambridge University Press, Cambridge, pp. 311–327.

International Council of Nurses (ICN), 2021. SDGs. ICN, Geneva. Online. Available: www.icn.ch/nursing-policy/icn-strategic-priorities/sustainable-development-goals.

International Network of Health Promoting Hospitals and Health Services, 2021. Online. Available: www.hphnet.org/about-us/.

Iroz-Elardo, N., Adkins, A., Ingram, M., 2021. Measuring perceptions of social environments for walking: A scoping review of walkability surveys. Health Place, 67 (102468). Online. Available: https://doi.org/10.1016/j.healthplace.2020.102468.

Larcombe, D.L., van Etten, E., Logan, A., et al, 2019. High-rise apartments and urban mental health—Historical and contemporary views. Challenges, 10 (2), 1–15. Online. Available: https://doi.org/10.3390/challe10020034.

Lees, R.A., Niner, A., 2021. Tracing the impacts of the COVID pandemic on Australia's fastest-growing migrant group. Politics Soc. Online. Available: https://lens.monash.edu/@politics-society/2021/04/12/1383007/tracing-the-impacts-of-the-covid-pandemic-on-australias-fastest-growing-migrant-group.

Logan Together, 2018. Logan's Community Gateways: A discussion paper. Logan Together, Logan.

McAuliffe, M., Khadria, B. (Eds), 2019. World migration report 2020. International Organization for Migration, Geneva.

Moyes, A., 2019. Exploring the experiences of secondary school nurses who encounter young people with mental health problems: A grounded theory study. Unpublished PhD thesis. Curtin University, Perth. Available: Curtin library e-space.

National Council of State Boards of Nursing, Inc. (NCSBN), 2018. A nurse's guide to the use of social media. NCSBN, Chicago.

National Rural Health Alliance (NRHA), n.d. The health of people living in remote Australia. NRHA, Canberra.

National Rural Health Alliance (NRHA), 2021. House Select Committee on Mental Health and Suicide Prevention. NRHA, Canberra.

Nelson, H.J., Burns, S.K., Kendall, G.E., et al, 2019. Preadolescent children's perception of power imbalance in bullying: A thematic analysis. PLoS ONE, 14 (3), e0211124. Online. Available: https://doi.org/10.1371/journal.pone.0211124.

Office of the High Commissioner, Human Rights (OHCHR), 2021a. About extreme poverty and human rights. United Nations, Geneva.

Office of the High Commissioner, Human Rights (OHCHR), 2021b. Homelessness and human rights. United Nations, Geneva.

Organisation for Economic Co-operation and Development (OECD), 2020. OECD Policy responses to coronavirus (COVID-19). Cities policy responses. OECD, Paris.

Parker, S., Fruhen, L., Burton, C., et al, 2018. Impact of FIFO work arrangements on the mental health and wellbeing of FIFO workers. Centre for Transformative Work Design, Perth.

Public Health England, 2021. Place-based approaches for reducing health inequalities: main report. United Kingdom Government, London. Online. Available: www.gov.uk/government/publications/health-inequalities-place-based-approaches-to-reduce-inequalities/place-based-approaches-for-reducing-health-inequalities-main-report.

Rural Health Information Hub (RHIhub), 2021. Social determinants of health for rural people. RHIhub, Grand Forks, ND.

Safe Work Australia, 2020. FIFO and DIDO. Online. Available: https://covid19.swa.gov.au/covid-19-information-workplaces/industry-information/fifo-dido.

Shonkoff, J.P., Slopen, N., Williams, D.R., 2021. Early childhood adversity, toxic stress, and the impacts of racism on the foundations of health. Annu. Rev. Public Health, 42, 115–134.

Smith, T., McNeil, K., Mitchell, R., et al, 2019. A study of macro-, meso- and micro-barriers and enablers affecting extended scopes of practice: the case of rural nurse practitioners in Australia. BMC Nurs., 18 (14), 1–12. Online. Available: https://doi.org/10.1186/s12912-019-0337-z.

Taylor, J., O'Hara, L., Talbot, L., et al, 2021. Promoting health: The primary health care approach, seventh ed. Elsevier, Sydney.

The Commonwealth Fund, 2021a. International healthcare system profiles. Australia, The Commonwealth Fund, Washington, DC.

The Commonwealth Fund, 2021b. International healthcare system profiles. New Zealand. The Commonwealth Fund, Washington, DC.

Thomas, J., Barraket, J., Wilson, C.K., et al, 2020. Measuring Australia's digital divide: The Australian Digital Inclusion Index 2020. RMIT and Swinburne University of Technology, Melbourne, for Telstra.

United Nations High Commissioner for Refugees (UNHCR), 2010. Convention and protocol relating to the status of refugees. UNHCR, Geneva.

United Nations High Commissioner for Refugees (UNHCR), 2021. Statelessness. UNHCR, Geneva.

United Nations Population Fund, 2020. Urbanization. United Nations, New York.

Van Otten, G., Dutton, J.A., 2020. The importance of place. College of Earth and Mineral Sciences, The Pennsylvania State University, Pennsylvania.

Victoria State Government, 2020. Tackling climate change and its impact on health. Victoria State Government, Melbourne. Online. Available: www2.health.vic.gov.au/about/health-strategies/public-health-wellbeing-plan/tackling-climate-change.

Victorian Ombudsman, 2020. Investigation into the detention and treatment of public housing residents arising from a COVID-19 'hard lockdown' in July 2020. Victorian Ombudsman, Melbourne.

Wettasinghe, P.M., Allan, W., Garvey, G., et al, 2020. Older Aboriginal Australians' health concerns and preferences for healthy ageing programs. Int. J. Environ. Res. Public Health, 17 (20), 7390. Online. Available: https://doi.org/10.3390/ijerph17207390.

World Bank, 2021. Poverty. World Bank, Washington, DC. Online. Available: www.worldbank.org/en/topic/poverty/overview.

World Health Organization (WHO), 2019. Promoting the health of refugees and migrants—Draft global action plan, 2019–2023. WHO, Geneva.

World Health Organization (WHO), 2021a. Globalization. WHO, Geneva.

World Health Organization (WHO), 2021b. Millennium Development Goals (MDGs). WHO, Geneva.

World Health Organization (WHO), 2021c. Urban health. WHO, Geneva.

World Health Organization (WHO), 2021d. Healthy Cities vision. WHO, Geneva.

World Health Organization (WHO), 2021e. Age-friendly cities and communities. WHO, Geneva.

World Health Organization (WHO), 2021f. What is a healthy city? WHO, Geneva.

World Health Organization and the United Nations Educational, Scientific and Cultural Organization (WHO & UNESCO), 2020. Report of the first Virtual Meeting of the External Advisory Group (EAG) for the development of Global Standards for Health Promoting Schools and their implementation guidance. WHO & UNESCCO, Geneva.

World Health Organization—Regional Office for the Western Pacific (WHO/WPRO), 1996. Health Promoting Schools. Regional guidelines. Development of health-promoting schools. A framework for action. WHO/WPRO, Manila.

World Health Regional Office for Europe, 2021. Nature, biodiversity and health: an overview of interconnections. WHO, Copenhagen.

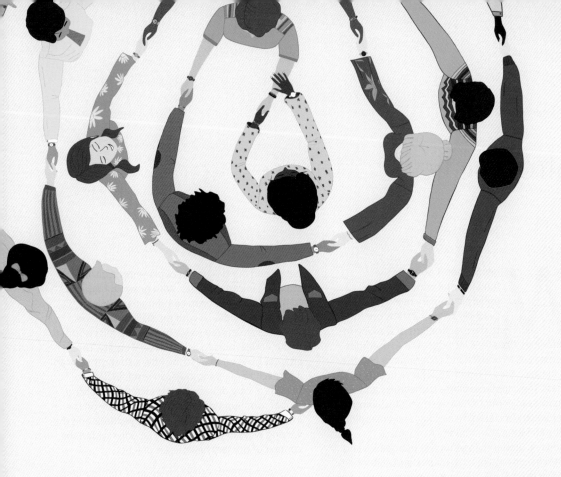

Section 2

Primary health care in practice

Introduction to the section

While Section 1 outlined the fundamental principles that underpin primary health care practice, Section 2 shifts our focus to the practicalities of working in communities. Chapter 4 introduces us to methods that enable us to understand communities and the ways in which they function to achieve health and wellness. The chapter explores frameworks and approaches to community assessment including epidemiology, social epidemiology, asset mapping and the McMurray Community Assessment Framework. Global change such as pandemics and *climate change* require us to understand community need in ways that are different from in the past. With *equity* and *sustainability* underpinning our approach, our sources of information and development of appropriate interventions are changing too. The chapter discusses the different sources of assessment information health practitioners can access and introduces a range of community interventions for health and wellbeing including partnership and engagement, community development, community infection prevention and public health interventions such as contact tracing and communicable disease prevention.

Chapter 5 provides the framework for our work in communities, exploring models of care that are informed by the principles of primary health care. Working in and with communities requires us to work with individuals, families and communities to achieve health, each requiring different approaches and skill sets. In this chapter, we provide a framework for exploring structured approaches to planning care with individuals and families and examples of how the framework can be used in practice. Importantly,

we extend our discussion of planning to project planning in communities. With growing demand for health promotion in communities, project planning provides us with the skills to manage work in a structured way, ensuring we miss nothing in our endeavours to achieve social equity. The chapter goes on to describe how a strengths-based approach to planning care can result in flexible models of care delivery across local, national and global communities. We also touch briefly on the importance of evaluating our interventions and the varying ways in which this can be done within the context of primary health care practice.

Chapter 6 extends our knowledge of communities by examining the wide range of nursing and other health practitioner roles present in communities and the many ways in which we can enable community capacity. We can all assist communities using a *comprehensive primary health care* approach, which supports all aspects of community life, helping to conserve what is special and helpful, and assisting them in countering what is not. Other activities are aimed at *selective primary health care*, which is a more targeted approach, where specific groups or issues are given priority attention. Because primary health care has become integral to professional practice in both Australia and New Zealand, we examine primary health care roles in the context of various models of practice for nursing and other community-based health practitioners, and the situations that guide role development including: rural and remote nursing; child, school and occupational health nursing; community mental health; and the more generic roles of practice nurses and nurse practitioners. In today's healthcare environments nurses undertake a range of these traditional roles and some that have evolved in response to contemporary lifestyles. We describe some of these new roles and examine their effectiveness in a range of health service contexts. We highlight the importance of interdisciplinary practice and ensuring teamwork in practice. We also discuss a range of allied health roles and their contribution to interdisciplinary teams and to community health and wellness. At the end of each chapter we revisit the Smith and Mason families, using our case study to demonstrate how nurses can work effectively within communities.

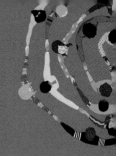

CHAPTER 4

Assessing the community

Introduction

This chapter discusses the importance of assessment in the context of primary health care practice and the types of interventions—both systemic and local—that are needed to achieve community health and wellness. The chapter will: explore community assessment; introduce the practitioner to public health interventions such as contact tracing, case management and community infection prevention; and provide the practitioner with the tools to partner with a community to achieve change. We outline a range of existing assessment tools and focus on the McMurray community assessment framework as a comprehensive approach to community assessment founded on the principles of primary health care and the social determinants of health (SDH). We emphasise the importance of

working in partnership with the community in the assessment process.

Assessment is the foundation for planning to meet the needs of the community. These needs are identified on the basis of any known risks, hazards and strengths, as well as the priorities and preferences of community residents. To plan effective, efficient, adequate, appropriate and acceptable health interventions we need both scientific data gathered by health planners (top-down information) and community perspectives (bottom-up information). As we mentioned in Chapter 1, an 'assets' approach to promoting health focuses on community strengths as well as needs. To generate a list of community assets and needs it is important to create an asset 'map' of geographic, demographic and social information. Geographic data indicate what features or hazards exist or may exist in the future in

OBJECTIVES

By the end of this chapter you will be able to:

1. compare a range of assessment approaches and their usefulness in developing programmes and policies to promote community health

2. describe the importance of working in partnership with communities in the assessment process

3. identify a range of sources of information about communities

4. outline a range of interventions with communities relevant to the current context

5. assess a community using the McMurray community assessment framework.

the natural and built environment, the patterns of health and illness among various groups defined by age or gender, and what social conditions require health promotion interventions for community residents. Simultaneously, the assessment involves finding out from members of the community how they assess their health strengths and needs in terms of personal perspectives and experiences. Once this information has been gathered, the next stage of planning is to develop intervention strategies for improvement, or measures that can be taken to sustain positive aspects of community life. Global pandemics and climate change are changing our focus with communities but the fundamental principles of primary health care as well as equity and sustainability still underpin our interventions. The advantage of conducting a comprehensive assessment is that it allows us to forecast patterns of health or potential changes that may impact on people's lives or the lives of their children in the future. In the final analysis the information should produce a snapshot of strengths, weaknesses, opportunities and threats to community health.

General knowledge of the community has limited usefulness unless it is analysed in terms of subsequent steps that can be taken in partnership with community members to strengthen community resources and enable health and wellbeing. Selecting an assessment strategy should therefore be *goal directed*, so that the assessment information is linked to promoting and sustaining community health and wellness.

Community assessment

Many decades ago, community assessment was predominantly a checklist approach to assessing communities and their ability to support the needs of residents. A number of tools were developed to ensure that assessments took into account vital information on personal as well as community health hazards and risks. This information was then used to predict people's exposure to diseases or the risk of accidental ill health from such things as bushfires, drowning or other events common to the area. Many of these tools focused on the population and age-specific risks (e.g. asthma in children), with only

cursory evaluation of the relationship between health and place, or the assets (e.g. health services) that could help maintain better health. Some of those tools remain useful in assessing community health and the risk of ill health, but in the context of today's primary health care approach, we recognise that people are quite knowledgeable about their needs and the needs of their communities, and community assessment is incomplete without their input.

One of the earliest approaches to assessment was the epidemiological model, which focused on the determinants and distribution of health and disease. The epidemiological approach was embraced by all health professions on the basis that it reflected a whole-of-population approach and included comprehensive assessment of the person, host and environment, called the 'epidemiological triad'. Epidemiological assessments continue to be useful today in developing a base of scientific evidence on health and its determinants in specified populations. Epidemiology is essential for tracking communicable diseases such as COVID-19, measles or tuberculosis.

EPIDEMIOLOGICAL ASSESSMENT

Epidemiology can be defined as 'the study of the distribution of health and diseases in *groups of people* and the study of the factors that influence this distribution' (Wassertheil-Smoller & Smoller 2015, p. 83). The classic model of epidemiology is to examine specific aspects of the host (biology), the agent (a causative factor) and environment (factors that exacerbate or moderate the effects of the agent on the host), to see how each of these affects the spread of a disease or ill health in the population. The objective of epidemiological researchers is to collect data on the incidence of individuals 'at risk' of developing a particular disease in order to inform development of a vaccine or treatment for that disease. Data from epidemiological analyses are presented in terms of *incidence* and *prevalence*. Incidence is calculated by dividing the number of *new* cases in a population by the population at risk, then multiplying this by a base number (1000 or 100 000). This estimates the likelihood that a condition would occur in the population. The prevalence of a certain condition is the number of *new and existing* cases divided by the

---

BOX 4.1

....

EXAMPLE OF EPIDEMIOLOGICAL RATES

....

Population at risk

$$\text{Incidence} = \frac{\text{No. of new cases}}{\text{Population at risk}} \times 1000 \text{ (or } 100\,000\text{)}$$

$$\text{Prevalence} = \frac{\text{No. of existing cases (new and old)}}{\text{Population at risk}}$$
$$\times 1000 \text{ (or } 100\,000\text{)}$$

The group of people who are susceptible to a disease or condition (e.g. non-immunised children) or who have been exposed to an agent that could cause disease (e.g. occupational dust).

---

population at risk multiplied by 1000 or 100 000 (see Box 4.1). Box 4.2 provides a case study of classic epidemiology in action.

KEY POINT

....

Rate

A measure of the frequency of a disease or condition, calculated by dividing prevalence by the incidence multiplied by a population base number (1000 or 100 000).

Incidence

The number of *new* cases of a disease or health issue in a specific period of time, divided by the population at risk multiplied by the base number.

Prevalence

The *total number* (new plus existing) of cases of a disease or health issue in a population at any one time, divided by the population at risk multiplied by the base number.

If an occupational group is exposed to a certain toxic substance, a measure of the 'relative risk' of becoming ill from that exposure can be calculated by comparing a group (called a cohort) who were exposed to the hazard with a cohort who were not exposed. If the group exposed to the hazard has a higher rate of the illness, that hazard is declared a risk factor. To confirm that it is a risk factor we would then assess its effect over a longer period of time in the entire population, which would provide greater insight. An example of how relative risk can be used to identify inequity is found in a study that examined the differences in disability outcomes between Māori and non-Māori 24 months after experiencing an injury (Wyeth et al 2019). The study collected data from 375 Māori and 1824 non-Māori on pre-injury, injury-related and early post-injury characteristics 3 and 24 months after injury. At 24 months after injury, 26% of Māori and 10% of non-Māori were experiencing disability. The authors found that the variables predicting disability 24 months after injury were the same for Māori and non-Māori with one noticeable difference—trouble accessing healthcare services. Trouble accessing healthcare services for injury placed Māori (but not non-Māori) at increased risk of disability at 24 months (RR = 2.58; 95% CI 1.4–4.9). The relative risk (RR) was 2.58. If RR is near to or equals 1, there is no or little association. If RR is greater than 1, then there is a positive association meaning the risk in the exposed population (in this case Māori with injury) is greater than the risk in non-exposed people. If RR is less than 1, there is a negative or inverse association (the risk from exposure is less than the risk in non-exposed people). The authors recommend that significant work has still to be done to improve access to healthcare services for Māori in New Zealand.

The findings from Wyeth and colleagues' 2019 study are important for providing insight into the inequities that exist in our health systems for some sectors of the population. Relatively small sample sizes make it difficult to draw definitive conclusions so further work is needed, but these findings add to the already substantial research identifying inequities in outcomes for Māori and Indigenous people in Australia (see Chapters 2 and 9). Studies like this help pinpoint where and how interventions can be made to improve health services to address inequity.

BOX 4.2

EPIDEMIOLOGY CASE STUDY

Australia and New Zealand's response to COVID-19 provides a classic example of epidemiology in action. As the world began to recognise the risk posed by the new corona virus emanating from Wuhan in China known as COVID-19, Australia's and New Zealand's public health units responded quickly and efficiently. First, the biology of the virus itself was identified enabling scientists to understand better the way in which it worked and how it might be counteracted (in this case through the development of a vaccine). Second, work was undertaken to identify how the virus was transmitted from person to person and what the risk was that a person would develop the disease if they were exposed to it. Third, factors that exacerbated or moderated the effects of the virus were identified so that risk of disease could be reduced; for example, using masks, physical distancing and good hand hygiene were all factors that reduced the risk of contracting the disease. While this work was underway, traditional approaches to communicable disease prevention were also underway to reduce the incidence (the number of new cases) of the disease in the population. In Australia and New Zealand this involved quarantine, isolation, testing and contact tracing. As a result, in both countries, the prevalence of the disease (i.e. the number of people actually with the disease in the population) was kept to a minimum.

- Quarantine occurs when a person or animal arrives from a place where they may have been exposed to an infectious agent or pest and spend a period of time isolated from others in order to prevent the spread of a disease or pest.
- Isolation is when a person or animal is kept separate or isolated from others in order to protect others from a disease or pest.
- Testing is undertaken to determine if a person or animal has an infectious agent or carries a pest.
- Contact tracing is the process of identifying all people or animals that may have been exposed to an infectious agent or pest. People or animals that are identified by contact tracing may be required to isolate from others for a period of time in case they carry the infectious agent or pest.

KEY POINT

Relative risk is a measure of the extent to which a group exposed to a risk has a higher rate of illness than those not exposed, calculated by dividing the incidence rate among those exposed by those not exposed. If the rate is higher among those exposed, it is called a *risk factor*.

Because traditional epidemiological measurements of an agent, host and environment are somewhat limited in terms of what we know about the causes of illness, an expanded model known as the web of causation, which includes the interconnections between each of these, provides a more comprehensive basis for analysis (see Fig 4.1). The web of causation is also inclusive of demographic and social features such as age, gender, ethnicity and social circumstances, which is more closely aligned with a socio-ecological model of health and the SDH.

POINT TO PONDER

If the rate of asthma in preschool children was increasing in a community, how would you go about investigating whether the cause was a risk factor unique to that community, unique to only certain neighbourhoods or unique to only certain types of families?

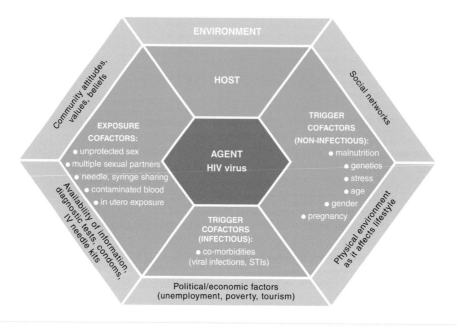

Figure 4.1 Web of causation

METHODS THAT SUPPORT EPIDEMIOLOGY

Contemporary methods to support epidemiological and other community assessment approaches enable information to be quickly and accurately compiled, presenting more quantitatively accurate assessments. For example, geographical information systems (GIS) are being commonly used to plan, administer and analyse community assessment information. Geospatial analysis in particular is being increasingly used to manipulate large and complex datasets according to location using GIS and global positioning systems (GPS) (Liu et al 2021). Liu and colleagues (2021) used geospatial analysis to identify the gaps in public dental service locations for people living with disability in Australia, identifying specific geographic locations where people with disabilities lived further than 5 km from public dental services. In another study, Hobbs and colleagues (2021) used geospatial analysis to show that over a 10-year period, there was a decrease in distance and time to both fast-food outlets and supermarkets but the biggest decrease in distance to a supermarket was seen in the most deprived areas.

These types of studies improve our understanding of how geography is related to health; however, the risks of the GIS approach mean that some smaller population cohorts within a community may not have their needs identified (Fowler et al 2020). For example, the different needs of a small pocket of refugee families in a community or a group of families with children who have Down syndrome and are spread across a wider geographical area may not have their particular needs identified. Statistics from the geographic analysis reveal what is *typical* and what *trends* exist in the community, rather than what special needs exist for various segments of the population. This aggregated information contributes to the risk of 'ecological fallacy'; that is, when correlations between measures based on aggregate or combined data do not apply to individuals within the combined or aggregated group (Fowler et al 2020). To gain a more realistic picture of the community, a combination of information should be used concurrently, such as combining GIS and traditional epidemiology.

Where to find more...

On how to analyse your community using GIS ...

The United States (US) Environmental Protection Agency's community-focused exposure and risk screening tool (C-FERST) is a good example of how GIS can be used in real time, providing easy access to maps, locally specific environmental data and other information in a user-friendly format (www.epa.gov).

New Zealand's Department of Statistics (www.stats.govt.nz) and Australia's Bureau of Statistics (www.abs.gov.au.) provide useful local data but are yet to develop the complexity of the US tool. However, like population trends, none of these tools capture the breadth of variation in human behaviour, which is a limitation of many systematic approaches.

KEY POINT

The ecological fallacy is the risk of misunderstanding individual risk in terms of the overall population risk. Some people's health is determined by unique factors rather than those that are typical of the group or community.

CHALLENGES OF THE EPIDEMIOLOGICAL APPROACH

Epidemiological approaches to community assessment have traditionally struggled to reconcile the scientific approach with the broader contextual factors that impact on people's lives and contribute to their health status. Some of the challenges include the struggle to integrate epidemiologically or scientifically determined risk factors with behavioural and social strengths or risk factors, or an inability to identify risk factors whose origins lie in the interactions between individuals or between individuals and their environment. Epidemiological models are also unable to predict the effects of alternative interventions, which are frequently non-Western in origin (e.g. acupuncture), because all interventions tend to be assessed on the basis of traditional Western scientific approaches. Epidemiology also struggles to articulate the experiences of those with multiple co-morbidities, tending once again to focus on an individual disease rather than the impact of multiple co-morbidities on a person or group. So, for example, a person who has worked in an occupation with a hazardous exposure to dust (such as in a flour mill), and who also has lived in a bushfire area, may develop pulmonary disease. The pulmonary condition may also predispose the person to a number of other risks (cardiac, renal, stress-related diseases). In this case it would be difficult to pinpoint the cause of ill health to the workplace, the natural environment or the lack of preventative programs that would have provided protection from agents that can cause respiratory problems. The message is that epidemiological data provides only part of the picture. It is also necessary to search for causes of ill health in the social and political factors that impact on health (Goodman et al 2019).

As researchers have become aware of epidemiological limitations, many have become committed to analysing community input in a way that would capture people's experience of certain risks. For example, some epidemiologists have identified that not all people on low incomes experience their life as deprived. This has led them

KEY POINTS

Limitations of epidemiology

- No contextual information
- Human behaviour
- People's preferences
- Individual experiences
- Social and political factors ignored

to conclude that using income solely as a determinant of health may not be the most appropriate way to judge needs or risks. In fact, it is more helpful to health promotion planning to understand how people experience deprivation, and the ways deprivation may impinge on their health, than to simply link low income to poor health (Chung et al 2018). These types of studies provide useful information on population health status contributing to our knowledge of communities and their needs.

Social epidemiology

In a comprehensive primary health care context, assessment information should reveal where inequities exist in the community, what levels of disadvantage exist for which groups in the community, what links there are between community attitudes, local and centralised decisions and health outcomes, and myriad other relationships relevant to the SDH. One approach to collecting this information is to adopt a 'social epidemiological' approach. Social epidemiology is a subset of epidemiology that focuses on the health effects of social institutions, structures and relationships over time and the social factors that contribute to the distribution of disease (Kim 2021, Robinson & Bailey 2020). The goal of social epidemiology is to test associations between the socio-ecological aspects of community life and population health outcomes (Kim 2021). This approach is closer to the goals of both primary health care and the SDH than the types of assessment outlined earlier, in that it is aimed at resolving issues of inequity. Used in conjunction with community-based participatory research (CBPR) (see more details later this chapter), social epidemiology yields a depth and breadth of information that can be helpful for planning.

KEY POINT

Social epidemiology is an approach to assessing associations between the socio-ecological aspects of community life and population health outcomes.

A social epidemiological assessment begins with demographic and epidemiological data, mapping the main indicators of community life. Concurrently, a CBPR study can provide information on what people believe community life is like, what could be done to improve the community, what would improve health, how the health department could help and how the community nurse and other health practitioners can effectively participate in enabling health and wellbeing (Brush et al 2020, Hulen et al 2019). Next, the social epidemiological data will show the balance between resources and demand, strengths and needs. Among the information collected would be indicators of social capital such as indicators of cohesiveness and bonding, health behaviours, illness indicators and community perceptions. Integral to the process is evaluation of the power structures and how they affect certain groups, to provide policy planners with the information to challenge these conditions, including issues of racism, discrimination or other forms of social exclusion (Kim 2021). Identifying community assets or strengths can help community members develop empowering strategies to gain mastery and control over health decision-making— particularly in communities that have experienced social exclusion such as lesbian, gay, bisexual, transgender, intersex (LGBTI+) and other diverse groups. In this way, information can be inspiring, helping people participate fully in their community and expand their ability to negotiate, influence, control and hold accountable the institutions and decision-makers that control their lives.

Asset mapping

In order to provide a comprehensive picture of a community, and in particular when working with Indigenous communities, it is essential to include assessment of positive community features or 'assets' (Adcock et al 2019, Bank of I.D.E.A.S. 2020). (See Fig 4.2.) Asset mapping is a more resourceful, inclusive approach that can help identify health inequities in the community, particularly if the assessment includes information on the capability of communities to identify problems and activate solutions. This approach to assessment is therefore responsive to the goals of primary health care and the

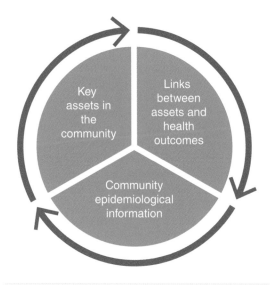

Figure 4.2 The asset model

SDH. An asset map is intended to build an inventory of community strengths in relation to the SDH. Data consists of epidemiological information on: the population; their key assets at each stage of life; the physical, environmental and social assets that exist within the community; and the links between these assets and health outcomes (Bank of I.D.E.A.S. 2020). Asset mapping aligns well with an Indigenous approach to understanding communities, one that recognises that the most important asset within a community is the people (Adcock et al 2019). This assessment information can provide a foundation for planning strategies to reduce health inequities. Categories of information include primary building blocks (assets and capacities of residents; their skills, talents and experiences; the presence of community associations under neighbourhood control); secondary building blocks (assets in the community controlled primarily by outsiders, such as physical resources, land, waste, energy, public institutions and services); and potential building blocks (resources outside the community controlled externally, such as public capital and expenditures) (Bank of I.D.E.A.S. 2020). From this base of evidence members of the community can work with health practitioners to identify actions to improve health that will be evaluated for their effectiveness. In particular, the use of asset-based community development can help mobilise a community to address identified needs using identified assets (Adcock et al 2019, Mathie et al 2017).

However, in using this approach to assessment, consideration must be given to the way data are aggregated. As noted earlier in the chapter, if the information represents an epidemiological approach that focuses only on the total assets within each of these building blocks, it would be difficult to identify pockets of inequity among subgroups, even within a particular neighbourhood. As a guide for planning to meet the goals of primary health care, it would be necessary to ensure that information was *stratified*, or categorised according to groups such as the homeless, young people, older citizens and those with disabilities. Examples of how this can be achieved are growing. For example, researchers in New Zealand worked with local Iwi (Māori tribal group) to use asset mapping (Aka Matua) along with other Kaupapa Māori approaches (see Chapters 9 and 10) to address health inequities experienced by Māori women and pēpē (infants) in Te Wairoa. The approach has strengthened relationships within the community and resulted in development of a community-led maternity care pathway (Adcock et al 2019).

Community-based participatory research (CBPR)

The strength of asset mapping is that it is a community-based approach to assessment intended to respond to the SDH, and it continues to evolve. A related assessment approach is encompassed in community-based participatory research (CBPR). CBPR is designed to equitably involve all partners in the research process and is increasingly used by community members and researchers to examine health inequities within a community and co-design approaches to addressing these (Brush et al 2020). One of the key elements of CBPR as an approach to community research is the engagement of the community at the earliest possible moment in the process. This ensures that community members are involved in identifying the most appropriate approach to data collection, analysis and reporting, that they have a say in how the information is interpreted, that they are encouraged to share their knowledge and skills with the researchers and that they can gain increased knowledge and skills in return. This reciprocal process aligns well with Indigenous approaches to health and wellness and contributes to community and individual improvements in health literacy reflecting the primary health care principle of community participation. Further information on CBPR can be found in Chapter 10.

The evolution of community assessment tools in nursing

Assessment tools to gather information on community health have evolved over time to incorporate more appropriate representation of the social characteristics of communities. This refinement of approaches to assessment is useful in prompting nurses and other health practitioners to base health policies and programs on knowledge of the SDH and to include community input. As far back as the 1980s several models of assessment were developed to be used in combination with epidemiological data. West (1984) devised an assessment tool based on the interaction between people and their environments in a small community. The tool included analysis of interactions, actions and awareness, and, although it was comprehensive, it was somewhat diffuse and was not validated with larger communities. Its strength was that it was intended to capture extensive information about how people felt about their community, which was helpful in encouraging the primary health care principle of community participation. Another community assessment tool of the 1980s was developed to correspond to functional health assessment of individuals living in the community (Fritsch Gikow & Kucharski 1987). However, this tool did not reflect a primary health care approach, and instead was focused on structured assessment of community health patterns that corresponded to personal health patterns, such as health perception and management, intersectoral role relationships and social issues. The assessment was very 'top-down', and based on health practitioners' presumptions about health patterns among the population. Some of these patterns may be relevant to particular communities, but the assessment approach implied that we could use a 'one-size-fits-all' approach to community assessment. The major limitation of this type of tool is that it is inefficient and ineffective without valuable community input from which planners could predict the relative success of their interventions on the basis of community acceptability. In addition, simply assessing patterns of health and ill health fails to consider inequities between different groups of people, which is important to achieving the primary health care goal of social justice.

KEY POINT

Simply assessing patterns of health and ill health fails to consider inequities between different groups of people, which is important to achieving the primary health care goal of social justice.

The assessment tool just mentioned, and other assessment tools of the 1980s, reflected the commitment of nursing to the systematic approach of the nursing process. The nursing process revolves around making nursing diagnoses, typically described as 'deficits' that nurses can address. Clark's 1984 model of assessment is a comprehensive tool specifically aimed at facilitating a nursing diagnosis. It was originally described as the 'epidemiologic prevention process model', and has more recently been known as the 'dimensions model of community health nursing' because of its later focus on the determinants of health and the dimensions of nursing (Bigbee & Issel 2012, p. 373). Categories of information include general information about the community, epidemiological information such as population characteristics and health status indicators, attitudes towards health, environmental factors and community relationships with society. Box 4.3 provides a case study of the development of Clark's assessment model over time.

Like Clark's model, Anderson and McFarlane's (1988, 2014, 2019) assessment model is based on the nursing process and their philosophy of 'community as partner', which is congruent with primary health care, and a 'systems' approach to the community. Systems approaches are derived from the notion that a community is a living system that is more than the sum of its parts because of numerous and ongoing internal and external interactions that help maintain homeostasis (Neuman 1982, Neuman & Fawcett 2010). In Anderson and McFarlane's (2014, 2019) adaptation

---

BOX 4.3

. . . .

THE EVOLUTION OF A COMMUNITY ASSESSMENT TOOL

. . . .

Clark's assessment tool arose from having to undertake an assessment of health needs at a summer day camp in 1995. She began the task by categorising the various needs of campers, then identifying a set of primary and secondary interventions designed to address these needs. The process was intended to identify a series of nursing diagnoses that would illuminate the physical risks and service deficits that could potentially impact on camp participants. As was accepted practice at the time, there was no dialogue with staff or campers regarding their perspective on needs and means of addressing these. Nearly 10 years later, Clark (2003, p. 457) critiqued the model in terms of new ideas on community health, following feedback from a research project she was undertaking, where community members reported feeling 'researched to death'. She and her colleagues recognised the need for a community engagement process to round out the assessment information (Clark et al 2003). By using focus groups with community members, the researchers identified a range of community health needs and assets. The major needs identified by community members were housing, environmental and safety needs, followed by access to health care. The major assets included the proximity of the community to the larger metropolitan area, its mild climate and recreational opportunities. From the findings of this research, Clark and her colleagues were able to identify a number of community-led initiatives to address some of the needs. Clark's most recent text updated the model further (Clark 2015).

So what does this tell us?

The development of models helps guide nursing practice with communities, and this case study demonstrates how models evolve over time as new knowledge is gained. Being aware of the history of model development helps nurses understand past practice in the context of contemporary practice and encourages us to explore new models and practices based on our previous experiences and knowledge.

What do you see as the next phase in community assessment model development?

BOX 4.4

A COMPARISON OF COMMUNITY ASSESSMENT: ANDERSON AND MCFARLANE, AND CLARK

Anderson and McFarlane (1988, 2011, 2014, 2019)

- Physical environment
- Economics
- Education
- Safety and transportation
- Health and social services
- Politics and government
- Communication
- Recreation

Clark (1984, 2003, 2015)

- Physical
- Biophysical
- Sociocultural
- Behavioural
- Health system

involvement in the early stages of the process. Communities should be involved as early as possible, as we underline throughout the chapter.

POINT TO PONDER

Early assessment models included person–environment interactions and were not always inclusive of what we now call the SDH. They were also intended to provide a nursing diagnosis as a basis for systematic health planning.

What are the strengths and weaknesses of these early approaches?

of Neuman's systems model, assessment is guided by an assessment wheel with eight subsystems, which include similar categories of information to those used by Clark with some expansion of the areas assessed (see Box 4.4). Despite the differences, the assessment processes remain the same. Nurses assess each of the categories or subsystems to diagnose the health of the community in order to inform implementation plans based on each.

Anderson and McFarlane's community assessment wheel has been one of the more widely used models of community assessment in nursing with adaptations of their wheel developed for Canadian, Australian and New Zealand users (Francis et al 2013, Vollman et al 2016). While providing a useful framework for community assessment, the model is limited by its 'top-down', deficit approach; that is, the identification of community problems rather than strengths, and seeking community input after problem identification. An existing concern with many community assessment approaches is a lack of community

Although the early assessment tools were devoid of community input, they did help advance nursing's scientific agenda, by recognising the processes of assessment. Over time, those using the tools began to recognise the importance of social and interactive factors that are so important to community health. However, by being prescriptive about categories of assessment data, sometimes critical information was overlooked, including the need to assess cultural factors within various community neighbourhoods and groups. Subsequent community assessment models have contributed to a deeper understanding of the cultural domain of assessment, following the lead of Leininger (1967) and other nursing theorists (Giger & Davidhizar 2002, Jirwe et al 2006, Leininger & McFarland 2006, Ramsden 2002, Tripp-Reimer et al 1984). Cultural assessment is now a major focus in community assessment, integrating cultural information with other assessment information. Cultural assessment strategies are intended to provide the depth and breadth of locally identified information that is crucial to ensuring their acceptability in the context of the nurse–client relationship.

KEY POINT

All cultural assessments must include the perspectives of members of the cultural groups on their assets, strengths and needs.

Cultural assessment information can include community members' perspectives on their worldview and relevant issues related to ethnicity, values, beliefs, history and social orientation. For refugee and migrant groups, information on pre-movement, migration and post-migration events is also collected to assess the combination of social, environmental, cultural and medical factors that determine health. Despite the often traumatic experiences of refugees prior to resettlement, a strengths-based approach to assessment enables the identification of resilience in the face of adversity, mediating factors that enable or constrain the ability to cope with adversity, and the facilitators that enable positive coping (Lewis et al 2021). Comprehensive assessment of refugee populations, which includes detailed information on family factors, family reactions to the transition to a new country, the impact of changes and aspects of the host community that cause or exacerbate the trauma and stress of dislocation is essential. An important element of the cultural assessment involves assessing healthcare providers, as some researchers have found that accessibility and use of services depends on the cultural and language competencies of staff members (Neilly et al 2019, Tyrrell et al 2016). Including cultural assessment in all community assessments is congruent with the work of Ramsden (2002) in highlighting cultural safety in all professional interactions. Cultural information also provides a more realistic picture of the community and its sociocultural environment, and shifts the emphasis from the deficit model of the nursing process to the more positive 'asset mapping' model of assessment

Assessment tools specific to health education planning

Among the most specific, goal-directed tools is the PRECEDE-PROCEED tool for health education planning (Green & Kreuter 2005) (see Fig 4.3).

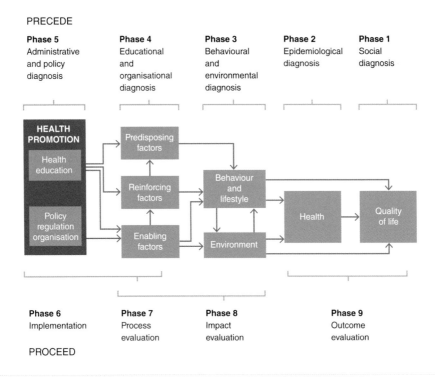

Figure 4.3 PRECEDE-PROCEED model

The objective of the tool is to provide a framework for planning and evaluating behaviour change programs among members of a community or group (Parker & Baldwin 2019). Like the nursing process models, Green and Kreuter's model revolves around gathering diagnostic information. First, a social diagnosis is undertaken which includes examining community issues such as crime, population density, education, unemployment and other aspects that are similar to the SDH. Second, an epidemiological diagnosis is made. This identifies rates of morbidity, mortality, disability and fertility and is aimed at determining the extent and nature of the determinants of health in the community (Green & Kreuter 2005). Third, a behavioural and environmental diagnosis is undertaken to identify factors related to actions people might take and how interactions with their physical and social environments might affect these (Green & Kreuter 2005). Included are preventative actions such as safe sexual behaviour, self-care indicators, dietary patterns and coping skills. The environmental diagnosis includes geographic and economic indicators of community health, as well as how people connect and relate to health services.

Fourth, an educational and organisational diagnosis is undertaken resulting in identification of Predisposing, Reinforcing and Enabling factors. Predisposing factors include knowledge, attitudes, values and perceptions of community members, making it essential to assess health literacy at this stage. Reinforcing factors include the attitudes and behaviours of others that can affect behaviour and environments for change (Green & Kreuter 2005). Enabling factors are those skills, resources, assets or barriers that may either support or obstruct wanted change. Finally, an administrative and policy diagnosis is undertaken to clarify what strengths and resources are present in the community to enable it to respond to needs. Once complete, such a detailed assessment allows implementation of changes to begin (Green & Kreuter 1991, 2005).

Examples of the PRECEDE-PROCEED model in action include developing strategies to address dental caries in Aboriginal children living in rural and remote communities in New South Wales (Dimitropoulos et al 2018) and exploring knowledge and attitudes towards physical activity among older

adults living in a North West England community (Sanders et al 2018). The PRECEDE-PROCEED model has been used for many years to make a community diagnosis, but like some of the other models, it is limited by the top-down perspective of the health practitioner on what a community needs or prefers. In this respect, it is limited in providing a comprehensive assessment that includes input from community members who feel empowered to participate in charting the course of community health.

Streamlining community assessment—the McMurray community assessment framework

It should be evident from the assessment models described so far that most community assessment tools combine epidemiological data with psychosocial, sociocultural and environmental indicators, including information about the health system and its use. The most useful tools are those that combine the multidimensional and dynamic nature of community life as well as capturing individual and family strengths and constraints (McMurray 2014). Community assessment does not need to be a complex process, although the more information that is included in the assessment, the more likely it will be that the interventions will be appropriate and acceptable to the community. Figure 4.4 shows the McMurray community assessment framework. The framework describes a step-by-step process for undertaking a community assessment. The difference between the McMurray community assessment framework and other models of community assessment is that each step in the McMurray model ensures community members are engaged in the process, which ultimately results in community empowerment.

1. ENGAGE with the community

Approach key community members to identify how you can work with their community to undertake a

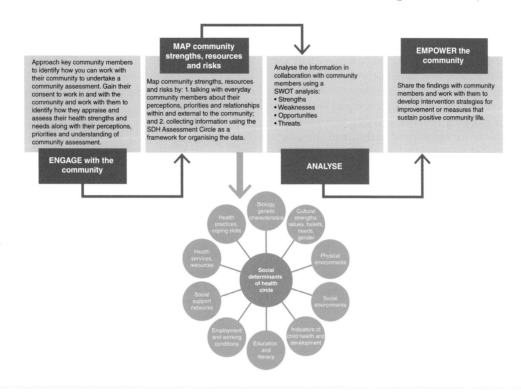

Figure 4.4 McMurray community assessment framework

community assessment. Gain their consent to work in and with the community and work with them to identify how they appraise and assess their health strengths and needs along with their perceptions, priorities and understanding of their community. Key community members are those who hold positions of respect and/or authority in the community, either through formal or informal leadership. These people may be community elders, local healthcare providers, teachers, social workers, town council or community board members and/or others who may provide services in the community. While speaking with some of these people may simply be a formality, speaking with community elders and gaining their consent to work with you in the community is an essential first step to community assessment. Talk to them about what *you* want to find out and what *they* want to find out, and let them tell you where to find the information. They will know who to talk to, where to look for

information and what not to do as you undertake your community assessment. This process will also help establish trust between you and the community and keeps everyone 'in the loop' as you go about your assessment.

2. MAP community strengths, resources and risks

Mapping is a two-step process (although both steps can occur concurrently). First, talking with community members yields a wide range of information that shows the demographic 'mix' in the community: how many people in which population groups may require certain specific services (e.g. older persons, young children), the mix of cultures in the community, what people think about their lives, opinions about environmental strengths that may support healthy lifestyles, or barriers to health. Find out about people's perceptions, priorities and relationships—these are the relationships that exist between people, and between people and their environment. Once this information is obtained, the second part of this step involves mapping resources—trying to understand the capacity for supporting health, and the assets and support systems that may be mobilised for certain interventions. The SDH assessment circle outlined in Figure 4.5 comprises part of the McMurray community assessment framework and enables the mapping of these resources. The SDH assessment circle gathers information within the 10 categories of the SDH shown. The circle incorporates all the elements of community assessment, epidemiological data and social epidemiological information in one cohesive place. Appendix A shows the McMurray community assessment framework with the SDH assessment circle broken down into separate sections with accompanying questions. These questions will guide you as you undertake your review and many can only be answered by speaking with community members.

Further information on sources of assessment information can be found later in the chapter.

The following list outlines the SDH as found in the SDH Community Assessment Circle.

- Indicators of child health and development
- Biological or genetic population indicators
- Cultural strengths, values, beliefs, history and needs; gender
- Health services and resources and patterns of accessing these by various population groups
- Health practices, coping skills in the context of recreation and leisure, which may support or compromise health, such as drop-in centres, places that encourage health literacy and capacity, or drug and alcohol misuse
- Physical environments, including geographical factors such as climate change or transportation barriers to care, or activity-friendly neighbourhoods
- Social environments, indicators of social inclusion or exclusion
- Employment and financial status of the population, including unemployment rates, working conditions, types of employers, availability of workplace support
- Education and literacy indicators
- Social support networks, access for vulnerable groups, volunteer networks

3. ANALYSE the information in collaboration with community members using a strengths, weaknesses, opportunities and threats (SWOT) analysis

The third step is to analyse the information gathered using a SWOT analysis to identify strengths, weaknesses, opportunities and threats to community health. Included in the SWOT analysis will be a deeper level of analysis of the community that provides information on the SDH. This analysis should be done in collaboration with community members to ensure the way you interpret and make

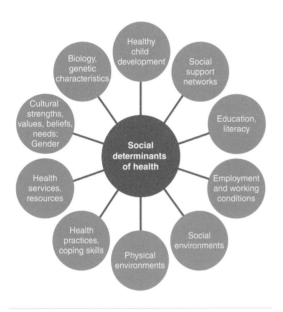

Figure 4.5 The SDH Community Assessment Circle

sense of the information is aligned with community members' understanding of the data. This action will help build trust with the community and serve to facilitate the development of the community-led interventions that make up the final step in the process.

4. EMPOWER the community by sharing the findings with community members and working with them to develop intervention strategies for improvement or measures that sustain positive community life

The final step is where you work with the community to identify, develop and implement interventions to support the needs of the community. Interventions may be as simple as lobbying local government for a new pedestrian crossing or as complex as a multifaceted diabetes prevention program. Engaging with communities throughout the assessment process is key to empowering community members to identify, seek and implement solutions to their own issues and concerns. An example of the importance of community engagement can be found in a study that used participatory action research to engage with an Aboriginal community to develop localised, culturally appropriate stroke health resources. While the resources were an important outcome from the study, it was the engagement and sense of community ownership that arose from the project that is likely to have most tangible long-term outcomes (Peake et al 2021).

Sources of assessment information

For health practitioners who are new to a community, comprehensive assessments can be daunting, and the sources of information a bit confusing. Some information will be available online in government documents. For example, Australian data on morbidity, mortality and age-related conditions are included in the document 'Australia's Health', which is updated every 2 to 4 years. This can be found at www.aihw.gov.au/reports-data/australias-health. Australian Government census and health department reports on a variety of topics are also available online. The New Zealand Ministry of Health has a range of publications that provide background data on the health status of New Zealanders. The New Zealand Health Survey is now a continuous study and provides the most up-to-date information on population health in New Zealand. Findings are published on the Ministry of Health website: www.health.govt.nz. Statistics New Zealand (www.stats.govt.nz) is also a useful portal for accessing any statistical data on communities and publishes many existing community profiles developed from census data. For the more enthusiastic practitioner, it is also possible to manipulate Excel data tables to find the specific statistics required for a geographical area. The Yellow Pages (www.yellowpages.com.au) are another source of community information, as are community business directories. Some of the most useful information for community assessment comes from local surveys that may have been conducted in recent years, or from observations of community life. A search of websites like Google or PubMed, or any of the research databases (see Chapter 10) may also reveal whether there have been any research studies in the community, which may provide additional information.

Most community nurses and other health practitioners have their own strategies for collecting various types of information, depending on whether they are responsible for the whole community, or practising in specific areas, such as: general practice; child, school or occupational health; or in a visiting nurse service. In the first instance health practitioners can become familiar with a community by conducting a 'windscreen survey', driving around to gain a sense of the community—a big picture of life in that context. Such a survey can yield information about: spaces for recreation; transportation and access; childcare services; the location of schools, clinics, hospitals and other health services; places of employment; the state of available housing such as whether there are affordable homes; or whether certain sections of the community seem to be in decline. This type of information can also be confirmed by speaking to various community groups or by analysing records of community activities such as immunisation rates, public health indicators and data from other policy documents that indicate activities of the local council or other authorities (fitness programs, elder daycare facilities). Community assets, strengths and risks can also be identified by being attentive to people's visible

health behaviours such as observing people out walking, older persons engaging in Tai Chi, and/or parent get-togethers.

KEY POINT

A windscreen survey is an effective way of gaining an understanding of the 'lay of the land' in a community.

On completion of a community assessment, presentation of your work to the community and/or to your colleagues and peers is a useful way of disseminating the information you have gathered. These groups may have useful ideas on where further information can be obtained, how the information can be used and what the next steps in the process may be. In the context of community student placements, discussion of assessment information with community nurses or the teaching staff supervising your placement can also provide locally relevant information for health promotion.

Conclusion

Assessment of the community enables a deeper understanding of strengths, weaknesses, opportunities and threats to community health. The McMurray community assessment framework provides us with a structure to grow our understanding of a community and work alongside community members to identify and develop interventions to empower communities to address their own health and social needs. Chapter 5 builds on our assessment knowledge to help us plan interventions with individuals, families and communities. Before we move on, take some time to consider how the McMurray community assessment framework may help the Mason and Smith families.

Reflecting on the Big Issues

- Community assessment includes mapping strengths, resources, risks and needs with input from members of the community.
- Epidemiological data provide information on the determinants and distribution of risks and diseases

in the population, usually defined as incidence and prevalence rates.

- Quantifying rates of health risks and diseases is useful in some ways, but is not inclusive of community

Reflecting on the Big Issues—cont'd

perspectives and preferences or the particular needs of subgroups in the population.

■ Socio-ecological assessment tools have evolved over the years to reflect an increasing emphasis on the SDH.

■ Asset mapping is a tool for assessment that outlines primary, secondary and potential features and resources that can be mobilised for community health.

■ CBPR can be combined with asset mapping to provide a realistic assessment of community health needs.

■ Social epidemiological assessment integrates demographic and epidemiological assessment data with information from the community, often in the context of CBPR.

■ The McMurray community assessment framework is an ideal way to ensure data are collected on all the SDH in a community.

CASE STUDY

Assessing community needs for the Mason and Smith families

We now return to the Smith and Mason families to provide an example of some of the information you may collect as part of assessing their communities' strengths, weaknesses, opportunities and threats to health. There are distinctive differences in the three communities that influence health and wellness for both families. The mining camp where Colin works is sparse and functional, approximately 1000 km from Perth, the capital of Western Australia and the epicentre of the 'resources boom'. In the area surrounding the mining camp are several small towns, where each community is composed of a mix of long-term residents and newcomers. Many of the townspeople live in caravan parks because of the shortage and high cost of housing. Some are service workers who service the mine and the local population. The physical environment is challenging, with extreme dry, dusty heat during the day and little rainfall.

Maddington is known as a family-friendly but diverse community with many young families, some of them migrants, and older residents. The Smith family has ready access to the train station and the shopping centre, which they can reach by bus from the stop on their street. There is moderate unemployment in the suburb because there are so many opportunities across a range of jobs to work in the mines, and access to the airport is ideal, within 10 km of Maddington. The Smiths' neighbourhood has a large number of fly-in fly-out (FIFO) families, and an informal mining wives' club that meets regularly at the community centre. There is a shortage of GPs in the area, but several child health clinics, and a school health nurse attends the public school. The day care is staffed by accredited early childhood educators.

Papakura is a low socioeconomic community with moderate levels of unemployment and a high multicultural population. The area has a large number of young families, single-parent households and older retired people. There is also a large number of state houses and private rental properties, and some home ownership. The community has a local integrated family health centre which offers general practice, pharmacy and physiotherapy services. There is a local Plunket room and a playground near the shops.

Reflective questions: How would I use this knowledge in practice?

1 Using the McMurray community assessment framework, identify the most important priorities for promoting health in the mining community.

2 What information will you use to assess the Maddington community in relation to its strengths, weaknesses, threats and opportunities for socio-ecological support for the Smith family?

3 What strengths, weaknesses, threats and opportunities are readily identifiable in Papakura?

4 What information do you need to glean from Rebecca and Huia on their family and community needs? Compile a list of questions to prompt your assessment interview with each of the women.

5 What gaps in assessment data did you find from your assessment interviews?

6 What extra sources of information did you use to complete the assessments in both communities?

7 From the assessment data of all three communities, what provisional plans would you put in place for health promotion?

8 Group exercise: Community assessment

Working in small groups, brainstorm the various ways you think information about your community can be collected. Make a list of where you will find this information locally.

9 Group exercise: SDH assessment

Working in groups of two to three, undertake a windscreen survey in your local community. Make notes on what you observe. Consider how the notes you have made (the data you collected) fit into the McMurray community assessment framework and where. Make some notes on how useful you found this exercise and what you learned. Share your findings with the wider group.

References

Adcock, A., Storey, F., Lawton, B., et al, 2019. He Korowai Manaaki: mapping assets to inform a strengths-based, Indigenous-led wrap-around maternity pathway. Aust. J. Prim. Health, 25 (5), 509–514. Online. Available: https://doi.org/10.1071/PY19029.

Anderson, E., McFarlane, J., 1988. Community as partner: Theory and practice in nursing. JB Lippincott.

Anderson, E., McFarlane, J., 2014. Community as partner: Theory and practice in nursing, seventh ed. Lippincott, Williams & Wilkins.

Anderson, E., McFarlane, J., 2019. Community as partner: Theory and practice in nursing. Anderson, E., McFarlane, J. (eds.), eighth ed. Wolters Kluwer.

Bank of I.D.E.A.S., 2020. A guide to asset mapping. Online. Available: https://boifiles.s3-ap-southeast-2.amazonaws.com/2020/Asset+Mapping+A+Guide%5B14734%5D.pdf.

Bigbee, J.L., Issel, L.M., 2012. Conceptual models for population-focused public health nursing interventions and outcomes: The state of the art. Public Health Nurs., 29 (4), 370–379. Online. Available: https://doi.org/10.1111/j.1525-1446.2011.01006.x.

Brush, B.L., Mentz, G., Jensen, M., et al, 2020. Success in long-standing community-based participatory research (CBPR) partnerships: A scoping literature review. Health

Educ. Behav., 47 (4), 556–568. Online. Available: https://doi.org/10.1177/1090198119882989.

Chung, R.Y.-N., Chung, G.K.-K., Gordon, D., et al, 2018. Deprivation is associated with worse physical and mental health beyond income poverty: A population-based household survey among Chinese adults. Qual. Life Res., 27 (8), 2127–2135. Online. Available: https://doi.org/10.1007/s11136-018-1863-y.

Clark, M., 1984. Community nursing: Health care for today and tomorrow. Reston Publishing.

Clark, M.J., 2003. Community health nursing: Caring for populations, fourth ed. Pearson Education Inc.

Clark, M.J., 2015. Population and community health nursing, sixth ed., Pearson.

Clark, M.J., Cary, S., Diemert, G., et al, 2003. Involving communities in community assessment. Public Health Nurs., 20 (6), 456–463. Online. Available: https://pubmed.ncbi.nlm.nih.gov/14629677/.

Dimitropoulos, Y., Holden, A., Gwynne, K., et al, 2018. An assessment of strategies to control dental caries in Aboriginal children living in rural and remote communities in New South Wales, Australia. BMC Oral Health, 18 (1), 177. Online. Available: https://doi.org/10.1186/s12903-018-0643-y.

Fowler, C.S., Frey, N., Folch, D.C., et al, 2020. Who are the people in my neighborhood? The 'contextual fallacy' of measuring individual context with census geographies. Geogr. Anal., 52 (2), 155–168. Online. Available: https://doi.org/10.1111/gean.12192.

Francis, K., Chapman, Y., Hoare, K., et al, 2013. Community as partner: Theory and practice in nursing (Australasian edition), second ed. Lippincott, Williams & Wilkins.

Fritsch Gikow, F., Kucharski, P., 1987. A new look at the community: Functional health pattern assessment. J. Community Health Nurs., 4 (1), 21–27. Online. Available: https://doi.org/10.1207/s15327655jchn0401_4.

Giger, J., Davidhizar, R., 2002. Culturally competent care: Emphasis on understanding the people of Afghanistan, Afghanistan Americans, and Islamic culture and religion. Int. Nurs. Rev., 49, 79–86.

Goodman, R.A., Buehler, J.W., Mott, J.A., et al, 2019. Defining Field Epidemiology. In: Rasmussen, S.A., Goodman, R.A. (Eds.), The CDC field epidemiology manual, third ed., pp. 3–20. Online. Available: https://doi.org/10.1093/oso/9780190933692.003.0001.

Green, L., Kreuter, M., 1991. Health promotion planning: An educational and environmental approach. Mayfield Publishing Company.

Green, L., Kreuter, M., 2005. Health program planning: An educational and ecological approach, fourth ed. McGraw-Hill Higher Education.

Hobbs, M., Mackenbach, J.D., Wiki, J., et al, 2021. Investigating change in the food environment over 10 years in urban New Zealand: A longitudinal and nationwide geospatial study. Soc. Sci. Med., 269, 113522. Online. Available: https://doi.org/10.1016/j.socscimed.2020.113522.

Hulen, E., Hardy, L.J., Teufel-Shone, N., et al, 2019. Community Based Participatory Research (CBPR): A Dynamic Process of Health care, Provider Perceptions and American Indian Patients' Resilience. J. Health Care Poor Underserved, 30 (1), 221–237. Online. Available: https://doi.org/10.1353/hpu.2019.0017.

Jirwe, M., Gerrish, K., Emami, A., 2006. The theoretical framework of cultural competence. J. Multicult. Nurs. Health, 12(3), 6–16.

Kim, D., 2021. New horizons in modeling and simulation for social epidemiology and public health. Wiley.

Leininger, M., 1967. The culture concept and its relevance to nursing. J. Nurs. Educ., 6 (2), 27–37.

Leininger, M., McFarland, M., 2006. Culture care diversity and universality: A worldwide theory of nursing, second ed. Jones and Bartlett Publishers.

Lewis, F.J., Tor, S., Rappleyea, D., et al, 2021. Behavioral health and refugee youth in primary care: An ecological systems perspective of the complexities of care. Child. Youth Serv. Rev., 120. Online. Available: https://doi.org/10.1016/j.childyouth.2020.105599.

Liu, N., Kruger, E., Tennant, M., 2021. Identifying the gaps in public dental services locations for people living with a disability in metropolitan Australia: a geographic information system (GIS)-based approach. Aust. Health Rev., 45 (2), 178–184. Online. Available: https://doi.org/10.1071/AH19252.

Mathie, A., Cameron, J., Gibson, K., 2017. Asset-based and citizen-led development: Using a diffracted power lens to analyze the possibilities and challenges. Prog. Dev. Stud., 17 (1), 54–66. Online. Available: https://doi.org/10.1177/1464993416674302.

McMurray, A., 2014. Healthy communities: The evolving roles of nursing. In J. Daly, S. Speedy, D. Jackson (Eds.), Contexts of nursing, fourth ed., pp. 305–324. Elsevier Inc.

Neilly, C.-H., Rader, A., Zielinski, S., et al, 2019. Using transcultural nursing education to increase cultural sensitivity and cultural assessment documentation by staff in an in-home chronic disease self-management program. J. Dr. Nurs. Pract., 12(1), 16–23. Online. Available: https://doi.org/10.1891/2380-9418.12.1.16.

Neuman, B., 1982. The Neuman systems model. Appleton-Century-Crofts.

Neuman, B., Fawcett, J., 2010. The Neuman systems model, fifth ed.. Pearson.

Parker, E., Baldwin, L., 2019. Contemporary practice. In M. Fleming, E. Parker, I. Correa-Velez (Eds.), Introduction to public health, fourth ed., pp. 184–196. Elsevier.

Peake, R.M., Jackson, D., Lea, J., et al, 2021. Meaningful engagement with Aboriginal communities using participatory action research to develop culturally appropriate health resources. J. Transcult. Nurs., 32 (2), 129–136. Online. Available: https://doi.org/10.1177/1043659619899999.

Ramsden, I., 2002. Cultural safety and nursing education in Aotearoa and Te Waipounamu. Doctoral thesis. Victoria University of Wellington.

Robinson, W.R., Bailey, Z.D., 2020. Invited commentary: What social epidemiology brings to the table—reconciling social epidemiology and causal inference. Am. J. Epidemiol., 189 (3), 171–174. Online. Available: https://doi.org/10.1093/aje/kwz197.

Sanders, G.J., Roe, B., Knowles, Z.R., et al, 2018. Using formative research with older adults to inform a community physical activity programme: Get Healthy, Get Active. Prim. Health Care Res. Dev., 20, 1–10. Online. Available: https://doi.org/10.1017/S1463423618000373.

Tripp-Reimer, T., Brink, P., Saunders, J., 1984. Cultural assessment: content and process. Nurs. Outlook, 32 (30), 78–82.

Tyrrell, L., Duell-Piening, P., Morris, M., et al, 2016. Talking about health and experiences of using health services with people from refugee backgrounds. Victorian Refugee Health Network, Melbourne.

Vollman, A., Anderson, E., McFarlane, J., 2016. Canadian community as partner: Theory and multidisciplinary practice, fourth ed. Lippincott, Williams & Wilkins.

Wassertheil-Smoller, S., Smoller, J., 2015. Mostly about epidemiology. In: Biostatistics and epidemiology: A primer for health and biomedical professionals. Springer New York, pp. 83–132. Online. Available: https://doi.org/10.1007/978-1-4939-2134-8_4.

West, M., 1984. Community health assessment: The man-environment interaction. J. Community Health Nurs., 1 (2), 89–97. Online. Available: https://doi.org/10.1207/s15327655jchn0102_3.

Wyeth, E.H., Samaranayaka, A., Lambert, M., et al, 2019. Understanding longer-term disability outcomes for Māori and non-Māori after hospitalisation for injury: Results from a longitudinal cohort study. Public Health (Elsevier), 176, 118–127. Online. Available: https://doi.org/10.1016/j.puhe.2018.08.014.

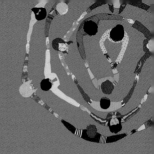

CHAPTER 5

Planning for intervention

Introduction

Chapter 5 provides the framework for our work with individuals, families and communities. We have explored community assessment tools and introduced the McMurray community assessment framework as a tool for working with communities. In this chapter we will extend our understanding of assessment to consider individuals and families more closely and the steps needed to work at the individual and family level. We explore care planning for individuals and families, and project planning for communities, both informed by the principles of primary health care and incorporating the impacts of social determinants of health. We describe how strengths-based approaches to the development of care and project planning can result in flexible delivery of interventions across local, national and global communities. The importance of evaluating our interventions and the varying ways in which this can be done within the context of primary health care practice is also reviewed.

Overview

In order to provide a high standard of care, community health nurses and other health practitioners use several tools to assist them in developing relevant and appropriate intervention strategies. One of these foundational tools is planning for intervention, which guides practice by identifying and developing community, family and person-centred diagnoses, objectives and strategies for care, followed by evaluation criteria. The aim is to develop a systematic approach to evidence-based, customised care relevant to need and involves

OBJECTIVES

By the end of this chapter you will be able to:

1 outline current and potential nurse-led primary health care models of practice for health and wellness

2 identify strategies for working in partnership with individuals and families to develop sustainable people-centred care plans and interventions

3 describe an approach to project planning with communities

4 describe the contribution of the socio-ecological approach to health improvement

5 outline the role of primary health care practitioners in managing chronic disease in the community

6 develop a comprehensive evaluation strategy for a primary health care program.

four steps: assessment, development of objectives, implementation and evaluation (Toney-Butler & Thayer 2020).

Community health nurses and other health practitioners need to plan for interventions in environments that are less structured or controlled than those in hospitals. Practitioners must be able to understand the implications of the social determinants of health (SDH), screen clients for their psychosocial needs and design meaningful objectives and implementation strategies. Planning requires an understanding of impacting contextual factors to enhance the most effective interventions (Jain & Chandrashekar 2020).

As discussed in previous chapters, planning for intervention should be undertaken within a socio-ecological model of health, in collaboration with individuals, families and communities, and have an interdisciplinary approach with other health and non-health practitioners. Community health nurses facilitate acceptable, accessible evidence-based primary health care goals and objectives. Their family and person-centred approaches focus on health inequalities and enhancing meaningful, equitable and sustainable strategies which maximise community, family and individual self-management and resilience (Australian Primary Health Care Nurses Association [APNA] 2021a). However, several factors cause interference with these considerations, including the marginalisation of concerns relating to perspectives of community members' lived experiences and social perspectives, in addition to impacts of neoliberal influences on health policies which focus on cost constraints, rigorous activity measurement and uncoordinated service contracting, all of which do not take into account the SDH (Javanparast et al 2020). Across Australian and New Zealand, it is essential to include legally designated strategies that promote people's health and wellbeing, such as mandatory reporting for child and senior abuse (Australian Human Rights Commission [AHRC] 2019, World Health Organization [WHO] 2020a). The Australian guidelines for mandatory reporting differ between states and territories and there is no national legislation in New Zealand, although there is some regulation by district health boards (CFCA 2020, New Zealand Ministry of Health [NZMOH] 2018).

Where to find out more on ...

Mandatory reporting guidelines

- Australia: www.aifs.gov.au/cfca/publications/mandatory-reporting-child-abuse-and-neglect
- New Zealand: www.health.govt.nz/our-work/preventative-health-wellness/family-violence/family-violence-questions-and-answers

Models of care and project planning

A model of care is the way in which services are optimally designed and delivered to meet evolving healthcare requirements. Primary health care nursing practice models are client centred, working in partnership with individuals, families and communities to support self-management and develop pathways for health and wellbeing. The best models use a multidimensional approach with nurses able to work as equal interdisciplinary partners across differing health structures and settings (Australian College of Nursing [ACN] 2020). A defining feature of models is the quality affiliations fostered between nurses and clients, of which empowering relationships are a key goal for community health nursing practice (ACN 2019). Models need to be underpinned by evidence-based practice utilising critical-thinking skills to ensure development of appropriate implementation and evaluation strategies (Toney-Butler & Thayer 2020). Within nursing and midwifery practice, there are several examples of models of care including nurse/midwife-led clinics, family/women-centred care, transitional care and case management. A primary health care approach can be used to develop a range of models within healthcare settings, such as general practice, hospital and community care and specialist health services in tertiary centres. The following elements have been identified as providing comprehensive care delivery for individuals, families and communities across these varying models of care (Australian Commission on Safety and Quality in Health Care [ACSQHC] 2018, p. 17):

- client goals of care guide health decisions and the client journey

- diversity and equity are respected and supported
- transparency is a core element of safety and quality care.

Each of these elements is underpinned by the principles of primary health care outlined in Chapter 1: accessible healthcare, appropriate technology, health promotion, cultural safety, intersectoral collaboration and community participation.

Flexible models of care acknowledge that people, whether individuals, families or whole communities, may need different strategic approaches to optimally provide for their needs. Comprehensive primary health care approaches recognise that flexible models and strategies are needed to develop strengths-based, culturally sensitive healthcare services and relationships within Aboriginal communities (Munns & Robson 2020) and with Māori people. Home visiting is an approach to engage people in their own settings, which enables community practitioners to develop plans with them to suit their unique needs. Of note is the emerging collaboration between peer support workers and community health nurses to develop culturally acceptable support strategies for Aboriginal parents through home visiting or in a range of community venues. The peer support workers' abilities to understand local SDH through lived experience is a source of strength-based strategies, helping parents to cope with health and social inequalities (Munns & Walker 2018).

New models of care will be required to meet the challenges currently facing health systems, particularly during epidemics and pandemics such as COVID-19. A growing population, growing diversity, increasing prevalence of long-term conditions and an ageing population will continue to challenge the ways we provide care, and nurses and other health practitioners will need to develop new models to address these needs. Changing technology will enable more flexible delivery of care and disruptive innovation such as that seen by the advent of new technology-based providers like Airbnb, Uber and Babylon, which challenge traditional approaches. Babylon, for example, provides internet-based access to general practitioner services with no requirement for the bricks-and-mortar models we currently use. It is important we think carefully about the value of current models and the changes we will need to make to improve health outcomes among the most vulnerable families and communities with whom we work. Others are already considering new approaches and we need to be ready to join them or, at a minimum, understand them, as the people we currently work with will want to know more about them whether we like it or not. Models of care inform care planning that addresses requirements for individuals, families and whole communities. The approaches that are most suitable for each setting will incorporate a range of elements according to need, cultural environments and changing SDH (Martin et al 2021).

CARE PLANNING FOR INDIVIDUAL CLIENTS AND FAMILIES

Community health nurses need to work in partnership with individuals and families to develop plans of care for a range of physical and psychosocial prevention, early intervention activities and chronic disease management. Developing positive relationships with clients and understanding their needs and preferences underpin plans of care that are realistic and achievable within their capabilities (Gordon 2021). Creating objectives, intervention strategies and evaluation of care will be explored further in this chapter.

CARE PLANNING FOR COMMUNITIES

Care planning for communities is likely to be undertaken as project planning. Projects can be undertaken as stand-alone activities or incorporated into continuous improvement or long-term strategic programs. Similar to planning for care with individuals and families, a health practitioner partnership approach with communities assists in identifying needs and priorities for projects. Interdisciplinary teams are common, with their range of different strategies often requiring a program logic map to demonstrate the evidence-based sequence of steps needed for a particular plan. This also helps to facilitate consensus among all team members (Parker & Baldwin 2019). Further details on goals, objectives, strategies and evaluation will be discussed in the following sections of the chapter.

Guiding approaches for effective planning

Two approaches underpin effective planning for individuals, families and communities: strengths-based approaches and the principles of primary health care.

STRENGTHS-BASED APPROACHES

Remembering our previous discussions on empowerment, self-efficacy and self-determination, it is important for strengths-based approaches to be used when formulating intervention plans. This enables issues for individuals, families and communities to be considered within broader, holistic contexts that impact on both strengths and challenges. Strengths-based practice enables community health nurses and other health practitioners to work in partnership with all clients to identify their abilities, interests and skills, and help them navigate choices and control to develop their own health and wellbeing goals (McKillop & Munns 2021).

PRIMARY HEALTH CARE PRINCIPLES

Integration of primary health care principles into planning is essential for effective and sustainable outcomes. Comprehensive primary health care encourages partnerships between health practitioners, people and their communities to improve their health and wellbeing through equitable access to a range of accessible preventative, health-promoting, culturally safe and socially acceptable services. Appreciation of the influence of the SDH is vital along with the ability of these determinants to enhance or diminish health and wellbeing of individuals, families and communities (Javanparast et al 2020). Contemporary care is shifting from disease models to a focus on health and wellbeing, particularly in relation to

prevention, health promotion and quality outcomes for tertiary levels of disease progression. Community health nurses and other practitioners are well positioned within interdisciplinary teams to contribute their primary health care expertise to facilitate multi-focused approaches in order to develop quality community, family and person-centred intervention planning (Taylor et al 2021).

Planning for intervention: steps

CLIENT ASSESSMENT

A comprehensive assessment of the individual, family or community using appropriate evidence-based or evidence-informed tools, with effective communication and observation, will allow you to identify and validate holistic health and wellbeing issues. It is important to remember that these can be potential or actual issues where you can recognise both deficit and strengths-based areas affecting people and communities. It is also crucial to use standardised and validated assessment tools. These can facilitate systematic implementation of the tools thereby making sure the most appropriate data is collected. Findings can be analysed in a logical manner with valid comparison of results. Consideration of which tools are appropriate for specific psychosocial and cultural settings, such as perinatal mental health screening for Indigenous Australian women, are central to quality planning of care (Health.vic 2020, Kotz et al 2020).

POINT TO PONDER

Review the primary health care principles in Chapter 1. Consider how you could use these in care planning for individuals, families and communities. Remember that communities may be geographical or virtual.

The previous chapter has given an extensive overview of assessment tools for use with communities and we now extend this to family and individual assessments. Examples include the

Calgary Family Assessment Model (Leahey & Wright 2016, Shajani & Snell 2019; see Appendix B), Friedman's Family Assessment Model (Friedman et al 2003), Bristol Breastfeeding Assessment Tool (Ingram et al 2015), the HEEADSSS adolescent assessment tool (Klein et al 2014; see Appendix C) and the Edinburgh Postnatal Depression Scale (Cox et al 1987). Complementing these tools is the use of genograms and ecomaps. Assessments of families is integral to community health practice as their functioning, parenting capacity and access to social and family supports influence child and family health, wellbeing and resilience. Exploring family functioning can be challenging, as issues are complex and multidimensional, with the SDH impacting on family members' abilities to cope in times of physical and psychosocial stress (Australian Institute of Health and Welfare [AIHW] 2019). Of note is recent research highlighting the self-identified need for healthcare providers to partner with families to facilitate decision-making, goal setting and effective communication in order to provide holistic care strategies that address the SDH (Oldland et al 2020).

A comprehensive framework for family assessment is the Calgary Family Assessment Model, comprising three major classifications: the structural, developmental and functions aspects of families (Leahey & Wright 2016, Shajani & Snell 2019). The model is found in Appendix B. You will note there are several subcategories within each of the classifications. However, professional expertise can be used to decide which of these are relevant for discussion. It is important to be aware of how families cope with the process of exploring their lives. If they are feeling overwhelmed or challenged, it may be beneficial to collect the data over a period of time. Community health nurses need to be cognisant of families' individual situations and their own personal belief systems and biases. Reflexive practice is important in order to develop trust and accurately appreciate family circumstances, particularly in cross-cultural contexts (Kaihlanen et al 2019, Wright & Leahy 2013).

Additional strategies to assist with family assessment are the use of the Family Partnership model of interaction along with genograms and ecomaps (see box below). The Family Partnership approach facilitates non-expert, partnership communications between nurses and families (Centre for Parent and Child Support [CPCS] n.d.), with genograms and ecomaps providing visual representations of family structures and their significant relationships between the family and the social support interactions in their communities. A genogram is a chart of the family constellation and is similar to the genealogical trees known from genetics. An ecomap is a diagram of the family's connections outside the core family, assisting in enhancing client engagement and visualising the significant relationships between the family and the world (Roenne et al 2021).

Where to find out more on ...

Genograms

- https://practice-supervisors.rip.org.uk/wp-content/uploads/2019/11/Drawing-a-genogram.pdf

Ecomaps

- www.strongbonds.jss.org.au/workers/cultures/ecomaps.html

Consider how these tools can be used across a range of family environments. Try drawing a genogram and ecomap for your own family.

Individual members of families require assessments for a range of issues. The HEEADSSS adolescent assessment tool (Klein et al 2014) and the Edinburgh Postnatal Depression Scale (EPDS) (Cox et al 1987) are two tools frequently applied in community midwifery, child and school health settings. We discuss the HEEADSSS assessment in detail in Chapter 8. The EPDS can be used to assess the risk of anxiety and depression for women in the antenatal and postnatal periods. It can also be used with male partners. Using a partnership approach, this tool has the potential to enhance safe communication about sensitive topics with parents (CAHS 2019a).

Effective communication is vital to the assessment process, with community health nurses and other health practitioners needing to be aware of any issues, such as the effects of culture on language expression, how questions are best communicated, whether people are being interviewed in their primary language and what effects people's views on health and wellbeing have on the assessment information. It is important to note any subjective information which illustrates people's perceptions of topics under discussion, along with objective evidence which the nurse or other health practitioner identifies from observations of individuals and families and how they are functioning within their community (Potter et al 2021). A point of difference between collecting information from individuals and families, as compared to communities, is the greater range of strategies used in community assessments, including one-on-one interviews, focus groups and questionnaires. Optimal outcomes from these processes are achieved when practitioners have experience in undertaking research (Taylor et al 2021).

Following comprehensive data collection, presenting issues can be identified. Within nursing, these are referred to as nursing diagnoses but will be referred to here as issues as they encompass a wide range of psychosocial strengths and challenges.

KEY POINT

Presenting issues can relate to:

- individuals
- families
- communities

When documenting issues, it is important they are community, family or person centred and include all the information that allows the factors affecting the issue to be understood. They can have four parts.

- A label. What is the issue affecting the community, family or person? For example, 'ineffective breastfeeding' (individual); 'dysfunctional family processes' (family); and 'ineffective activity planning' (community) (Herdman 2021). This describes the actual issue.

- The related factors. These contribute to or are associated with the issue and can include a wide range of physical, psychosocial and developmental factors. For example, 'ineffective breastfeeding *related to lack of maternal self-confidence*' (individual); 'dysfunctional family processes *related to maternal anxiety*' (family); 'ineffective activity planning *related to lack of recreational space*' (community) (Herdman 2021).

- Signs supporting the issue. This part is supported by the subjective and/or objective evidence. For example, 'ineffective breastfeeding related to lack of maternal self-confidence *as evidenced by the mother's anxiety and stating she is not sure about how to breastfeed*' (Lippincott Williams & Wilkins 2013, p. 59, Herdman 2021); 'dysfunctional family processes related to maternal anxiety *as evidenced by the father stating that his wife is too nervous to take the children to school*' (family); 'ineffective activity planning related to lack of recreational space *as evidenced by 100% of resident responses in community assessment*' (community) (Herdman 2021). As discussed in Chapter 4 when exploring the McMurray community assessment framework, it is important to ensure community members are engaged in identifying issues important to them along with their predisposing factors. This facilitates a partnership approach which is central to empowering individuals, families and community members to further investigate and implement sustainable and meaningful solutions, with the use of appropriate resources.

- Evidence supporting the issue. This may not be a well-understood component of your documentation, but it is important to demonstrate evidence-based practice by supporting your clinical reasoning and judgment with research evidence.

Discussion to identify which issues are a priority is necessary as there will be reduced acceptance of any interventions unless strategies are meaningful and co-designed with clients. Short-, medium- and long-term priorities may need to be set.

DEVELOPMENT OF OBJECTIVES

Setting objectives provides a focus for direction in care planning that addresses the unique needs of clients and communities, and sets benchmarks for evaluation (Toney-Butler & Thayer 2020). When addressing the needs of communities while undertaking project planning, there may also be overall goals or aims that indicate planned, long-term changes. A common problem is for objectives to be written outlining what the health practitioner will do. In partnership with individuals, families and communities, it is important to co-design objectives, setting key steps towards targets they want to achieve (Taylor et al 2021). To be effective, objectives need to be SMART (Taylor et al 2021, p. 202):

- **S**pecific, with one idea per objective
- **M**easurable, with each objective having an action verb that can be measured
- **A**chievable, ensuring that the activities associated with the objective will be realistic for the individual, family or community and health practitioner
- **R**elevant, ensuring that the objectives are clearly linked to the identified issue and any overall goals or aims
- Include a **T**imeframe, stating a realistic time for each objective to be achieved.

They also need to be fiscally and ethically responsible. The evaluation measures the objectives, so it is crucial that they address all the areas above to ensure effective measurement.

Where to find out more on ...

Developing measurable objectives

- Guidance for writing behavioural learning objectives, American Psychological Association (APA): www.apa.org/ed/sponsor/resources/objectives.pdf

IMPLEMENTATION

Implementation strategies are the activities planned to enable the objectives to be achieved (Taylor et al 2021). They will have credibility if they are supported by evidence-based research and address a holistic range of activities such as physical, psychosocial, spiritual and financial strategies. Incorporation of primary health care principles enhances their effectiveness and acceptability, thereby facilitating sustainability of outcomes. Additionally, with the aim of developing self-efficacy, health literacy and empowerment for all clients, embedding health education and health promotion within care plan implementation strategies is a crucial step. Theoretical models help guide the planning of these strategies and influence the way in which we apply them. Modes of intervention provide tools for how we may work in partnership with people and whole communities. We will now give some examples of different types of theoretical models and modes of intervention to help build our understanding of planning for interventions. Recall our previous discussion on models of care.

Theoretical models underpinning care planning implementation strategies

The ecological model which was discussed in Chapter 1 recognises that health and wellness are influenced by both biological and environmental factors. Use of the term 'socio-ecological' identifies that social influences are also included in the environmental domain. The interactions between individual, family, organisational, community and public policy factors highlight the range of factors influencing the ability of people and communities to maintain health and wellbeing. Figure 5.1 demonstrates the influences each factor has on the other.

Individual factors relate to biological and personal histories that enhance and present challenges to maintaining health and wellness. SDH involving age, gender, socioeconomic status and genetics influence people's abilities for self-efficacy, health literacy and self-management of health. Interpersonal factors recognise that a person's peers such as family members shape their health-seeking behaviours, influencing their physical and psychosocial environments to enable or inhibit health and wellbeing activities. Organisational and community factors investigate the

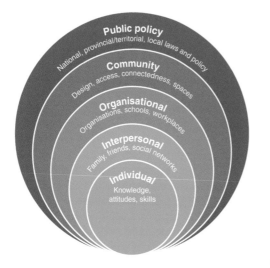

Figure 5.1 Socio-ecological model of health

Source: Adapted from Centers for Disease Control and Prevention, Social Ecological Model. Online. Available: www.cdc.gov/violenceprevention/about/social-ecologicalmodel.html.

quality of settings in which people work, learn and live, examining the characteristics that enable or counter healthy lifestyles. SDH such as housing, transport and economic considerations influence these opportunities. Public policy factors relating to health, economic and social policies can influence social inequalities by supporting accessible, affordable, equitable and culturally appropriate ways of assisting individuals or groups in the community (Centers for Disease Control and Prevention [CDC]) 2021). When planning strategies, community health nurses and others working in the community need to understand the characteristics of each factor within the model and how they interrelate and influence each other.

As you can see, the impacts of the SDH need to be recognised when developing implementation strategies within individual, family and community project care plans. Each level in the socio-ecological model of health can be positively influenced by primary health care approaches, particularly in relation to health education and health-promoting activities.

The Ottawa Charter for Health Promotion outlined in Chapter 1 is a further model or framework for guiding planning of strategies for care and project planning. The five core strategies of the Charter (build public health policy, create supportive environments, strengthen community action, develop personal skills, re-orient health services) are underpinned by the principles of primary health care to enhance health promotion approaches within community health, thereby assisting clients in all settings to be empowered and supported to make changes to their health and wellbeing (Guzys 2021, WHO 2021). The Ottawa Charter identifies the fundamental conditions and resources for community health, and using the Charter to guide care planning ensures a comprehensive approach to improving health.

KEY POINT

Inequalities and inequities

The implementation strategies encouraged by the Ottawa Charter are aimed at overcoming inequalities (bias and disadvantage) and inequities (unfair distribution of healthcare and other resources) through action on the SDH at all levels of society.

The ultimate goal is social justice.

Modes of intervention

As health services change as we move into the future, the types of interventions we use will also change. Traditional approaches still have a place and we will consider these first. The use of groups as a flexible model of care delivery has been discussed in Chapter 4. This model can be used for a wide range of people and settings, such as seniors' groups, men's groups, young parents' groups, health fairs and primary and adolescent health groups in urban, rural and remote areas. Planning care for men in the community can be challenging, but connecting and developing strategies through innovations such as Men's Sheds have the potential to deliver practical and social activities that encourage positive health behaviours (Kelly et al 2021). Health and wellbeing expos or fairs can use novel methods of presenting health education and health promotion across a wide range of topics. Strategies such as demonstrations, personal use of health products and the availability of health promotion material can be made available to large numbers of people (Men's Health Information & Resource Centre n.d., Northern NSW Local Health District 2021). As previously highlighted, adapting group work to virtual online engagement is an emerging strategy that is being used by community health nurses for people preferring this type of approach and for isolated population groups (Taylor et al 2021).

Primary health care practitioners, including community health nurses, have an integral role in the prevention and management of chronic diseases using a primary health care approach within the socio-ecological model of care. Chronic diseases are long lasting with continuing effects and include cardiovascular conditions, cancers, mental illness, diabetes, respiratory diseases, musculoskeletal conditions, chronic kidney disease and oral diseases. Of note is the presence of multimorbidity, where there are two or more concurrent conditions. Adding to these complexities are recent findings highlighting that around 45% of people in these health situations live in very low socioeconomic conditions. As such, the physical, psychosocial and economic impacts of chronic conditions affecting quality of life for people and their families are increasingly becoming a healthcare priority (AIHW 2021a).

Most morbidity and mortality is caused by chronic diseases which are significant global, national and individual health burdens, causing approximately 3 in 4, or 42 million deaths worldwide in 2019, an increase of 7% over the previous nine years (AIHW 2021b, Global Burden of Disease Collaborative Network 2020). Risk factors such as tobacco and alcohol consumption, along with intake of illicit drugs, significantly increase the incidence of chronic disease, injury and premature death and are of urgent concern for adults and children in Australia and New Zealand. Notably, smoking tobacco is considered to be the leading cause of preventable morbidity and mortality with smoking rates linked to poor SDH and disadvantage (AIHW 2021c).

As part of care planning across individual, family and community groups, community health nurses are taking a lead role in helping clients engage in health-protective behaviours while understanding and advocating in relation to underlying SDH. Health education, health promotion and case management are all fundamental to primary health care practice. Nurses and other health practitioners need to be cognisant of how the SDH are influencing clients' behaviours and responses to prevention and management strategies, thereby influencing their ongoing participation in their own health and wellbeing outcomes. They can work in partnership with other agencies and entire communities to creatively facilitate population-level changes to help individuals and families maintain health and wellbeing (Taylor et al 2021).

Interdisciplinary practice is a strong feature of chronic disease management, with a range of strategies such as group work, general practice management plans and motivational interviewing being utilised in care planning to support ongoing client health management and behaviour change. These may be facilitated through face-to-face modes or by the increasing use of telehealth (Allen & Brown 2020). The aim of brief intervention through motivational interviewing is to use a range of approaches to promote positive health and wellbeing, and lessening probability of harm. Motivational interviewing is a credible strategy to encourage behaviour change, with community health nurses and other health professionals working in partnership with individuals and families, offering non-judgmental information and strategies appropriate to their needs. Based on an understanding of clients' SDH, the interventions aim to intrinsically help them to develop skills and knowledge that address their unique personal difficulties, potentially enhancing their resilience and capacity for change (CAHS 2019b). It is important not to push too much information into a brief intervention which has the potential to reduce successful outcomes (Randell & Scanlen 2018). Central to quality engagement and outcomes are the principles of working in partnership with clients and their families.

Where to find out more on ...

Motivational interviewing

- Royal College of Nursing (RCN), How motivational interviewing works: www.rcn. org.uk/clinical-topics/supporting-behaviour-change/motivational-interviewing

New and innovative modes of engagement and intervention during care planning are also starting to become more prevalent, most notably in the areas of digital health technologies and health informatics. Digital health can engage people through flexible, integrated digital care technologies to support and enhance a range of healthcare strategies, while health informatics is described as the storage, retrieval, sharing, use and management of health data from the digital interface to facilitate decisions for health issues (Health Informatics New Zealand [HiNZ] n.d.). Telehealth can reduce geographical inequities across rural and remote regions of Australia and New Zealand through audio and video communications, supporting clients in their homes, sole practising nursing staff and medical practitioners needing specialist assistance (Butler-Henderson 2020). Of note has been increasing use of telehealth services internationally in urban as well as rural areas during COVID-19 restrictions on population movements, including management of chronic conditions (Bhaskar et al 2020).

Everyday use of personal health trackers is increasing in the community, enabling constant measurement of heart rate, oxygen saturation, stress levels and blood sugar. This data has the potential to be uploaded automatically to an individual's personal health record, enabling a nurse or other health practitioner to monitor health from a distance. Diabetes care has seen smartphone apps becoming popular for tracking data such as blood glucose, insulin doses and factors affecting good diabetes control such as exercise and sleep (Cafazzo 2019).

While there are benefits to digital health technologies and health informatics, there are also issues with their use in the community. Individuals, families, communities and health professionals require reliable broadband internet services and need to understand how to use these technologies. Accessible and easily understood education materials and technology support are necessary. Additionally, there are privacy, confidentiality and security implications for services such as group sessions, along with sharing and storage of data (Hoffman 2020).

An example of an innovative digital health activity includes serious games to support dementia care. Serious games are a range of activities, including board, video and virtual reality games. Clients can engage through a variety of devices such as somatosensory technology, 3D graphics and sensor technology, which can also be used in collaboration with additional activities such as music therapy (Ning et al 2020).

Planning for care needs to take into account the growing demands of individuals, families and entire communities for flexible, innovative client-centred approaches to care. It is important to facilitate empowering environments that enable people and community groups to make decisions regarding their own health and wellbeing in partnership with community health nurses and other health professionals.

Research evidence is crucial for substantiating strategies that are used for planning, establishing evidence-based models of care and government-funded models with a flexible range of implementation. It is also imperative to ensure a primary health care approach underpins these strategies to ensure they are realistic, achievable, affordable and culturally safe for all population groups. Just a reminder for your documentation: it is important to list all resources needed for your strategies in a single document, particularly for community project group activities. This enables you to consider costs more effectively and remember requirements such as booking venues and guest speakers. It also allows other health practitioners to quickly understand all that is needed if they are undertaking the strategies in your absence.

Examples of care plans and project planning approaches are available online at http://ws.elsevier.com/AU/Clendon/community/.

EVALUATION

A care plan allows objectives to be measured, observing and documenting responses to interventions to assess effectiveness. It is a continual, cyclic process where strengths and challenges of objectives and intervention strategies can be highlighted, and different approaches can be developed when necessary (Douglas & Crisp 2021). It is important to take a strengths-based approach, reviewing what went well, what contributed to the success and how these factors may be incorporated into future care planning. Giving praise to people for achievements is integral to feelings of self-efficacy and self-determination. Even when outcomes have not met anticipated objectives, commending them for their efforts, for 'giving it a go', is fundamental for ongoing confidence.

The processes of evaluation have similarities and differences for individuals, families and community projects. Individuals and families have a more personalised approach than whole communities with the following steps being carried out:

- comparing evaluation findings with the care plan objectives
- assessing if the objectives and intended results have been met, partially met or not met
- helping to understand what worked and under what conditions
- assessing if there are any unintended effects (SECO & OECD n.d.).

Using critical reflection and judgment, evaluation findings can be reviewed to consider if the original care plan remains relevant to the presenting issues and whether there has been partial or no progress. This reassessment requires critical-thinking skills, with clinical judgments and client partnership feedback to inform more specific, tailored objectives and intervention strategies. As such, evaluation can determine the appropriateness of interventions and resources, and client responses to plans of care (Douglas & Crisp 2021).

Evaluation of planning for community projects is required for identifying strengths and challenges in addition to informing reports for funding agencies and stakeholders. To inform a comprehensive approach, both quantitative and qualitative data are collected, enabling collection of both statistical results and the lived, contextual experiences of program participants. The primary health care and health promotion aspects can be challenging to evaluate as issues such as the impact of the SDH and behavioural changes are developmental and complex. It is recognised that the achievement of overall program aims can be long term, with direct association of strategies to outcomes being problematic (Taylor et al 2021).

Three basic types of evaluation underpin the assessment of community project programs: process, impact and outcome evaluation.

- Process evaluation assesses the type, quantity and quality of program strategies implemented.
- Impact evaluation assesses the immediate program effects on participants. A crucial factor is whether the program's objectives have been met.
- Outcome evaluation considers if the long-term program aims or goals have been achieved. Measures may reveal changes in health behaviours and indicators (RHIHub 2021, Taylor et al 2021).

There is a range of tools that can be used to collect quantitative and qualitative data for each of these types of evaluation. Process evaluation assesses the degree to which the community group has been engaged with the program and participant satisfaction. Feedback on the number of participants completing a program, and their feedback on the organisation of activities and strategies such as suitability and accessibility of venues, length of session times, availability of child activities, availability of refreshments, suitability of program content, and facilitator presentation and interpersonal skills, are important for their ongoing engagement. Paper-based or online questionnaires are the most commonly used data-collection tools (RHIHub 2021, Taylor et al 2021).

Impact evaluation reviews whether project program objectives were met. Critical analysis of the evaluation also reveals the reasons for successful objectives and strategies within project planning along with details on why they may not have been achieved. Unexpected project outcomes may be learned, all of which help improve their design and supporting policies. Quasi-experimental and non-experimental evaluation designs are generally used for data collection with experimental designs that are not considered optimal for participatory community health promotion activities. Non-experimental designs do not include a control or comparison group. Quasi-experimental designs can use comparison groups, while both are frequently used for pre-test/post-test assessment. A variety of data-collecting strategies can be applied such as pre- and post- paper-based and online questionnaires and spider web diagrammatic representation of findings. It is important that strategies for confidentiality of data are implemented, with each participant choosing the degree to which their information and their identity are publicly disclosed. This requires informed consent prior to participation in evaluation activities (RHIHub 2021, Taylor et al 2021). An economic evaluation to measure program costs may be included as part of impact evaluation strategies (Parker & Baldwin 2019).

Outcome evaluation frequently utilises statistical indicators such as quality of life, health status and morbidity and mortality indices to assess if aims or goals have been achieved. Measurements of behavioural changes are difficult as successful outcomes may be attributed to a number of integrated strategies. The same tools as detailed for impact evaluation can also be used for outcome evaluation (Taylor et al 2021).

Once the evaluation of community project programs has been completed, development of an information dissemination strategy is an important step. This is seen as a community development process, supporting community members in their empowerment, health literacy and health and wellness capacity building (Taylor et al 2021). It is also recognition of the partnership approach within care and project planning and community health practice. Reports on program outcomes potentially benefit ongoing program funding, contribute to the evidence base for care and project planning and demonstrate quality practice approaches.

Disability

The WHO (2020b) has recognised disability as the relationship that people experiencing ongoing or temporary health conditions have with their psychosocial, individual and SDH, which all impact on their functional ability. The rates of disability are increasing, with COVID-19 disproportionately affecting people's ability to access quality health services. As such, it is imperative for primary health care services to improve disability services in the community and to highlight the need to incorporate a socio-ecological perspective of health into models of care (Brown 2021).

Internationally, governments have developed and funded key strategies to improve care planning in identified chronic disease and disability priority areas. These include Disability Support Services (DSS) in New Zealand (NZMOH 2021) and the National Disability Insurance Scheme (NDIS) in Australia (NDIS 2019). A defining feature of NDIS in Australia is the ability of individuals and their families to have greater choice over their own planning and resources than in previous programs. Although the strategies are legislated, community health practitioners are encouraged to personalise the approaches as much as possible according to clinical need and preferences of individuals and families (Department of Social Services 2021). In New Zealand, individualised funding is helping people with disabilities make their own decisions regarding their care and who provides it. These funding mechanisms enable nurses to work with families and disability funding agencies to meet client needs more effectively through accessibility of appropriate and affordable support.

Advocacy groups

Advocacy groups also research and develop policy advice for governments and health practitioners for improved health and wellbeing strategies, thereby influencing funding and evidence for care planning. The Australian National Rural Health Alliance is an example of a national alliance of consumer and professional groups developing well-targeted, cost-effective, evidence-based strategies aimed at improving the health and wellbeing of people in rural and remote Australia (NRHA 2021). Similarly, the Rural Health Alliance Aotearoa New Zealand is an association of multiple rural sector consumer and professional organisations, identifying priority needs in rural health and providing government advocacy for equitable health and wellbeing care strategies (RHAANZ 2021). Community health nurses and other practitioners are encouraged to access these advocacy services and to actively participate in their professional organisations to keep current with policy development and to integrate contemporary strategies into practice. By so doing, they are also able to help advocate for their clients and primary health care policy and programs, critical to the needs of their clients across Australia and New Zealand (APNA 2021b).

Where to find out more on ...

Rural and remote health strategies

- The National Rural Health Alliance fact sheets and infographics: www.ruralhealth.org.au/factsheets/thumbs
- The Rural Health Alliance Aotearoa New Zealand information, resources and podcasts: www.rhaanz.org.nz
- The Australian Primary Health Care Nurses Association position and advocacy statements: www.apna.asn.au/profession/APNA-position-statements

Conclusion

Planning for care is an essential element of working with individuals, families and communities. The key elements of care planning have been identified across these contexts, highlighting the need to work in respectful partnership with clients and interdisciplinary groups. Evidence-based planning is essential for quality assurance, safety and credibility of strategies and outcomes. We have developed a set of care plans for the Smith and Mason families that are available online. These examples show how care plans can be used within the context of complex family lives. We also present two examples of project planning that can be implemented following community assessments.

Reflecting on the Big Issues

- Community healthcare nurses and other health practitioners use a range of tools to develop relevant and appropriate primary health care intervention strategies including care and project planning.
- Care and project planning is optimally undertaken in partnership with individuals, families, communities and interdisciplinary teams.
- Care and project planning is developed within a primary health care and strengths-based framework.
- The SDH have a significant role in determining aims/goals, objectives and strategies within care and project plans that work towards social justice for all.

- Care and project planning comprises assessment, development of evidence-based objectives, implementation and evaluation.
- Ecomaps, genograms and family assessment are useful tools in the assessment process.
- Theoretical models such as the ecological model and the Ottawa Charter underpin implementation approaches.
- Models of care describe the way in which services are designed and implemented.
- Modes of intervention, such as motivational interviewing and group work, are the types of

Continued

Reflecting on the Big Issues—cont'd

approaches we use in our work with individuals, families and communities.

■ Partnership approaches to disability support, such as individualised funding, enable individuals and families to work more closely with health practitioners to have their needs met.

■ Community health nurses and other health practitioners can work with advocacy groups to help develop care and project plans, in addition to enhancing primary health care policies and programs.

CASE STUDY

Care and project planning with the Smith and Mason families

• Care plans for the Smith and Mason families: http://evolve.elsevier.com/AU/Clendon/community/

• Community project plans: http://evolve.elsevier.com/AU/Clendon/community/

Reflective questions: How would I use this knowledge in practice?

1 Explain the importance of evidence-based care planning in community health nursing practice.

2 What conditions might affect culturally acceptable care plans?

3 Explain how to develop care and project plan objectives that are measurable and relevant.

4 Create a mind map with an overview of the differing implementation strategies that can be used across a range of individual, family and community situations. Consider their relevance to each situation.

5 Develop ecomaps for the Smith and Mason families.

6 What tools could you use to work with Colin to proactively encourage him to reflect on his drinking?

7 Reflecting on the project plans found online, what other approaches may be appropriate for developing breastfeeding support in a community?

8 Write a project plan designed to increase exercise among a group of teenage girls.

9 Develop a care plan designed to address Jake's asthma.

References

Allen, J., Brown, R., 2020. Home-based care. In: Guzys, D., Brown, R., Halcomb, E., Whitehead, D. (Eds), An introduction to community and primary health care, third ed. Cambridge, Port Melbourne, pp. 399–409.

American Psychological Association (APA), n.d. Guidance for writing behavioral learning objectives. Online. Available: www.apa.org/ed/sponsor/resources/objectives.pdf.

Australian College of Nursing (ACN), 2019. White paper: A new horizon for health services: Optimising advanced practice nursing. ACN, Canberra.

Australian College of Nursing (ACN), 2020. Value-based health care through nursing leadership. A white paper by ACN 2020. ACN, Canberra.

Australian Commission on Safety and Quality in Health Care (ACSQHC), 2018. Review of the key attributes of high-performing person-centred healthcare organisations. ACSQHC, Sydney.

Australian Human Rights Commission (AHRC), 2019. Children's Rights Report 2019. In their own right: Children's rights in Australia. AHRC, Sydney.

Australian Institute of Health and Welfare (AIHW), 2019. Australia's welfare 2019 data insights. Australia's welfare series no. 14. Cat. no. AUS 226. AIHW, Canberra.

Australian Institute of Health and Welfare (AIHW), 2021a. Chronic disease. AIHW, Canberra.

Australian Institute of Health and Welfare (AIHW), 2021b. Chronic condition multimorbidity. AIHW, Canberra.

Australian Institute of Health and Welfare (AIHW), 2021c. Alcohol, tobacco & other drugs in Australia. AIHW, Canberra.

Australian Primary Health Care Nurses Association (APNA), 2021a. What is primary health care nursing. APNA, Melbourne.

Australian Primary Health Care Nurses Association (APNA), 2021b. Advocacy. APNA, Melbourne.

Bhaskar, S., Bradley, S., Chattu, V.K., et al, 2020. Telemedicine across the globe: Position paper from the COVID-19 pandemic health system Resilience PROGRAM (REPROGRAM) International Consortium (Part 1). Front. Public Health. Online. Available: https://doi.org/10.3389/fpubh.2020.556720.

Brown, R., 2021. Exploring disability from a social model of health perspective. In: Guzys, D., Brown, R., Halcomb, E., Whitehead, D. (Eds), An introduction to community and primary health care, third ed. Cambridge, Port Melbourne, pp. 41–58.

Butler-Henderson, K., 2021. Health informatics. In: Guzys, D., Brown, R., Halcomb, E., Whitehead, D., (Eds), An introduction to community and primary health care, third ed. Cambridge, Port Melbourne, pp. 206–221.

Cafazzo, J.A., 2019. A digital-first model of diabetes care. Diabetes Technol. Ther., 21 (S2), 52–58. Online. Available: https://doi.org/10.1089/dia.2019.0058.

Centers for Disease Control and Prevention (CDC), 2021. The social-ecological model: A framework for prevention. CDC, Atlanta. Online. Available: www.cdc.gov/violenceprevention/about/social-ecologicalmodel.html.

Centre for Parent and Child Support (CPCS), n.d. Family partnership model. CPCS, London.

Child and Adolescent Health (CAHS), 2019a. Perinatal and infant mental health. Community Health Clinical Nursing Manual Government of Western Australia, Department of Health, Perth.

Child and Adolescent Health (CAHS), 2019b. Adolescent psychosocial brief intervention. Community Health Clinical Nursing Manual. Government of Western Australia, Department of Health, Perth.

Child Family Community Australia (CFCA), 2020. Mandatory reporting of child abuse and neglect. Australian Institute of Family Studies, Canberra.

Cox, J.L., Holden, J.M., Sagovsky, R., 1987. Detection of postnatal depression: Development of the 10-item Edinburgh Postnatal Depression Scale. Br. J. Psychiatry, 150 (6), 782–786. Online. Available: http://doi.org/10.1192/bjp.150.6.782.

Department of Social Services, 2021. National Disability Insurance Scheme. Australian Government, Canberra.

Douglas, C., Crisp, J., 2021. Gathering relevant information and making decisions. In: Crisp, J., Douglas, C., Rebeiro, G., Waters, D., (Eds), Potter and Perry's fundamentals of nursing, sixth ed. Elsevier, Chatswood, pp. 114–174.

Friedman, M.M., Bowden, V.R., Jones, E.G., 2003. Family nursing: Research, theory & practice. Prentice Hall, Upper Saddle River.

Global Burden of Disease Collaborative Network, 2020. Global Burden of Disease Study 2019 (GBD 2019). Results. Institute for Health Metrics and Evaluation, Seattle.

Gordon, C.J., 2021. Fostering sleep. In: Crisp, J., Douglas, C., Rebeiro, G., Waters, D., (Eds), Potter and Perry's fundamentals of nursing, sixth ed. Elsevier, Chatswood, pp. 1132–1156.

Guzys, D., 2021. Community and primary health care. In: Guzys, D., Brown, R., Halcomb, E., Whitehead, D., (Eds), An introduction to community and primary health care, third ed. Cambridge, Port Melbourne, pp. 3–18.

Health Informatics New Zealand (HiNZ), n.d. What is health informatics? Auckland, HiNZ.

Health.vic, 2020. Assessment process. State of Victoria, Melbourne. Online. Available: www.health.vic.gov.au/patient-care/assessment-process.

Herdman, T.H. (Ed.), 2021. NANDA International Nursing Diagnoses: Definitions & classification, 2021–2023. Thieme Medical Publishers, New York.

Hoffman D.A., 2020. Increasing access to care: Telehealth during COVID-19. J. Law Biosci., 7 (1), 1–15. Online. Available: https://doi.org/10.1093/jlb/lsaa043.

Ingram, J., Johnson, D., Copeland, M., et al, 2015. The development of a new breast feeding assessment tool and the relationship with breast feeding self-efficacy. Midwifery 31 (1), 132–137. Online. Available: http://doi.org/10.1016/j.midw.2014.07.001.

Jain, S.H., Chandrashekar, P., 2020. Implementing a targeted approach to social determinants of health interventions. Am. J. Manag. Care., 26 (12), 502–504. Online. Available: https://doi.org/10.37765/ajmc.2020.88537.

Javanparast, S., Baum, F., Ziersch, A., et al, 2020. A framework to determine the extent to which regional primary healthcare organisations are comprehensive or selective in their approach. Int. J. Health Policy Manag., 1–10. Online. Available: https://doi.org/10.34172/IJHPM.2020.182.

Kaihlanen, A-M., Hietapakka, L., Heponiemi, T., 2019. Increasing cultural awareness: Qualitative study of nurses' perceptions about cultural competence training. BMC Nursing, 18 (38). Online. Available: https://doi.org/10.1186/s12912-019-0363-x.

Kelly, D., Steiner, A., Mason, H., Teasdale, S., 2021. Men's Sheds as an alternative healthcare route? A qualitative study of the impact of Men's Sheds on user's health improvement behaviours. BMC Public Health 21, 553. Online. Available: https://doi.org/10.1186/s12889-021-10585-3.

Klein, D.A., Goldenring, J.M., Adelman, W.P., 2014. HEEADSSS 3.0: The psychosocial interview for adolescents updated for a new century fueled by media. Contemp. Pediatr. Jan, 16–28.

Kotz, J., Marriott, R., Reid, C., 2020. The EPDS and Australian Indigenous women: A systematic review of the literature. Women Birth, 34 (2), e128–e134. Online. Available: https://doi.org/10.1016/j.wombi.2020.02.007.

Leahey, M., Wright, L.M., 2016. Application of the Calgary family assessment and intervention models. Reflections on the reciprocity between the personal and the professional. J. Fam. Nurs. 22 (4), 450–459.

Lippincott Williams & Wilkins, 2013. Nursing care planning made incredibly easy, second ed. Wolters Kluwer/Lippincott Williams & Wilkins, Philadelphia.

Martin, M, Jones, K., Buliak, A., et al, 2021. Collaborating for integrated care. In: Crisp, J., Douglas, C., Rebeiro, G., Waters, D. (Eds), Potter and Perry's fundamentals of nursing, sixth ed. Elsevier, Chatswood, pp. 176–200.

McKillop, A., Munns, A., 2021. Working in primary and community health sectors. In: Crisp, J., Douglas, C., Rebeiro, G., Waters, D. (Eds), Potter and Perry's fundamentals of nursing, sixth edition. Elsevier, Chatswood, pp. 1413–1445.

Men's Health Information & Resource Centre, n.d. Men's health promotion kits. University of Western Sydney, Sydney. Online. Available: http://mengage.org.au/effective-male-health-promotion/aimhs-men-s-health-promotion-kits.

Munns, A., Robson, K., 2020. The early years. In: Biles, B., Biles, J. (Eds), Aboriginal and Torres Strait Islander peoples' health and wellbeing. Oxford, Victoria, pp. 136–164.

Munns, A., Walker, R., 2018. The relevance of Aboriginal peer-led parent support: Strengthening the child environment in remote areas. Compr. Child Adolesc. Nurs., 41 (3), 199–212. Online. Available: https://doi.org/10.1080/24694193.2018.1502534.

National Disability Insurance Scheme (NDIS), 2019. Overview of the NDIS operational guideline—About the NDIS. Canberra, NDIS.

National Rural Health Alliance Inc. (NRHA), 2021. About us—National Rural Health Alliance. NRHA, Canberra.

New Zealand Ministry of Health (NZMOH), 2018. Family violence questions and answers. NZMOH, Wellington.

New Zealand Ministry of Health (NZMOH), 2021. Disability services. NZMOH, Wellington.

Ning, H., Li, R., Ye, X., et al, 2020. A review on serious games for dementia care in ageing societies. J. Transl. Eng. Health Med., 8, 1400411. Online. Available: https://doi.org/10.1109/JTEHM.2020.2998055.

Northern NSW Local Health District (NNSWLHD), 2021. Health promotion. NNSWLHD, Lismore.

State Secretariat for Economic Affairs (SECO) & Organisation for Economic Co-operation and Development (OECD), n.d. Evaluation guidelines. Paris, OECD. Online. Available: www.oecd.org/dac/evaluation/seco_guidelines.pdf.

Oldland, E., Botti, M., Hutchinson, A.M., et al, 2020. A framework of nurses' responsibilities for quality healthcare—Exploration of content validity. Collegian, 27 (2), 150–163. Online. Available: https://doi.org/10.1016/j.colegn.2019.07.007.

Parker, E., Baldwin, L., 2019. Contemporary practice. In: Fleming, M.L., Parker, E., Correa-Velez, I., (Eds), Introduction to public health, fourth ed. Elsevier, Sydney, pp. 184–196.

Potter, P.A., Perry, A.G., Stockert, P.A., et al, 2021. Fundamentals of nursing, tenth ed. Elsevier, Missouri.

Randell A., Scanlan F., 2018. Evidence summary: How effective are brief motivational interventions at reducing young people's problematic substance use, second version. Orygen, The National Centre of Excellence in Youth Mental Health, (AU), Parkville.

Roenne, P.F., Esbensen, B.A., Broedsgaard, A., et al, 2021. Family nursing conversations with patients with chronic non-cancer pain and their selected family members: A protocol for the FANCOC-PAIN quasi-experimental trial. Medicine Case Reports and Study Protocols, 2 (5), e0103. Online. Available: http://doi.org/10.1097/MD9.0000000000000103.

Rural Health Alliance Aotearoa New Zealand (RHAANZ), 2021. Online. Available: www.rhaanz.org.nz.

Rural Health Information Hub (RHIHub), 2021. Evaluation design. RHIHub, Grand Forks, ND.

Shajani, Z., Snell, D., 2019. Wright and Leahey's nurses and families: A guide to family assessment and intervention, seventh edition, F.A. Davis, Philadelphia.

Taylor, J., O'Hara, L., Talbot, L., et al, 2021. Promoting health. The primary health care approach, seventh ed. Elsevier, Chatswood.

Toney-Butler, T.J., Thayer, J.M., 2020. Nursing process. StatPearls Publishing, Treasure Island, FL.

World Health Organization (WHO), 2020a. Elder abuse. WHO, Geneva.

World Health Organization (WHO), 2020b. Disability and health. WHO, Geneva.

World Health Organization (WHO), 2021. Health promotion. WHO, Geneva.

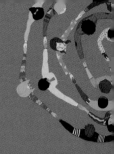

CHAPTER 6
Primary health care in practice

Introduction

Chapter 6 brings the focus onto the practitioner, exploring the various roles from which nurses, midwives and paramedics promote health and wellbeing in their communities. As you will see throughout the chapter, despite having common primary health care goals, they all use a variety of approaches to community health that are influenced by the context of community care, the population they assist, diverse and changing regulations, policy imperatives, employer requirements and their specialised preparation for practice. Because the models and processes of care differ between settings and between different groups of people, we describe both generalised and specialised practice in response to changing needs and different contexts. Although the focus is predominantly on nurses and nursing roles, we start by exploring interdisciplinary practice in some detail because of the importance of working in this way with colleagues and clients to improve health outcomes. We also look at strategies for working in teams and with groups, and leadership within the healthcare team. To provide context for the reader, the chapter also includes several community practice profile examples.

An interdisciplinary primary health care approach

Partnering with clients to achieve better outcomes is the mandate of all health practitioners. One

---

OBJECTIVES

By the end of this chapter you will be able to:

1 discuss the major factors influencing primary health care practice

2 explore how a variety of nursing and health/non-health practitioners can work in partnership to develop interdisciplinary primary health care approaches targeted at individuals, families and communities

3 identify the range of nursing, midwifery and paramedic roles within community settings and the ways these contribute to improving health outcomes

4 identify the most important elements of successful group work

5 explore the influences of practitioner delegation and leadership on primary health care practice.

approach to this is through interdisciplinary practice. Interdisciplinary practice occurs when multiple healthcare providers work with a client, integrating their knowledge and expertise with that of the client to develop an integrated strategy to achieve common health objectives. Holistic and integrated quality care occurs if all health practitioners integrate their strengths-based expertise and work in partnership with clients to facilitate a range of strategies supporting self-determination, health and wellbeing (Social Care Institute for Excellence 2018). Community health nurses and other health practitioners need to be integral members of interdisciplinary teams to improve clients' experiences of care and their health outcomes within sustainable, economically responsible environments (World Health Organization [WHO] 2018). The term 'interdisciplinary' is important. It can be used synonymously with interprofessional and you will also see the terms 'multidisciplinary' and 'multiprofessional' used. We prefer, and use throughout the book, the term 'interdisciplinary' due to its integrated approach to caring. Table 6.1 outlines the differences between multidisciplinary and interdisciplinary.

Interdisciplinary practice in the community is guided by the principles of primary health care: accessible healthcare, appropriate technology, health promotion, intersectoral collaboration, community participation and cultural safety. While these principles provide an underpinning context for interdisciplinary practice, a systematic review identified 12 characteristics required for effective interdisciplinary teamwork. These characteristics form a framework for interdisciplinary leadership with one of the most important elements being the presence of a team leader who is cognisant of the goals of interdisciplinary practice and how it can be achieved. Using the framework as a basis supports interdisciplinary practice and facilitates integrated practice across professions. The 12 characteristics are as follows:

- facilitation of shared leadership
- transformation and change
- personal qualities of team members
- goal alignment between team members
- creativity and innovation

TABLE 6.1 Practice models

Type	Definition
Uniprofessional practice	A single healthcare provider collaborates with a client to address a health issue.
Multiprofessional or multidisciplinary practice	Multiple healthcare providers from different professions work with a client to achieve the client's health objective. There is little collaboration with other professionals apart from information sharing.
Interprofessional or interdisciplinary practice	Multiple healthcare providers work with a client, integrating their knowledge and expertise with that of the client to develop an integrated strategy to achieve common health objectives.

Source: Adapted from Stadick, J.L., 2020, The relationship between interprofessional education and healthcare professional's attitudes towards teamwork and interprofessional collaborative competencies. Journal of Interprofessional Education and Practice 19 100320, 1–7. https://doi.org/10.1016/j.xjep.2020.100320; Social Care Institute for Excellence, 2018, Integrated care research and practice. Author, London. Online. Available: www.scie.org.uk/integrated-care/research-practice.

- communication
- team building
- leadership clarity
- direction setting
- external liaison
- skill mix and diversity
- clinical and contextual expertise (Smith et al 2018, p. 1)

International contemporary models of practice highlight the value of interdisciplinary approaches to enhance quality care for individuals, families and communities, and to reduce client risks, in addition to facilitating more positive and resilient work environments. Coordination and delivery of safe, high-quality care is dependent on well-organised policies and strategies across institutional, specialty and cultural parameters, recognising complexity and increasing prominence of preventive and chronic care (Rosen et al 2018). Combined professional expertise, in collaboration with individuals, families and communities, can create unique client-centred support strategies to lessen risk and enhance successful outcomes (Social Care Institute for Excellence 2018). Findings from a further review correlated evidence that the addition of new care providers into interdisciplinary teams, especially nurses, in addition to contemporary models of care, is associated with increases in delivery of preventive activities and an increase in community-based care and enhanced chronic disease management outcomes (Wranik et al 2019).

However, there are challenges for interdisciplinary team members which need to be recognised and addressed to maintain integrated approaches. Differences between professional perspectives on care management require all health professionals to be cognisant and respectful of each other's scope of practice, values and norms. Failure to do this may result in active or passive resistance to participation in interdisciplinary practice or under-utilisation of professional capabilities (Junod Peron et al 2019, Szafran et al 2019, McInnes et al 2021). Additionally, communication preferences need to be acknowledged and understood in terms of professional and personal requirements. Of note is how interdisciplinary teams are able to co-locate or regularly interact in order to negotiate their integrated practice and enhance team functioning and ways of working (Schot et al 2020).

Further, there is a requirement for ongoing team-based professional support, which is integral to maintaining optimal frameworks of interdisciplinary primary health care practice. Participation in regular reflective practice sessions enhances opportunities for teams to critically examine their collaborative responses to health and wellbeing issues in order to achieve health-promoting, client-centred care (McInnes et al 2021).

Overall, evidence indicates the value of interdisciplinary practice in improving primary health care approaches and enhancing individual, family and community outcomes. Community health nurses are integral members within these teams, and are well positioned to assist in the development of equitable and socially just healthcare through their use of primary health care frameworks to guide health and wellbeing activities (McInnes et al 2021, Munns & Robson 2020).

Types and categories of healthcare practitioners

Interdisciplinary care is undertaken by a range of healthcare practitioners, including nurses, doctors and allied health practitioners, such as social workers, occupational therapists, physiotherapists and paramedics. Some may be located within hospitals, while others are based in the community or work between both sectors of practice. Practice models for community-based nurses, midwives and paramedics are explored in this section while recognising the need for integration of their expertise with other professional personnel within a socio-ecological health perspective. At times, non-professional staff, such as peer-support workers and practice assistants, may be team members.

The World Health Organization (WHO) recently reiterated the importance of primary health care to address health issues globally, and unequivocally identified nursing and midwifery practice as critical drivers for transforming health service organisation and health care delivery. It is recognised that nurses and midwives comprise approximately 50% of the global health workforce and are frequently the sole health provider for communities across a diverse range of health situations (WHO 2020). The impact, range and expertise of community health nurses is increasing, with growing recognition of their ability to positively influence healthcare in traditional and non-traditional settings (International Council of Nurses [ICN] 2020, Australian Primary Health Care Nurses Association [APNA] 2021). Examples of community nursing roles include practice nurses, public health nurses, child health nurses, district nurses, rural and remote area nurses, occupational health nurses who work in industry, sexual health nurses, nurses providing care to specific groups (e.g. people with long-term conditions and people with disabilities), and nurses working in urgent care clinics. Community nurses work in well child services, youth health, occupational health, family planning/sexual health, mental health and addictions, prisons, health education/promotion, aged care, non-governmental organisations and for Māori and Iwi providers, Pacific health providers and Aboriginal and Torres Strait Islander health providers. Community nurses are also managers and leaders of community-based services. Community nursing covers a wide range of practice—some nurses have a very specific individual focus, while others have broad roles that encompass well and at-risk populations, health promotion, early detection, intervention, diagnosis and treatment across the lifespan. Central to primary health care nursing is partnership with people, individuals, families, whānau and communities, to achieve the shared goal of health for all.

Community nurses have had a long tradition of working relatively autonomously, with the safety net of supervision by employers and colleagues who help ensure they are engaging in best practice informed by the most recent, relevant and rigorous evidence to support their work. In recent times, many have been required to move to different roles as part of rapid responses to issues such as the COVID-19 pandemic, bushfires and political unrest. These additional and demanding roles impact on nurses and other health professionals who experience difficulty in prioritising and accessing their own professional support (Martin & Snowdon 2020). Support and mentoring of community practice can take place through face-to-face or online individual or group meetings with peers, supervisors and managers. This is important for all practitioners to enable them to meet the high standards of nursing practice and educational currency required for their roles (Guzys 2021a). Later in this chapter we discuss reflective practice which is another strategy for managing the challenges of autonomous practice in the community.

The following sections provide a deep dive into just a few examples of community nursing, midwifery and paramedic practice. As already noted, there are multiple roles and specialties and subspecialty areas of practice for practitioners in the community and there is no way we could do justice to all of them. We hope these examples will give you a taste of community practice and pique your interest in exploring others in more depth. We encourage you to talk to practitioners working in community roles to understand in more detail the extent of their work and their individual career pathways. Given the diversity of roles and career pathways that practitioners can follow, we also encourage you to use your searching skills to uncover more about fundamental competencies and standards of practice for community nurses (e.g. see the Aotearoa New Zealand Primary Health Care Nursing Standards of Practice available at www.nzno.org.nz/Portals/0/publications/Primary%20Health%20Care%20Nursing%20Standards%20of%20Practice%202019.pdf?ver=XYUZI2v-cpVH28Oy1rhfdw%3d%3d or the National School Nursing Standards for Practice: Registered Nurse available at https://anmf.org.au/documents/reports/ANMF_National_School_Nursing_Standards_for_Practice_RN_2019.pdf). These standards provide a starting point for understanding the skills required for community nursing practice and provide still more detail than we can provide in the following sections.

ADVANCED NURSING PRACTICE

Internationally, there is no consistent interpretation of advanced nursing practice with a range of meanings relating to the term. The title 'advanced practice nurse' incorporates a number of advanced practice roles where registered nurses are extending their traditional scope of practice, supported by further postgraduate education and research activities. Although advanced practice skills have improved client outcomes, there is no agreement on the specific criteria for these roles or for regulation of this level of practice (Chief Nursing and Midwifery Officers [CNMO] Australia 2020). A range of professional designations are used, such as advanced practice nurse (APN), nurse practitioner (NP), nurse consultant (NC), clinical nurse specialist (CNS) and nurse anaesthetist (NA) (Ohio Association of Advanced Practice Nurses [OAAPN] 2020).

In the United Kingdom, four core pillars integral to advanced practice have been identified as:

- clinical/direct care
- leadership and collaborative practice
- improving quality and developing practice

- developing self and others (Royal College of Nursing [RCN] 2021, p. 4).

These align with the identification of advanced practice in the Australian context which recognises five domains:

- direct comprehensive care
- support of systems
- research
- education
- publication and professional leadership (Gardner et al 2016, Mick & Ackermann 2000).

In Australia, it is recognised that advanced nursing practice is not a role but is specific to an individual practitioner within their scope of practice, whether they are enrolled nurses, registered nurses or nurse practitioners. Their higher recognisable levels of competence allow them to manage clients with complex care needs through their relevant expertise and critical thinking (Nursing and Midwifery Board of Australia [NMBA] 2020). Advanced practice has been acknowledged by the Nursing Council of New Zealand through the development of the nurse practitioner role that reflects highly developed clinical skills and judgments, working across diverse settings to enhance health service delivery and support the wider profession (Nursing Council of New Zealand [NCNZ] 2021). In New Zealand, nurse prescribing is also considered an element of advanced nursing practice and nurse prescribers are identified separately on the register of nursing.

Internationally, it is recognised that there is a need to improve health service delivery to individuals, families and communities, particularly vulnerable populations. Access to primary health care is vital for issues of health equity and justice but there are challenges of continuity and fragmentation within current models of care across Australia and New Zealand (Taylor et al 2021, McInnes et al 2021, New Zealand Nurses Organization [NZNO] 2018). Central to innovative, client-centred care at the advanced practice level is the evolving role of nurse practitioners who employ high levels of interdisciplinary, evidence-based health promotion and intervention approaches in their clinical practice (CNMO Australia 2020).

The first nurse practitioners were registered in Australia in 2000 (ACNP 2021) and in New Zealand in 2001 (NCNZ 2017). The scopes of practice for New Zealand and Australian nurse practitioners

have many similarities, with both requiring master-degree educational preparation for the role. They have specific codes of practice and are able to work autonomously and collaboratively within their legally designated scope of practice.

POINT TO PONDER

Review the professional requirements for Australian and New Zealand nurse practitioners, particularly noting both their scopes of practice and competencies.

- New Zealand: www.nursingcouncil.org.nz/public/nursing/scopes_of_practice/nurse_practitioner/ncnz/nursing-section/nurse_practitioner.aspx
- Australia: www.nursingmidwiferyboard.gov.au/Registration-and-Endorsement/Endorsements-Notations.aspx#nurse

---

Internationally, the nurse practitioner role has steadily evolved, gradually gaining acceptance as a viable contribution to primary health care systems. There is agreement on the positive enabling impact of nurse practitioners in the populations they serve, enhancing affordable, accessible and proficient care for individuals, families and communities across diverse population groups. Of note is the positioning and expertise of nurse practitioners in understanding the importance of primary health care and translating this knowledge into effective strategies and policies for change through holistic and interdisciplinary approaches (Tori 2021). In all levels of practice, community nurses in Australia and New Zealand have forged important links with the communities they serve, especially in creating models of primary health care. In rural and remote areas, cities and general practices, all nurses have a common commitment to health equity through empowering partnerships with their clients. Roles and responsibilities to strengthen the health and wellbeing of individuals, families and communities are undertaken within diverse practice positions, a number of which are discussed in the next section and are supplemented by the practice vignettes found throughout the text (e.g. Box 6.1).

BOX 6.1

NURSING ROLE PROFILE: DISTRICT NURSING

Kia Ora. My name is Di Johnston and I am a registered nurse working for a district nursing service in New Zealand.

What the role entails:

This is a diverse role and entails working alongside a wide cross-section of the community in people's own homes. I work as a primary nurse and have approximately 30 patients whom I see on a regular basis. Currently, my oldest patient is 103 and the youngest is 22.

A large majority of people that I work alongside are well and living independently (or with support from various care agencies or close whānau/family). The role encompasses care planning and coordination with a strong emphasis on interdisciplinary communication and networking. My day may include managing chronic wounds, providing post-surgical care at home, supporting home intravenous therapy, providing stomal care, supporting enteral feeding, providing palliative care and supporting catheter care among many other interventions in the home.

How I came to be in the role:

Prior to my current position I was employed in a very busy emergency department working around the clock. According to my beloved family, night shifts make me grumpy! District nursing is an absolute privilege. To be able to visit people in their own homes enables easier assessments as their living environments give plenty of clues as to how they are managing and the dynamics of perceived power imbalances are less evident than in a hospital environment.

What I find most interesting about the role:

The most interesting thing about the role is the relationships with all the people I am involved with. Establishing, maintaining and concluding relationships can be challenging and complex. District nurses often see people over extended periods of time, and it takes real skill to continue to look with fresh eyes and maintain warmth, professionalism and clear boundaries. A high proportion of the people I work with have multiple comorbidities and are in a higher age bracket. People are living longer, and it is a joy to assist people to live well in their own home for as long as possible. Liaising with other health providers is integral as is building relationships with family and those close to them.

The transition times—for example, a person who is nearing the end of their life or a person moving from their own home into hospital level care—can be a challenging time for family and for the individual concerned. Knowing when to have conversations about advanced care planning and sowing strong seeds to encourage people to consider the future and put good plans in place requires excellent communication skills, and the development of trust and rapport.

Advice for anyone wanting to become a district nurse:

Strong assessment skills are vital, as is the ability to form therapeutic relationships to ensure people's needs are met and goals of care are achieved. Willingness to meet people where they are, a well-developed sense of humour and the ability to be with the REAL rather than the IDEAL is also extremely helpful.

COMMUNITY HEALTH PRACTICE

General practice nursing

General practice nursing is a rapidly expanding area of community nursing with an increasingly pivotal role in delivering continuous care to clients, especially to those with chronic diseases. The role includes organising client care, managing quality and risk activities, solving problems within the general practice, providing education for clients and staff and being an agent of connectivity for interdisciplinary practice (APNA 2021). General practice nurses in Australia and New Zealand are able to plan and implement client care, and undertake health promotion and prevention activities for a range of population groups including managing emergency situations, lifestyle education, aged care, women's health, men's health, anti-smoking programs, infection control, chronic disease management (including cardiovascular, asthma and other respiratory conditions), immunisation, cancer management, mental health, maternal and child health, sexual health, population health, diabetes and wound management (APNA 2021, Halcomb & Ashley 2019). Practice nurses work autonomously to manage patient care, frequently specialising in areas such as cervical screening, respiratory health or refugee health. Practice nurses run nurse-led clinics for people with a range of conditions from acute presentations to management of long-term conditions. They often run immunisation clinics, with many taking on responsibility for COVID-19 vaccination for their practice population. Legislative and regulatory amendments have enabled nurses in New Zealand to add prescribing to their toolkit and many practice nurses are expanding their scope to include this intervention within their practice.

Many general practice nursing roles revolve around the primary care activities that are common in general practice, such as chronic illness management. However, there are increasing opportunities for primary health care activities in conjunction with primary care within Australia and New Zealand (Halcomb 2021). Practice nursing in Australia and New Zealand is a specialist strand of primary health care practice, complementary to the role of the GP (APNA 2021, Halcomb 2021). The role is expanding and becoming more diverse, with the scope of practice varying according to the nurse's expertise and experience, practice arrangements, the GP's understanding of the role and the needs and understanding of the role by the local population (Halcomb 2021).

As noted earlier, practice nurses play an important role in supporting people with long-term conditions and other acute and emerging health conditions. It is predicted that there will be a shortfall in the practice nurse workforce in Australia of around 814 full-time practice nurses by 2025 (Heywood & Laurence 2018) without accounting for the impact of the Covid-19 pandemic on general practice. This shortage will impact substantially on the ability of Australian general practices to develop new models of nurse-led care. In New Zealand, a nursing workforce shortage has been predicted for many years (Nursing Advisory Group 2022) and will have a similar impact on New Zealand general practice. See Chapter 1 for a practice profile written by a practice nurse.

Child health nursing practice

Child health nursing is a specialised area of nursing in the community. Working within a primary health care framework, child health nurses work in a diverse range of settings, delivering universal and targeted services to children and their families. In partnership with parents/caregivers and communities, child health nurses facilitate multidisciplinary and interdisciplinary approaches, to promote optimal developmental health for children from birth to 4 to 5 years through primary, secondary and tertiary activities conducted in homes and community locations (Wightman et al 2021). Additionally, they provide assessment and support for parental physical and psychosocial issues and can facilitate referrals to other interdisciplinary care providers (MCFHNA 2021).

In Australia there are differences in titles for these nurses within each state, such as Maternal Child and Family Health Nurse in Victoria and Community Child Health Nurse in Western Australia (WA) (Hooker 2021, Child and Adolescent Health Service (CAHS) 2021). Internationally, the term 'health visitors' is used in the United Kingdom (Public Health England 2020), and Plunket/Well Child/Tamariki Ora/public health nurses in New Zealand (NZMOH 2018). Currently, child health nurses in Australia and New Zealand are registered nurses, some with midwifery competencies, and postgraduate studies are generally required for their role (Health and Human Services 2019).

Internationally, there are wide scopes of child health practice, which are needed to address the complexity of the roles when developing appropriate care for families and children undertaken by child and family health nurses when caring for infants and children. As such, knowledge of the social determinants of health (SDH) and their effect on families are integral to child health nursing practice with a particular focus on prevention and early intervention activities. Of note, contemporary practice has identified the increasing need for these approaches to be more inclusive of children's mental health (Wightman et al 2021). As a result, contemporary practice has become more aligned with global primary health care goals, focusing on family strengths and assets as well as risks. The unique developmental health and wellbeing challenges experienced by a range of population groups across Australia and New Zealand, particularly Indigenous clients, are ideally addressed through strength-based approaches, which enable child health nurses

and parents to recognise and build on the families' expertise (Munns & Robson 2020).

What all child health nurses have in common is working in partnership with parents in a way that encourages their health literacy and participation in health decisions that will sustain their family's health and wellbeing throughout the family life cycle. Additionally, they have an expanding role in supporting vulnerable families. The New Zealand Well Child Tamariki Ora Schedule provides the framework for child health service provision for children under 5 years of age in New Zealand (NZMOH 2013). The schedule outlines a universal service that all New Zealand families can access and provides for a series of health assessments with a child health nurse up until the child turns 5, also including health promotion and specialist referrals (NZMOH 2013) (see Box 6.2). A review of the Well Child Tamariki Ora Programme undertaken in 2020 identified the need for a more targeted approach to early child health with a specific focus on achieving

---

BOX 6.2

....

NURSING ROLE PROFILE: CHILD HEALTH NURSE/PUBLIC HEALTH NURSE

....

Hi. My name is Karen Aitken and I am a public health nurse (PHN), rural Well Child Tamariki Ora (WCTO) nurse and hepatitis C community nurse.

What the role entails:

The role entails working with vulnerable populations in all three roles and having equity in mind at all times. These are specific to the following.

WCTO: Conversations with parents around breastfeeding, sleeping, mobility, safety, immunisation, teething and oral health, starting solids and solids progression, behaviour, vision and hearing, growth and development (including weight, height and head circumference); screening for postnatal depression, family violence and smoking; analysis around child, parent and family health determinants; facilitating links to community support; anticipatory guidance, health education and health promotion, early detection of any negative influences that may impact on child health outcomes.

PHN: School-based vaccination program, before-school checks for 4 year olds, personal referral follow-up into service and more recently COVID-19 response (contact tracing and case management of those in isolation; attending to COVID-19 vaccination clinics in aged and residential care facilities, home visits and public community settings).

Hepatitis C: Engaging with vulnerable populations and stakeholders for point of care (POC) testing, completing POC, follow-up of referrals to the service, FibroScanning of liver and reporting back to

Continued

BOX 6.2

NURSING ROLE PROFILE: CHILD HEALTH NURSE/PUBLIC HEALTH NURSE—cont'd

referrer, part of a mobile hepatitis C service about to be launched in the South Island, following through hepatitis C positive point from POC (obtaining a definitive hepatitis C viral load, primary provider for Maviret treatment, blood test check post treatment).

Knowing referral pathways is essential for all roles plus collaboration with service providers.

How I came to be in the role:

After 20+ years of being a surgical nurse, it was time to change direction (my passion for nursing continues) and transitioned to working in the community while taking on the postgraduate certificate training required to fulfil the WCTO role. Learning, orientating and studying concurrently all consolidated my knowledge and understanding of my position as a PHN and WCTO nurse. The hepatitis C role is a new addition just this year following a good understanding and empathy towards vulnerable populations, and collaboration with service providers throughout the community work I have engaged in.

What I find most interesting about the role:

The variety in my working week keeps me motivated, engaged and enjoying being a community nurse. It's such a privilege to be allowed into patient homes and welcomed in such a way that I feel like I am making a difference for these families/whānau.

Being with a baby/child for 5 years (WCTO) and watching them grow into little beings is very special—it's like a graduation when they head off to school and are discharged from the well child service provision!

Working with vulnerable populations is also a privilege; I certainly don't take this for granted. Being able to support an individual or family/whānau towards improved health outcomes for themselves is an amazing feeling.

Advice for anyone wanting to become a ...

PHN/WCTO/hepatitis C nurse

- Know that your assessment skills, knowledge and understanding are all transferable from one role to the next throughout your career.
- Concentrate on your head-to-toe assessment skills and be able to succinctly document your assessment results.
- Know your referral pathways.
- Your empathy and understanding towards vulnerable populations is essential, especially around equity.
- Confidence in having those 'hard conversations' (this can only be learned with practice).

equity for Māori, Pacific and high need/vulnerable children (Well Child Tamariki Ora Review Advisory Rōpū and Steering Group 2020). Nurses can also work in an interdisciplinary role with vulnerable children and families in specialist programs such as in Children's Teams as part of The Children's Action Plan for children at risk of abuse or neglect; and Family Start which is intensive home visiting support, focusing on improving children's developmental health, parent–child relationships and family physical and psychosocial environments. In Australia, child health nurse practice is guided by individual state and territory government policies. However, there is a high degree of commonality of services, including universal home visits for all families with new babies, facilitation of new parent groups, provision of well child clinics for developmental health assessments from birth to preschool and outreach services.

Enhanced and sustained home visiting for families with additional needs are available through programs such as right@home (ARACY 2021). Some programs are aimed at assisting families with culturally specific needs (Munns & Walker 2018), while others are part of outreach programs such as the Western Australian, New South Wales, South Australian and New Zealand Family Partnership training programs, all of which are aimed at developing parenting capacity. Of note are emerging models of practice incorporating partnerships between child health nurses and community peers in order to offer universal and targeted parent support relevant to families' needs, particularly for vulnerable families (Munns & Walker 2018). Another more specialised type of child health practice involves acting as the expert resource person in special schools for children with disabilities. In this context, the nurse's health promotion activities extend from primary and secondary care of the child to ongoing tertiary care for the entire family. On occasion, this includes hospital visiting and grief counselling for family members and fellow students.

KEY POINTS

Maternal, child and family health nurses, Plunket nurses, Tamariki Ora nurses and public health nurses provide:

- primary, secondary, tertiary prevention
- child and family case management
- postnatal home visiting
- care coordination
- parenting group work
- telephone and telehealth support
- interdisciplinary collaboration
- peer-support partnerships
- outreach.

School health nursing practice

School nurses use a primary health care approach to work in partnership with school-age children and their families to foster the health, wellbeing and learning potential of each child (Community Health Nurses Western Australia [CHNWA] 2021). Combining primary and secondary prevention, school nurses manage safety and protective strategies in the educational environment, promoting mental and physical health, screening children for developmental and health conditions and intervening early when concerns are detected and also providing immunisation services. In so doing, they are able to link students and their families, schools, health and social support services to facilitate intersectoral referrals, in addition to nurse-led brief interventions. Working in partnership with students, their families and the school communities, principles of care include family-centred practice, respectful communication, culturally secure service delivery and interdisciplinary collaboration with the aims of optimising health and wellbeing outcomes. School nurses can be based in secondary schools while others engage with a number of primary and preschools to conduct developmental assessments and anticipatory guidance (CAHS 2020, CHNWA 2021, Sanford et al 2021). In New Zealand, school nurses who work in preschool, primary and intermediate schools are usually public health nurses. Children with special needs can be enrolled in mainstream school education or within education support schools, requiring school nurses in these practice areas to be able to undertake health procedures such as percutaneous endoscopic gastrostomy (PEG) feeding in addition to their prevention activities (New Zealand School Nurses 2021).

In recent years, school nurses are being increasingly recognised for their expertise in the area of youth health, which is integral for maintaining the physical and psychosocial health and wellbeing during this vulnerable life transition period (New Zealand School Nurses 2021). In a recent youth health survey, young Australian people between 15 and 19 years were asked about their most concerning personal issues, with education (34.2%), mental health (17.2%) and COVID-19 (9.3%) being the top three issues. In addition, 42.6% of the respondents reported feeling stressed either all or some of the time. These statistics highlight the need for school nurses to have a focus on psychosocial assessment, prevention and early intervention strategies using a comprehensive primary health care approach (Tiller et al 2020).

As part of interdisciplinary teams within schools, school nurses assist in the management of student health and welfare policies in addition to being an important resource person for parents and teachers. It is important for them to advocate for contemporary policies, including social inclusion, food security, safe housing and gender and racial equality (Tiller et al 2021). The school nurse role is therefore complex, a specialised advanced practice role that revolves around promoting students' physical and psychosocial wellbeing.

KEY POINTS

. . . .

School nursing roles

- Primary, secondary and tertiary prevention and early intervention to enable children's capacity for academic achievement and their ongoing health and wellbeing
- Health promotion for students, families, staff and the school community

There are several emerging issues impacting on the health and wellbeing of young children and youth that are being addressed through interdisciplinary practice, with the role of the school nurse pre-eminent. Responding to children's needs for support in relation to online and face-to-face bullying and coping with transition issues during school changes are contemporary areas of need, even in very young children. As an example, the necessity to support students moving from primary to secondary schools has been well established (Sustainable Health Review 2019) with risk of adverse psychosocial wellbeing and declining academic standards being acknowledged during this time of rapid adolescent developmental change. There is a need for school nurses to identify students at psychosocial risk using evidence-based psychosocial assessment tools and facilitating appropriate interventions and referrals to interdisciplinary pathways (Gaskin & Dagley 2018).

Bullying can be overt and covert, resulting in a threat to physical and psychosocial health and wellbeing, with appearance and athleticism featuring as the main causes of power imbalances influencing aggression in preadolescent children. Empathy was recognised as a protective factor (Nelson et al 2019). The ability for school nurses to undertake developmentally appropriate engagement with students and their families demonstrates how meaningful and respectful confidential conversations can be facilitated, encouraging disclosure of bullying. Nurses can establish prevention and early intervention health promotion activities that aim to help students to confidently address stressful situations and also enhance bystander participation in helping bullying victims (Nelson et al 2018).

School nurses are pivotal in establishing positive cultures within schools, promoting healthy behaviours and facilitating trusting engagement with students and their families. Health promotion is vital during primary and secondary school years as behaviour problems underpinned by complex psychosocial issues are associated with decreased long-term health and wellbeing. Health promotion is a fundamental aspect of their practice, particularly in relation to specific identified needs such as bullying, self-harm, sexual health, body image and healthy lifestyles. A variety of approaches can be tailored to student preferences and needs, including one-on-one, group and online activities (Guzys 2021a).

In helping students to address issues of concern, one of the most important interactions school nurses have with primary and secondary students is in helping them develop health literacy, particularly with the many challenges associated with accessing health information through the internet. Higher levels of health literacy influence students' and families' capacities to modify personal behaviours and make healthy decisions. Nurse-led and interdisciplinary approaches need to be linked to specific developmental stages such as primary and secondary school environments, with health literacy messaging tailored for the specific needs of individuals, families and groups (International Union for Health Promotion and Education [IUHPE] 2018). School nurses are a credible source of information to assist with the use of appropriate internet sites and guiding students towards making positive health decisions. They are also in a position to recognise the SDH impacting on their judgments, and the need to work within a primary health care framework to facilitate positive outcomes.

POINT TO PONDER

Taking a psychosocial history is integral to health assessments for young people as psychosocial and physical wellbeing are closely linked (RCH 2021). Review the use of the HEEADSSS assessment tool for psychosocial screening. Consider the questions you could use to introduce each section. (See also Appendix C.)

The Health Promoting Schools (HPS) framework developed by WHO provides an evidence framework to strengthen health promotion in schools and provide guidance on key principles and practical actions for effective outcomes (WHO 2021). The guidelines for health promotion are based on the socio-ecological approach to health, with school nurses encouraged to use this framework in their own scope of practice and when working in collaboration with the school community in planning, implementing and evaluating school health promotion programs (CAHS n.d.).

School nurses must carefully balance the need to build effective relationships with students to promote health, responding quickly to any health needs arising in the school. Many see their role as helping children and young people develop resilience by encouraging them to develop self-awareness and the ability to find solutions and options to the issues that challenge them. Their approach is one of deliberate engagement, active listening, building trust and using evidence-based guidelines to provide an optimal school environment for students and their families. School nurses engage with students during critical developmental periods. By working in partnerships with schools, families and community agencies, they are able to facilitate strengths-based, effective and acceptable primary health care support (Guzys 2021a).

Community mental health nursing practice

The prevalence of mental health issues in our societies has created renewed awareness of the importance of community mental health nursing. Mental health nurses work in partnership with clients and interdisciplinary colleagues to enhance physical and mental health and prevention of physical and mental illness for individuals, families and whole communities (Australian College of Mental Health Nurses [ACMHN] 2020). Community-based services are better able to provide improved quality of life and social outcomes (New South Wales Ministry of Health 2021). This approach is particularly important for Indigenous Australians and other culturally diverse groups, where strengths-based integrated and culturally appropriate models of social and emotional wellbeing are demonstrating potential for success (Bainbridge et al 2018). However, taking into account the SDH, there are complex psychosocial issues that impact on the ability of mental health clinicians, including nurses, in their planning and implementation of culturally safe mental health care. A recent Australian study highlighted feelings by these practitioners of being unprepared to provide this level of cultural care to Aboriginal clients and their families. Key impacts related to lack of understanding about Aboriginal people's historical journeys since colonisation and the impact of unacknowledged racism on Aboriginal clients' mental health. Recommendations for reflective practice were highlighted in addition to co-design with practitioners and Aboriginal families and communities to enhance a primary health care approach to developing appropriate, acceptable and sustainable mental health care (McGough et al 2018).

Evidence has demonstrated that deinstitutionalisation (shifting people with mental health and learning and other disabilities from institutions into the community) and early discharge into community mental health care for clients hospitalised with mental illnesses are cost-effective (New South Wales Ministry of Health 2021), placing a focus on the ability of community mental health nurses to work in partnership with clients, their families and communities to manage and promote positive mental health (Brown 2021). They are able to provide support and care during life crises and transition periods at clients' homes or residential care, liaise with interdisciplinary teams and provide client-centred education on self-care and mental health maintenance (ACMHN 2020). They also provide acute care as members of community psychiatric response teams, increasingly working collaboratively with emergency service personnel in critical events (Heslop et al 2016, Western Australian Office of the Chief Psychiatrist 2017).

Community mental health nursing is a complex, specialised, multidimensional role; one that combines primary, secondary and tertiary prevention with individual and family case management for all age groups. This breadth of activities and age groups distinguishes the role of community mental health nurses from that of other community nurses whose practice is focused on young children in the context of child or school health, or domiciliary services with a primary responsibility for older people. In some cases, they may be working in an interdisciplinary role with other health practitioners. They are able to work with community child health and school nurses to support infants, children and youth with mental health issues and parents with perinatal anxiety and depression (Brown 2021, State of Victoria 2021). In Australia and New Zealand, postgraduate qualifications are required for mental health nursing practice. Importantly, a credentialling process for nurses working in general practice who wish to include mental health care in their practice has been established by Te Ao Māramatanga New Zealand College of Mental Health Nurses Inc (NZCMHN 2021). The Australian College of Mental Health Nurses has developed a similar accreditation program for nurses specialising in mental health (ACMHN 2020). Additionally, community mental health nurses have recognition within legislative acts, and in Australia are registered to act as responsible clinicians within their scope of practice (Western Australian Office of the Chief Psychiatrist 2021).

In 2016, the Australian Government transitioned an incentive funding package from the Commonwealth Department of Health to GP Primary Health Networks.

The Mental Health Nurse Incentive Program (MHNIP) was developed in 2007 to provide clients with severe mental illness timely access to mental health nursing care through general practices, psychiatrists and Aboriginal Community Controlled Health Services. A professional benefit has seen mental health nurses able to extend their practising competencies from acute to community sectors with the ability to focus on the wellbeing of their clients. Further evaluation outcomes have highlighted strong client benefits when credentialled mental health nurses are working in partnership with eligible medical practitioners, with the program also being highlighted as an economically accessible service (Happell & Platania-Phung 2019).

KEY POINTS

Community mental health nurses provide:

- primary, secondary, tertiary prevention
- specialised case management
- integration of physical and mental health
- counselling
- care coordination
- home visiting for clients across the lifespan
- family teaching, support, health literacy
- community support for vulnerable people.

A major challenge to the accessibility of community mental health nurses is the limited access to care across rural and remote areas of Australia and New Zealand. Inequitable distribution of mental health nurses is indicated in Australia by 35% of local government areas having no nurses, with the majority of the workforce being in cities and inner regional areas. As such, primary health care strategies are urgently needed to address the barriers to timely and appropriate mental health nursing services. Recent recommendations for improvement have included improving supply of mental health nurses through student placements and enhancing policies and funding for upskilling, primary degrees and retraining, in addition to exploring innovations in service delivery, including the use of technology for nurses and clients (Sutarsa et al 2021).

The mental health and wellbeing of Australian and New Zealand populations has been challenged due to the onset of the COVID-19 global pandemic and resulting social isolation restrictions. Mental health nurses are well placed to address the psychological issues related to reduced social interaction, online environments for schooling and work, and sudden unemployment. Referral pathways to digital and online crisis lines such as Lifeline, Beyond Blue and the Kids Helpline have been valuable means of support (Australian Institute of Health and Welfare [AIHW] 2021). An emerging concern during the COVID-19 pandemic has been an increase in suicide risk and suicide-related behaviours underpinned by social isolation and loneliness from public health policies. As such, innovations to community mental health nursing practice are required including sensitive virtual suicide risk assessments along with use of smartphone and online tools for prevention and intervention strategies (Brenna et al 2021).

Medication management is an important part of the role of community mental health nurses, frequently undertaken in physically and cognitively demanding circumstances that have the potential to influence the administration process (Keers et al 2018). Their level of clinical decision-making, especially in relation to medications, is distinctive in being beyond the scope of practice of most other nurses working in the community. Their intensive long-term support for clients and families involves mobile support and treatment, including medication assessment, reviews and ongoing monitoring reviews. They also work in partnership with clients to facilitate understanding on medication treatment regimes with a focus on empowerment (Brown 2021). Other areas of responsibility include careful management of chronic mental health disease, with emerging recognition that physical comorbidities are inextricably linked and need to be taken into consideration as part of the community mental health nurse's scope of practice. Research suggests that social stigma and fragmented health service integration contribute to physical illness in addition to a lack of holistic approaches to clients' health and wellbeing (AIHW 2020a), which highlights the

benefits of an interdisciplinary primary health care approach to nursing models of care.

One of the major issues for those who have experienced mental illness is securing affordable, secure housing. Social isolation is a predominant issue for people experiencing mental illness, with accompanying poor physical health and reduced capacity to source safe appropriate housing. Australian specialist home support services recently reported that the number of clients with a current mental health issue seeking accommodation increased by 1800 clients in the previous year. Additional vulnerabilities contributing to mental health issues and homelessness include family and domestic violence, substance and alcohol use. As an SDH, housing security is instrumental in feelings of wellbeing and ability to build social connections (AIHW 2020b). The coordination role of the mental health nurse is therefore significant, with addressing the SDH through primary health care activities part of the continuum of care.

Community-based child health, school health and mental health nursing are three wide-ranging practice areas for community nurses. There are many more settings where nurses engage in primary health care approaches with individuals, families and communities, such as occupational health, diabetes care and education, district nursing, contact tracing for sexually transmitted infections, multiple sclerosis support and Hansen's disease guidance in urban, rural and remote areas. All are underpinned by a primary health care model, working in partnerships with interdisciplinary teams and clients to facilitate accessible, empowering and sustainable strategies.

COMMUNITY MIDWIFERY PRACTICE

Comprehensive midwifery care needs to be responsive to the needs and preferences of women and their families. This includes their ability through co-design and shared decision-making to enhance informed evidence-based contemporary choices in relation to birthing and care providers in the perinatal period (COAG Health Council 2019). The perinatal period describes the time from 22 weeks of gestation to 7 days following a baby's delivery, with the health and wellbeing of both mother and baby being taken into consideration (WHO, Regional Office for Europe 2021). It needs to be recognised that there are several definitions for the perinatal period in the literature.

Significant changes to the education, models of care and positioning of midwives in community practice have been undertaken across Australia and New Zealand in recent years. Recognition of midwifery as a discrete profession from nursing has been supported by direct-entry Bachelor of Midwifery programs (Australian Government Department of Health 2021). In Australia, service improvement in the past decade has seen midwives providing continuity of care in community, home and hospital settings depending on complexity and risk. Continuity of care refers to continuous midwifery care given to a woman by a known primary midwife across the continuum of their pregnancy journey during the antenatal, intrapartum and postnatal stages (RCM 2018). Continuity of care models that are led by midwives include three major categories: community midwifery group practice case load care, team midwifery and private midwifery care in the community. Midwifery-led care has demonstrated a high degree of interdisciplinary collaboration being initiated by midwives with benefits for women, midwives and service delivery agencies (Queensland Health 2021), with good-quality care being identified by clients and midwives as 'fostering connection, providing flexibility for women and midwives and having a sense of control'. Informed decision-making was enhanced through equality of control between women and midwives (Cummins et al 2020, p. 125). Publicly funded homebirths are also an option for low-risk women in most states of Australia.

Similar to Australia, New Zealand midwifery practice includes home, community and hospital settings. Lead maternity carers (LMCs), who can be midwives, general practitioners with specialist education or obstetricians with specialty qualifications, provide continuity of care throughout the perinatal period, including birth. Women can birth at home, birthing centres or in maternity hospitals (New Zealand College of Midwives [NZCOM] 2021). Midwifery practice is led by the New Zealand midwifery partnership model where the principles of equality, reciprocity, informed choice and shared decision-making facilitate empowering relationships for the women and their whānau and family across

hospital and community settings (Guilliland & Pairman 2019).

Promising outcomes are evident for Aboriginal and Torres Strait Islander peoples and Māori using a midwifery continuity of care model on country where clinicians are able to build on the strengths and values of local communities. Emerging results of a recent Australian study have shown reductions in the rates of preterm births (Kildea et al 2019). In WA, an interdisciplinary collaboration between community midwives, Aboriginal health workers and community agencies has demonstrated a credible primary health care approach to antenatal engagement within the community for Aboriginal women and their families. Research has highlighted the need for flexibility of client-preferred care settings and recognition of SDH within a primary health care framework of care as strong contributors to development of a culturally safe program (Munns 2021).

Lactation consultants

Midwives and child health nurses can hold qualifications and competencies as lactation consultants, providing accredited evidence-based lactation services to mothers and their families who are experiencing a wide variety of complex breastfeeding scenarios. An International Board Certified Lactation Consultant (IBCLC®) qualification is required for Australian and New Zealand lactation consultants, with re-certification every 5 years. With a focus on prevention and early intervention, lactation consultants are able to address issues such as low milk production, re-lactation and slow weight gain (LCANZ 2021). They also provide education and support to other health professionals and communities about breastfeeding and human lactation (IBLCE 2018).

Where to find out more on …

Providing nursing and midwifery care during pregnancy, birth and the postnatal period

- The Pregnancy, Birth and Baby website and helpline: www.pregnancybirthbaby.org.au
- The Royal New Zealand Plunket Society: www.plunket.org.nz

PARAMEDICINE PRACTICE

Internationally, paramedicine is a relatively new health discipline with paramedics working mainly in community settings such as retrieval and industrial sites. Their role description encompasses a wide range of primary care and primary health care activities. The following excerpt from the College of Paramedics summarises the role.

Paramedics are autonomous practitioners who undertake a wide range of diagnostic, treatment and management activities for service users across the lifespan, who present in either primary, urgent or emergency healthcare settings.

Their role is to holistically assess, and if required treat and manage service users presenting with physical or mental health complaints; either as the result of injury, illness or an exacerbation of a chronic illness.

They have responsibilities in health promotion and supporting proactive care for service users.

They contribute positively to the local and wider health and care services.

Paramedics work in a multitude of environments and care settings either as a sole clinician or as part of a wider health and care team.

(College of Paramedics 2018, p. 2)

There is a common set of competency standards for Australian and New Zealand paramedic practitioners. Their practice reflects an interdisciplinary approach with an understanding of the SDH and the social model of health. Australian paramedics are required to register with the Paramedicine Board of Australia within the Australian Health Practitioner Regulation Agency, while paramedics in New Zealand will soon need to be registered with the Paramedic Council (Australasian College of Paramedicine [ACP] 2021).

Where to find out more on ...

Developing the roles of paramedics in Australia and New Zealand

- How do we best incorporate non-traditional paramedic roles into health care delivery? Australian College of Paramedicine: https://paramedics.org/podcasts/12

Across Australia and New Zealand, paramedics are employed in a large number of acute and primary health care roles, with a range of different titles (see Box 6.3). In a recent review, their employment opportunities were through both road and flight paramedic scopes of practice in: armed offender teams; urban and wilderness search and rescue; chemical, biological, radiological, incendiary, nuclear and explosive incident teams; and mental health teams (Wilkinson-Stokes 2021). Mining companies, particularly in Australia, employ paramedics for onshore, offshore and international operations to provide emergency health responses in addition to primary health care and health promotion activities such as health and safety strategies, and chronic disease management (Jones et al 2019).

The roles of the paramedic across Australia and New Zealand share many characteristics, with similar professional standards. Paramedic roles are adapting to accommodate population demographics such as ageing and diverse employment across regional and remote geographical areas. Emerging response models of practice are changing to those of integrated health services with a greater focus on provision of interdisciplinary primary health care (O'Meara & Duthie 2018, Jones et al 2019).

RURAL AND REMOTE AREA PRACTICE

Although the context may differ, practising in rural and remote areas holds many common challenges for health practitioners around the world. Most of these challenges are related to the need to provide primary health care to a geographically defined community that is disadvantaged by distance from specialist services and support (McCullough et al 2021). The notion of 'remoteness' varies, with the Australian Bureau of Statistics (2021) utilising a Remoteness Areas framework to identify five classifications of remoteness across Australia relative to each area's ability to access a range of services. The socioeconomic status of individuals, families and communities is adversely affected by remoteness, with opportunities for employment and career choices, education, high-speed internet and mobile phone coverage, affordable transport,

---

BOX 6.3

....

PRACTICE PROFILE: PARAMEDIC

....

Hi. My name is Sam and I am a paramedic.

What the role entails:

Paramedics are usually the first on scene at road traffic collisions and other calls for help from the public. They attend public and private locations for people with complex medical cases as well as life-threatening conditions such as heart attacks (myocardial infarctions) and cardiac arrest. For some time now the role of the paramedic has been evolving and in many parts of the world paramedics can work outside of a traditional ambulance setting; for example, on a cruise ship or in a hospital.

How I became a paramedic:

I have always wanted to be a paramedic since a young age, having witnessed paramedics working at a scene of a road traffic incident. This inspired me to go to university, which I did in the United Kingdom. However, at first I did not have the grades to go straight to university so I spent 3 years at a local college gaining the qualifications first so I could apply to university.

What I find most interesting about this role:

The media portrays the role of the paramedic to be always dealing with urgent and acute cases; however, the cases we attend are mainly complex, chronic conditions that have deteriorated. This is why there has been a shift away from the traditional role of the paramedic by many ambulance services who now have additional education that paramedics can complete to play a role in managing chronic cases outside of a hospital setting. This frees up emergency ambulances to deal with acute emergencies.

Advice for anyone wanting to be a paramedic:

There are a number of universities that offer paramedic degrees, so take a look at all of them which you can find online by search for accredited paramedic degrees. It is also important to remember that gaining employment after qualifying can be a challenge so make sure you undertake activities that build your CV so you can be competitive. For example, try and get some voluntary experience where possible, or paid work in a caring field, and be part of the student committees while at university, which shows commitment to community work.

---

food security and access to health and social services being impacted. Across rural and remote Australia and New Zealand, population groups with Indigenous, migrant and refugee families are particularly vulnerable to these SDH (National Rural Health Alliance [NRHA] 2017, Association of Salaried Medical Specialists [ASMS] 2021).

Because of substantial differences in resources and access to other health practitioners, the degree of remoteness is therefore significant in determining the breadth of nursing, midwifery and paramedicine roles, which can range from being part of a team to being a sole practitioner. In order to engage in reflexive, sustainable and client-centred activities, practitioners engage in a primary health model of care. Rural and remote area nurses (in New Zealand these nurses are known as rural nurse specialists) are described as specialist generalists delivering acute and primary health care with reduced access to the range of interdisciplinary clinical supports available to urban practitioners. In some areas, nurses may be the sole health professional providing face-to-face health services, with assistance from colleagues via telehealth and fly-in-fly-out (FIFO) support (NRHA 2019). Additionally, nurses and other health professionals need to have specific competencies for community development in relation to communication, cultural skills and demonstrating respect. Of importance is active listening which enhances partnership, trust and co-design of care strategies reflecting clients' requirements rather than nursing priorities (Dunbar et al 2019, McCullough et al 2021).

KEY POINT

Rural and remote populations face unique health issues often compounded by a lack of geographic access to healthcare services. A lack of appropriately skilled and well-resourced health practitioners to meet the needs of these populations adds to the problem.

Internationally, rural and remote area nurses, rural nurse specialists, midwives and paramedics work in a range of geographical settings for organisations such as government health services, Aboriginal community-controlled health services, primary health care clinics and outreach services, multipurpose centres, non-government organisations and mining companies. Initiatives such as the Australian Rural Health Outreach Fund encourage improved access for rural, remote and regional individuals, families and communities to medical specialists, general practitioners, community health nurses and midwives, and allied health practitioners such as paramedics. Currently the four primary health care priorities are chronic disease management, eye health, maternity and paediatric health and mental health, with other areas being considered if necessary (Australian Government Department of Health 2020). Increasingly, due to workforce issues, FIFO services are being provided through agencies such as the Royal Flying Doctor Services, in particular dental and mental health services (Australian Government Department of Health 2018). Nurses and midwives working for the Royal Flying Doctor Service also undertake primary health care activities

through nurse- and midwife-led clinics and with interdisciplinary teams, facilitating services such as child and family health, women's health, Aboriginal and Torres Strait Islander health, social and emotional wellbeing and health promotion (Royal Flying Doctor Service [RFDS] 2021). A new and useful method for engaging with clients is videoconferencing or telehealth services, allowing community health nurses and other health practitioners to support their clients in rural and remote areas when it is not feasible to visit sites through distance or cost. This tool can also be used for professional development activities to support staff, especially in their expanded practice roles (Guzys 2021b, Bennett et al 2020).

The advantages of rural and remote area practice include feeling closely connected with the community on a social as well as professional level. Relationships with people, groups and organisations can be interdisciplinary, multi-institutional or intersectoral. However, geographic remoteness can present challenging issues for nurses and other health practitioners working in rural and remote areas. Stress, isolation, longer working and on-call hours, reduced opportunities for professional development and a lack of collegial support are among some of the concerns. In rural and remote areas, nurses work in advanced practice roles although this may not be formally recognised. Greater understanding of their practice is recommended to assess how their scope could be safely enhanced and to support development of appropriate educational strategies (Muirhead & Birks 2020, Guzys 2021b).

Rural and remote practitioners also have greater role diffusion than those working with non-rural populations, where the boundaries between personal and professional life can be indistinct. Relationships with colleagues outside work have an effect on the work dynamic as well as on social relationships. This type of role diffusion has both negative and positive effects: it can be difficult for the practitioner to maintain anonymity in the community, with the need to maintain confidentiality at times posing difficulties. On the other hand, their closeness to the community may also make them more effective because of the level of trust they have established (Guzys 2021b).

The health promotion role of rural and remote area nurses and other practitioners ranges from whole-of-community initiatives to health teaching to foster health literacy for certain individuals or groups. Indigenous people worldwide remain disadvantaged compared with non-Indigenous populations (WHO n.d.) meaning a priority role of rural and remote area practitioners is to focus on identifying and building on the strengths of these groups to facilitate health, remembering their contextual SDH. Through their primary health care approach, rural and remote area practitioners need to recognise the impacts of these adversities, working in partnership with individuals, families and communities to co-design acceptable, affordable and sustainable strategies. As such, cultural safety is an important consideration in their role. Developing good relationships and, when appropriate, shared models of care with other health practitioners, including Aboriginal and Torres Strait Islander peoples and Māori health workers and community volunteers, is an enabling approach to effective client outcomes (Munns & Walker 2018).

Nurses, midwives and paramedics have the competencies to improve health outcomes in rural and remote areas across Australia and New Zealand. Nurses are particularly well placed for this role and to lead interdisciplinary teams due to their educational preparedness in primary health care approaches and their ability to work in partnership with individuals, families, communities and professional colleagues (ACN 2018). (See Box 6.4.)

Practice strategies— ways of working

In order to enhance the health and wellbeing of urban, rural and remote area populations, community nurses and other practitioners employ a variety of evidence-based strategies either as sole practitioners or within intersectoral and interdisciplinary practice. Professional practice models and strategies have been influenced by contemporary health evidence, economic influences, population vulnerabilities and workforce fluctuations. Models such as progressive universalism have been developed to augment capacity and enhance equity within universal health service delivery to target the needs of those population members who need additional support, such as parenting skills (Higgins 2015). Strategies are underpinned by approaches that facilitate client self-determination and empowerment, including culturally safe care and a partnership approach.

WORKING WITH GROUPS

Along with individual and community-level approaches, community health practice includes group activities to help people create and maintain their health, change their health behaviours or enhance their community through capacity building. There are several advantages to undertaking group work as opposed to one-on-one interactions. Linking vulnerable people into a community's social networks and groups encourages a sense of belonging, self-esteem and wellbeing (Taylor et al 2021). Group work can be rewarding, particularly when group members energise and support one another, but it can also be challenging, especially where individuals overwhelm the ideas of others by dominating the group, or when group members find the topic difficult to share. To meet the goals of the group the facilitator must accommodate different cultures, attitudes, behaviours, experiences and styles of relating to other people.

The success of group work depends on two main elements: content and process. In some cases, the content of the group is pre-determined by the reason it was constituted, which can be to provide group therapy, to provide mutual support for a common issue or condition, to develop group or community solutions to problems or a combination of all of these goals. Group topics can be varied, such as new parent support groups, toddler behaviour and toilet training, sexual health, anaphylaxis management and drug education. Nurses may decide to be a member of a community group where political and policy decisions have compromised their ability to provide equitable, accessible services to the community. This type of action is often influenced by decisions that have created disadvantage for the most vulnerable in society and is where nurses use their advocacy skills to articulate to policymakers the difficulties people experience from decisions such as discontinued rural health services and housing for the mentally ill or victims of violence.

Contemporary community health nursing practice also includes working with virtual

BOX 6.4

NURSING ROLE PROFILE: RURAL AND REMOTE AREA NURSING

Hi. My name is Nicky Cooper and I am a rural nurse specialist/public health nurse.

What the role entails:

The rural nurse specialist (RNS) provides holistic, culturally appropriate, comprehensive and cost-effective nurse-led primary health care to a designated population.

The RNS role combines advanced nursing knowledge and skills in the rural setting. The RNS assesses, interprets diagnostics and implements treatment protocols for patients. The RNS works both independently and in collaboration to provide care with colleagues from other disciplines including primary care and secondary services. In this particular role, the following services are included:

- well child services
- school-based health services
- primary response in medical emergencies (PRIME)
- registered nurse activity covering all service provisions within the health centre and hospital
- community-based services that respond to local community need and fit within the district health board's model of care.

How I came to be in the role:

A little background about my professional journey. I arrived in the rural community of Murchison in 2006, and although originally was planning on staying short term, fate stepped in; 15 years and three sons later I am still there! I wear many professional hats, broadly encompassing vaccinating well child/school-based health services, practice nursing, aged care, palliative care and district nursing. I also work regularly on call as a PRIME nurse (intensive care unit, critical care unit and palliative care was my speciality before moving into this rural farming area). PRIME nurses provide rapid response to emergencies in rural communities.

What I find most interesting about the role:

The rural population of New Zealand has unique healthcare needs which have traditionally been provided by a general practitioner and in more recent times the addition of a nurse practitioner. The role of the rural nurse specialist is highly diverse throughout New Zealand, reflecting the very different needs of the differing populations that they serve, thus there is no 'standard' job description. In this rural population I found many triggers resulting in higher levels of postnatal depression and anxiety associated with social isolation. In 2016 I set up a Facebook page for my well child families, to supply electronic resources and support: That resulted in a reduction in diagnosed postnatal depression and 100% engagement and participation in the service. This virtual village enabled many mothers to benefit from the extended family of support from the other parents and me. Despite COVID-19 lockdowns, the results speak for themselves and make the extended effort worthwhile.

Advice for anyone wanting to become a rural nurse specialist:

Relationship! Relationship! Relationship! What my role evolved into was ultimately a parent/child-initiated service based on good relationships to increase engagement.

groups using a number of technologies such as email, teleconferencing, text, Skype, Facebook, Twitter, blogs, videoconferencing, telehealth and electronic meeting systems to connect with clients across urban, rural and remote contexts. These interactive tools present opportunities for people to participate in groups regardless of proximity. However, the nurse facilitator needs to be aware that not all group members may have the language and technology skills to be fully involved with the discussion or to be able to navigate online confidentiality issues (Taylor et al 2021, Bennett et al 2020).

Effective group facilitators understand the importance of group processes, and the need to develop a sense of shared purpose. They are also able to monitor group progress while maintaining personal boundaries, understanding what is appropriate in terms of self-disclosure, particularly when drawing on personal experiences. They create a safe space for conversation, maintaining a non-judgmental attitude and consistency in the way they approach conflict resolution. Communication strategies are crucial to effective group processes and problem-solving. These include launching discussions in ways that are informative but do not preclude others' ideas, controlling the fairness and flow of the discussions, ensuring that familiar language is used and ensuring a balance between guided discussion and self-direction. Understanding and developing appropriate child- and adult-centred learning are important group learning strategies where the learning environment is structured to enhance interactive opportunities for their unique participation and learning needs (Taylor et al 2021).

Many groups are facilitated by interdisciplinary teams, where the perspectives of other disciplines can collaboratively address the SDH, enhance problem resolution and promote holistic views (Taylor et al 2021). A similar dynamic occurs when groups combine professionals and peer-support workers (PSWs) from the same communities as their clients, where enabling strategies can be developed through a shared PSW understanding of impacting SDH and their ability to deliver culturally relevant support and advocacy (Munns & Walker 2018).

KEY POINTS

Group planning and management needs to be addressed through a range of strategies. The following points provide an overview of the steps required to set up a new group.

- Establish purpose, goals and leadership.
- Establish rules for confidentiality.
- Set the tone for communication.
- Discuss organisational issues.
- Decide on tasks and responsibilities.
- Decide on progress markers.
- Determine how conflict will be resolved.

REFLECTIVE PRACTICE

As discussed throughout this chapter, therapeutic relationships between community health nurses and other health practitioners and their clients are vitally important in order to facilitate community health and wellness. The SDH can present complex issues for both health practitioners and clients, particularly in rural and remote areas and for clients with vulnerabilities. A high degree of problem-solving and interdisciplinary case management are needed. As such, reflective thinking and practice are important elements of nursing models of care, allowing for reflections on philosophies, personal viewpoints and actions in order to improve ongoing delivery of care. In some settings, this is termed 'clinical supervision'. In peer groups or in individual meetings, nurses are encouraged to consider both strengths and challenges within their practice, particularly in relation to professional isolation in rural and remote nursing. This involves a high degree of critical thinking and enhances clinical reasoning. Groups may also be interdisciplinary, which have the potential to enhance deeper understandings of context and practice. Key considerations are whether clients and communities feel comfortable and engaged with health practitioners and their health services (Guzys 2021b, Linsley & Barker 2019, Saab et al 2020).

LEADERSHIP

Community health nurses working with individuals, families and communities are seen to have a leadership role in implementing and sustaining access to primary health care programs through autonomous practice and as part of a team. Their ability to work in partnership within a socio-ecological model of health enables them to advocate for members of their diverse communities, acknowledging impacts of the SDH and giving a voice to those accessing care. Community health nurses use evidence-based and evidence-informed expertise to guide clients and communities through complex health systems and how they are able to access credible health information (APNA 2021).

Strategic skills and enhanced leadership competencies allow advanced practice nurses, including nurse practitioners, to lead change through evidence-based interdisciplinary approaches to care. Within overarching organisational and government health policies, they are in a unique position to facilitate improved service options and health service reform, thereby enhancing client access to holistic care and reducing inefficiencies and duplication of services (ACN 2019, Maddern et al 2020).

Leadership can be described as central to influencing organisational culture and behaviour, in addition to steering reforms through complex health environments. Effective managers are able to facilitate opportunities for clients and colleagues to ensure safe, effective and high-quality ethical care (Ayeleke et al 2018). The theory of transformational leadership (Burns 1978) is recognised as an enabling approach within health practice. These nurse leaders have interpersonal approaches enabling them to motivate their colleagues to work beyond organisational expectations. Clear unambiguous communication is required, particularly in relation to organisational objectives and strong relationships based on supporting nurses' needs. In turn, these positively influence their commitment to transformational nursing leadership. This type of leadership encourages participation and empowerment for colleagues and clients rather than creating a culture of disempowerment and anxiety.

Ethical behaviours, integrity and value-based decisions are stimulatingly modelled and fostered by the leader whose competencies include emotional intelligence, effective communication, collaboration and mentoring, all of which contribute to the development of positive interpersonal relationships, work satisfaction and quality care (Asif et al 2019).

Nurse leaders need to be critically aware of the need to model and embed culturally safe models of care within their workplaces which facilitates optimal opportunities for Indigenous health and wellbeing across Australia and New Zealand. Working in partnership with these clients and communities to recognise their strengths and resilience, along with their needs, facilitates appropriate flexible and acceptable policies and strategies for care (Biles & Biles 2020).

A contemporary issue for community health nurse leaders is changes in role redistribution from registered nurses to health assistants in nursing. A variety of causes underpin these changes, with a prime role being to support registered health professionals such as nurses and midwives to better utilise their expertise. Assistants in nursing are always placed within a health-setting team, with a delegated scope of practice under professional supervision (New South Wales Ministry of Health 2019). With the registered nurse remaining accountable for the health assistant's competencies, there have been concerns raised internationally in relation to their clinical safety and client health outcomes, particularly when there are reduced numbers of registered nurses (Griffiths et al 2019). It is therefore vital that community health nurse leaders be at the forefront of the development of the health assistant-in-nursing position in the primary health care context, in order to establish clear understanding of their role with approved frameworks for delegation of tasks and activities. While acknowledging their role in evolving shared models of care, it has been recommended that health service providers establish documented duties specific to assistants-in-nursing which need to be clarified and ratified through the providers' legal policies (Department of Health, Western Australia 2022).

A strategy to assist in redesign of acute and community health clinical teams is the use of the Calderdale Framework which consists of a seven-step, clinician-led process which systematically reviews and improves the skill mix and functional abilities of nursing and allied healthcare teams. The framework has been implemented across Australia and New Zealand with outcomes of providing a flexible and competent health workforce (Queensland Health 2016, South Island Alliance 2021).

> ## Where to find out more on ...
>
> ### Application of the Calderdale Framework
>
> - New Zealand: www.sialliance.health.nz/ programmes/workforce-development-hub/ calderdale-framework/
> - Australia www.health.qld.gov.au/__data/ assets/pdf_file/0030/149655/calderdale-framework.pdf

Community health nurses are integral to helping people achieve their goals for health and wellness. Their ability to accommodate different cultures, attitudes, behaviours, experiences and learning styles of varying population groups highlight the nurses' expertise and leadership in primary health care practice. Guidance on direction and delegation may be helpful for the nurse, and the Nursing Council of New Zealand has published information accordingly. This can be found on their website at www. nursingcouncil.org.nz/Public/Nursing/Standards_ and_guidelines/NCNZ/nursing-section/Standards_ and_guidelines_for_nurses.aspx?hkey=9fc06ae7-a853-4d10-b5fe-992cd44ba3de.

Conclusion

Nurses and other health practitioners span the breadth of a community and can be found in a range of roles and practice settings. Each practitioner group has its own unique approach to primary health care practice, yet each is underpinned by the principles of primary health care to ensure equitable care that achieves social justice. Health practitioners work in interdisciplinary teams to provide leadership and the most effective care in a range of population groups and cultural settings, undertaking group work and reflecting on their practice to ensure it is safe and meets the needs of the community. We now finish the chapter by reflecting on the big issues and examining some of the ways nurses work with the Smiths and the Masons.

Reflecting on the Big Issues

- There is considerable overlap in nurses' and other health practitioners' roles in the community, with the need for population and place-based interactions that incorporate physical, mental and social needs.

- Primary, secondary and tertiary prevention activities are integral to all community roles.

- Many aspects of roles are related to the practice setting and the regulatory environment that determines scope of practice.

- Population ageing and increasing rates of chronic illnesses have a significant impact on the roles of nurses and other health practitioners in all community settings.

- All nursing specialties in the community would benefit from further research that would advance the knowledge base and help provide role clarity.

- Models of interdisciplinary collaboration in practice and research can provide better health outcomes in communities.

- Nurses' professional activities could be enhanced by standardising titles and expectations, and developing evaluation studies of the impact of their practice on community health and wellness.

CASE STUDY | ## Occupational health for the Smiths and Masons

The occupational health nurses (OHN) employed by the mining company that employs Colin have developed several employee programs to support healthy lifestyles. They are experienced nurses who understand the social and geographic problems faced by the mining community and who work closely with safety personnel to deal with injuries and risks to wellbeing. Colin has been fortunate in not requiring any primary care services, but is feeling the effects of isolation after 1 year of employment in the mine. Colin remains connected to his family via the internet and has had relatively stable internet access with few disruptions. Colin attended one of the sessions put on by the OHN for stress management but didn't attend a second. He tends to go to the pub when he has a break, but otherwise stays in the men's quarters instead of socialising with the others.

The Maddington child and school health nurses are familiar with the difficulties of FIFO families and run a number of support groups to help enhance families' capacity to cope with the lifestyle. Practice nurses (PN) in the area are also aware of the issues faced by the FIFO families in the communities, and the PN attached to Rebecca's GP practice had a discussion with her about her lifestyle the last time they met, which was at her exercise group, where both are trying to lose weight. Rebecca also expressed her concern for Colin's health to the PN.

In Papakura, the local PN has been able to help Huia manage Jake's asthma. In addition, the exercise group that Huia volunteers with at the local marae has been developed by a new Māori nurse practitioner in the area. She has identified access issues for the local Māori community and has been contracted by the local primary health organisation to provide services for local Māori. Jason had previously spent many years working in mining but found the long-distance travel and time away from his family stressful and his health was suffering. His new job working for a Māori land trust is a complete change and he now struggles with his weight and blood pressure. There is no OHN at Jason's new work so he sees his local PN for help with his health.

Reflective questions: How would I use this knowledge in practice?

1 What elements of primary health care are transferable across the range of nursing and other health practitioner roles?

2 As a practice nurse, what would be your role in working with Rebecca to help her, the children and Colin deal with his occupational situation?

3 As the school nurse, what would be your approach to assessing John's developmental progress?

4 With family disruption related to her father's FIFO schedules, what four major elements could Emily's school nurse be planning to help Emily become more engaged in her studies?

5 As a community practitioner, how could you help Jason keep his blood pressure under control?

6 As the child health nurse, to what resources would you refer Huia to manage Jake's asthma?

7 How would you research the impact of the OHN role on worker health in the mining community?

References

Asif, M., Jameel, A., Hussain, A., et al, 2019. Linking transformational leadership with nurse-assessed adverse patient outcomes and the quality of care: Assessing the role of job satisfaction and structural empowerment. Int. J. Environ. Res. Public Health, 16, 2381, 1–15. Online. Available: http://doi.org/10.3390/ijerph16132381.

Association of Salaried Medical Specialists (ASMS), 2021. Rural health at a crossroads: Tailoring local services for diverse communities. ASMS Research Brief, 28, 1–15. ISSN 2624-0335.

Atkins, S., Murphy, K., 1994. Reflective practice. Nurs. Stand. 8 (39), 49–56.

Australian Bureau of Statistics (ABS), 2021. Australian Statistical Geography Standard (ASGS) Edition 3. ABS, Canberra.

Australian College of Mental Health Nurses (ACMHN), 2020. What is mental health nursing? ACMHN, Deakin West.

Australian College of Nurse Practitioners (ACNP), 2021. Learn more about nurse practitioners. Author, North Melbourne. Online. Available: www.acnp.org.au/aboutnursepractitioners.

Australian College of Nursing (ACN), 2018. Improving health outcomes in rural and remote Australia: Optimising the contribution of nurses. Author, Deakin.

Australian College of Nursing (ACN), 2019. A new horizon for health service: Optimising advanced practice nursing. Author, Deakin.

Australasian College of Paramedicine (ACP), 2021. Advancing paramedicine. ACP, Umina Beach, NSW. Online. Available: https://paramedics.org/.

Australian Government Department of Health, 2018. Royal Flying Doctor Service (RFDS) Program. Author, Canberra.

Australian Government Department of Health, 2020. Rural Health Outreach Fund. Author, Canberra.

Australian Government Department of Health, 2021. Australia's Future Health Workforce Report—Midwives. Author, Canberra.

Australian Institute of Health and Welfare (AIHW), 2020a. Physical health of people with mental illness. AIHW, Canberra.

Australian Institute of Health and Welfare (AIHW), 2020b. Specialist homelessness services annual report. AIHW, Canberra.

Australian Institute of Health and Welfare (AIHW), 2021. Mental health services in Australia. AIHW, Canberra.

Australian Primary Health Care Nurses Association (APNA), 2021. Community health nursing. APNA, South Melbourne.

Australian Research Alliance for Children and Youth (ARACY), 2021. right@home. Author, Canberra.

Ayeleke, R.O., Dunham, A., North, N., et al, 2018. The concept of leadership in the health care sector. In: Göker, S.D., Leadership. Çanakkale Onsekiz Mart University, Turkey. Online. Available: http://doi.org/10.5772/intechopen.72755.

Bainbridge, R., McCalman, J., Jongen, C., et al, 2018. Improving social and emotional wellbeing for Aboriginal and Torres Strait Islander people: An evidence check rapid review brokered by the Sax Institute (www.saxinstitute.org.au) for Beyond Blue. Online. Available: www.beyondblue. org.au/docs/default-source/about-beyond-blue/policy-submissions/aboriginal-programs-for-sewb_final-4. pdf?sfvrsn=157bbfea_4.

Bennett, E., Simpson, W., Fowler, C., et al, 2020. Enhancing access to parenting services using digital technology supported practices. Australian Journal of Child and Family Health Nursing, 17 (1), 4–11.

Biles, B., Biles, J. (Eds), 2020. Aboriginal and Torres Strait Islander people's health and wellbeing. Oxford University Press, Docklands, Victoria.

Brenna, C.T.A., Links, P.S., Tran, M.M., et al, 2021. Innovations in suicide assessment and prevention during pandemics. Public Health Res. Pract., 31 (3), e3132111. Online. Available: https://doi.org/10.17061/phrp3132111.

Brown, R., 2021. Community mental health nursing. In: Guzys, D., Brown, R., Halcomb, E., Whitehead, D., An introduction to community and primary health care, third ed. Cambridge University Press, United Kingdom, pp. 284–297.

Burns, J.M., 1978. Leadership. Harper & Row, New York.

Chief Nursing and Midwifery Officers Australia (CNMO Australia), 2020. Advanced nursing practice. Guidelines for the Australian context. Office of the Chief Nursing and Midwifery Officer, Department of Health, Canberra. Online. Available: www.health.gov.au/sites/default/files/documents/2020/10/advanced-nursing-practice-guidelines-for-the-australian-context.pdf.

Child and Adolescent Health Service (CAHS), 2020. School-aged health services. Government of Western Australia, Department of Health, Perth.

Child and Adolescent Health Service (CAHS), 2021. Child health. Government of Western Australia, Department of Health, Perth. Online. Available: https://cahs.health.wa.gov.au/Our-services/Community-Health/Child-Health.

COAG Health Council, 2019. Woman-centred care: Strategic directions for Australian maternity services. Canberra, Author. Online. Available: www.health.gov.au/sites/default/files/documents/2019/11/woman-centred-care-strategic-directions-for-australian-maternity-services.pdf.

College of Paramedics, 2018. Paramedic—scope of practice policy. Author, Bridgewater, United Kingdom.

Community Health Nurses Western Australia (CHNWA), 2021. Community health nurse roles. CHNWA, Perth.

Cummins, A., Coddington, R., Fox, D., et al, 2020. Exploring the qualities of midwifery-led continuity of care in Australia (MiLCCA) using the quality maternal and newborn care framework. Women Birth, 33 (2), 125–134. Online. Available: https://doi.org/10.1016/j.wombi.2019.03.013.

Department of Health, Western Australia, 2022. Assistant in nursing duties (Nursing setting). Department of Health, WA, Perth.

Dunbar, T., Bourke, L., Murakami-Gold, L., 2019. More than just numbers! Perceptions of remote area nurse staffing in Northern Territory Government health clinics. Aust. J. Rural Health, 27, 245–250. Online. Available: http://doi.org/10.1111/ajr.12513.

Gardner, G., Duffield, C., Doubrovsky, A., et al, 2016. Identifying advanced practice: A national survey of a nursing workforce. Int. J. Nurs. Stud., 55, 60–70.

Gaskin, C., Dagley, G., 2018. Recognising signs of deterioration in a person's mental state. ACSQHC, Sydney.

Gibbs, G., 1988. Learning by doing: A guide to teaching and learning methods. Further Education Unit, Oxford Polytechnic, Oxford.

Griffiths P, Maruotti A, Recio Saucedo A, et al, 2019. Nurse staffing, nursing assistants and hospital mortality: Retrospective longitudinal cohort study. BMJ Qual. Saf., 28, 609–617. Online. Available: http://doi.org/10.1136/bmjqs-2018-008043.

Guilliland, K., Pairman, S., 2019. The midwifery partnership model: The foundation of continuity of care. In: Guilliland, K., Dixon, L. (Eds), Continuity of midwifery care in Aotearoa New Zealand. Partnership in action. New Zealand College of Midwives, Christchurch. pp. 16–22.

Guzys, D., 2021a. School and youth health nursing. In: Guzys, D., Brown, R., Halcomb, E., Whitehead, D. (Eds), An introduction to community and primary health care, third ed., Cambridge University Press, United Kingdom, pp. 311–327.

Guzys, D., 2021b. Rural health nursing. In: Guzys, D., Brown, R., Halcomb, E., Whitehead, D. (Eds), An introduction to community and primary health care, third ed., Cambridge University Press, United Kingdom, pp. 353–363.

Halcomb, E., 2021. Nursing in general practice. In: Guzys, D., Brown, R., Halcomb, E., Whitehead, D. (Eds), An introduction to community and primary health care, third ed., Cambridge University Press, United Kingdom, pp. 390–398.

Halcomb, E., Ashley, C., 2019. Are general practice nurses underutilized? An examination of current roles and task satisfaction. Collegian 29 (5), 522–527.

Happell, B., Platania-Phung, C., 2019. Review and analysis of the Mental Health Nurse Incentive Program. Australian Health Review 43, 111–119. Online. Available: https://doi.org/10.1071/AH17017.

Health and Human Services, 2019. Maternal and child health service guidelines. Victorian Government, Melbourne.

Haywood, T., Laurence, C., 2018. The general practice nurse workforce: Estimating future supply. Aust. J. Gen. Pract., 47 (11), doi: 10.31128/AJGP-01-18-4461. Online. Available: www1.racgp.org.au/ajgp/2018/november/the-general-practice-nurse-workforce.

Heslop, B., Wynaden, D., Tohotoa, J., et al, 2016. Mental health nurses' contributions to community mental health care: An Australian study. Int. J. Ment. Health Nurs. 25 (5), 426–433. Online. Available: https://doi.org/10.1111/inm.12225.

Higgins, D., 2015. A public health approach to enhancing safe and supportive family environments for children. Australian Institute of Family Studies, Canberra.

Hooker, L., 2021. Maternal, child and family health nursing. In: Guzys, D., Brown, R., Halcomb, E., Whitehead, D. (Eds), An introduction to community and primary health care, third ed., Cambridge University Press, United Kingdom. pp. 298–310.

International Board Certified Lactation Consultant Examiners (IBLCE), 2018. Scope of practice for International Board Certified Lactation Consultant® (IBCLC®) certificants. Author, Fairfax.

International Council of Nurses (ICN), 2020. Guidelines on advanced practice nursing 2020. ICN, Geneva.

International Union for Health Promotion and Education (IUHPE), 2018. IUHPE Position statement on health literacy: A practical vision for a health literate world. IUHPE Global Working Group on Health Literacy, IUHPE, Paris.

Johns, C., 1994. Nuances of reflection. J. Clin. Nurs., 3, 71–75.

Jones, R., Cattani, M., Cross, M., et al, 2019. Serious injuries in the mining industry: preparing the emergency response. Australas. J. Paramedicine, 16, 1–6. Online. Available: https://doi.org/10.33151/ajp.16.652.

Junod Perron, N., Le Breton, J., Perrier-Gros-Claude, O., et al, 2019. Written interprofessional communication in the context of home healthcare: A qualitative exploration of Swiss perceptions and practices. Home Health Care Serv. Q., 38 (3), 224–240. Online. Available: https://doi.org/10.1080/01621424.2019.1616025.

Keers, R.N., Placido, M., Bennett, K., et al, 2018. What causes medication administration errors in a mental health hospital? A qualitative study with nursing staff. PLoS ONE, 13 (10), e0206233. Online. Available: https://doi.org/10.1371/journal.pone.0206233.

Kildea, S., Gao, Y., Hickey, S., et al, 2019. Reducing preterm birth amongst Aboriginal and Torres Strait Islander babies: A prospective cohort study, Brisbane, Australia. EClinicalMedicine, 12, 43–51. Online. Available: https://doi.org/10.1016/j.eclinm.2019.06.001.

Lactation Consultants of Australia & New Zealand (LCANZ), 2021. Lactation consultants. Author, Crows Nest.

Linsley, P., Barker, J., 2019. Reflection, portfolios and evidence-based practice. In: Linsley, P., Kane, R., Barker, J.H. (Eds), Evidence-based practice for nurses and healthcare professionals. Sage, London. pp. 157–169.

Maddern, J., Lambert, A.C., Dwyer, J., 2020. Health care managers in a changing system In: Willis, E., Reynolds, L., Rudge, T. (Eds), Understanding the Australian health care system, fourth ed., Elsevier, Chatswood, pp. 327–343.

Martin, P., Snowdon, D., 2020. Can clinical supervision bolster clinical skills and well-being through challenging times? J. Adv. Nurs., 76 (11), 2781–2782. Online. Available: https://doi.org/10.1111/jan.14483.

Maternal, Child & Family Health Nurses Australia (MCFHNA), 2021. Become a maternal, child and family health nurse. Author, St Leonards.

McCullough, K., Whitehead, L., Bayes, S., et al, 2021. Remote area nursing: Best practice or paternalism in action? The importance of consumer perspectives on primary health care nursing practice in remote communities. Aust. J. Prim.

Health, 27, 62–66. Online. Available: https://doi.org/10.1071/PY20089.

McGough, S., Wynaden, D., Wright, M., 2018. Experience of providing cultural safety in mental health to Aboriginal patients: A grounded theory study. Int. J. Ment. Health Nurs., 27, 204–213. Online. Available: http://doi.org/10.1111/inm.12310.

McInnes, S., Peters, K., Halcomb, E., 2021. Interprofessional practice. In: Guzys, D., Brown, R., Halcomb, E., Whitehead, D. (Eds), An introduction to community and primary health care, third ed., Cambridge University Press, United Kingdom, pp. 121–138.

Mick, D.J., Ackermann, M.H., 2000. Advanced practice nursing role delineation in acute and critical care: Application of the Strong Model of Advanced Practice. Heart Lung, 29 (3), 210–221.

Muirhead, S., Birks, M., 2020. Roles of rural and remote registered nurses in Australia: An integrative review. Aust. J Adv. Nurs., 37 (1), 21–33.

Munns, A., 2021. Community midwifery: a primary health care approach to care during pregnancy for Aboriginal and Torres Strait Islander women. Aust. J. Prim. Health, 27, 57–61. Online. Available: https://doi.org/10.1071/PY20105.

Munns, A., Robson, K., 2020. The early years. In: Biles, B., Biles, J. (Eds), Aboriginal and Torres Strait Islander people's health and wellbeing. Oxford University Press, Victoria, pp. 136–164.

Munns, A., Walker, R., 2018. The relevance of Aboriginal peer-led parent support: Strengthening the child environment in remote areas. Issues Compr. Pediatr. Nurs., 41(3),199–212. Online. Available: http://doi.org/10.1080/24694193.2018.1502534.

National Rural Health Alliance (NRHA), 2017. Social determinants of health. Author, Deakin West.

National Rural Health Alliance (NRHA), 2019. Nurses in rural, regional and remote Australia. Author, Deakin West.

Nelson, H., Burns, S., Kendall, G., et al, 2018. The factors that influence and protect against power imbalance in covert bullying among preadolescent children at school: A thematic analysis. J. Sch. Nurs., 34 (4), 281–291. Online. Available: http://doi.org/10.1177/1059840517748417.

Nelson, H., Burns, S., Kendall, G., et al, 2019. Preadolescent children's perception of power imbalance in bullying: A thematic analysis. PLoS ONE 14(3): e0211124. Online. Available: https://doi.org/10.1371/journal.pone.0211124.

New Zealand College of Mental Health Nurses (NZCMHN), 2021. Credentialing. NZCMHN, Auckland.

New Zealand College of Midwives (NZCOM), 2021. New Zealand midwifery. NZCOM, Wellington.

New South Wales Ministry of Health, 2019. Assistants in nursing working in the acute care environment. Health service implementation package. Revised edition. Author, Sydney.

New South Wales Ministry of Health, 2021. PCLI fact sheet. NSW Health, Sydney.

New Zealand Ministry of Health (NZMOH), 2013. Well Child / Tamariki Ora National Schedule 2013. Ministry of Health, Wellington.

New Zealand Ministry of Health (NZMOH), 2018. Well Child Tamariki Ora visits. New Zealand Government, Wellington.

New Zealand Nurses Organization (NZNO), 2018. Strategies for nursing. NZNO, Wellington.

New Zealand School Nurses, 2021. School nursing in New Zealand. Author, Auckland.

Nursing Advisory Group, 2022. Nursing safe staffing review. KPMG, Wellington, New Zealand.

Nursing and Midwifery Board of Australia (NMBA), 2020. Advanced nursing practice and specialty areas within nursing. Author, Melbourne.

Nursing Council of New Zealand (NCNZ), 2021. Nurse practitioner. NCNZ, Wellington. Online. Available: www.nursingcouncil.org.nz/Public/Nursing/Scopes_of_practice/Nurse_practitioner/NCNZ/nursing-section/Nurse_practitioner.aspx?hkey=1493d86e-e4a5-45a5-8104-64607cf103c6.

Nursing Council of New Zealand, 2017. Competencies for mātanga tapuhi nurse practitioner. NCNZ, Wellington.

Ohio Association of Advanced Practice Nurses (OAAPN), 2020. What are the different types of advanced practice nurses? OAAPN, Ohio.

O'Meara, P., Duthie, S., 2018. Paramedicine in Australia and New Zealand: A comparative overview. Aust. J. Rural Health 26, 363–368. Online. Available: http://doi.org/10.1111/ajr.12464.

Public Health England, 2020. Official Statistics. Health Visitor Service Delivery Metrics (Experimental Statistics). Quarter 3 2019/20 Statistical Commentary (April 2020 release). Author, London.

Queensland Health, 2016. The Calderdale Framework. Information sheet. Queensland Government, Brisbane.

Queensland Health, 2021. Maternity care options in Queensland. Queensland Government, Brisbane.

Rosen, M.A., Diaz Granados, D., Dietz, A.S., et al, 2018. Teamwork in healthcare: Key discoveries enabling safer, high-quality care. Am Psychol., 73 (4), 433–450. Online. Available: http://doi.org/10.1037/amp0000298.

Royal Children's Hospital Melbourne (RCH), 2021. Clinical practice guidelines: Engaging with and assessing the adolescent patient. Online. Available: www.rch.org.au/clinicalguide/guideline_index/Engaging_with_and_assessing_the_adolescent_patient/.

Royal College of Midwives (RCM), 2018. Position statement. Midwifery continuity of carer (MCOC). RCM, London.

Royal College of Nursing (RCN), 2021. Advanced level nursing practice. Section 2: Advanced level nursing practice competencies. RCN, London.

Royal Flying Doctor Service (RFDS), 2021. Primary health care. Online. Available: www.flyingdoctor.org.au/qld/what-we-do/primary-health-care-services/.

Saab, M.M., Kilty, C., Meehan, E., et al, 2020. Peer group clinical supervision: Qualitative perspectives from nurse supervisees, managers, and supervisors. Collegian 28 (4), 359–368. Online. Available: https://doi.org/10.1016/j.colegn.2020.11.004.

Sanford, C., Saurman, E., Dennis, S., et al, 2021. 'We're definitely that link': The role of school-based primary health care registered nurses in a rural community. Aust. J. Prim. Health, 27 (2), 76–82. Online. Available: https://doi.org/10.1071/PY20149.

Schot, E., Tummers, L., Noordegraaf, M., 2020. Working on working together. A systematic review on how healthcare professionals contribute to interprofessional collaboration, J. Interprof. Care, 34 (3), 332–342. Online. Available: http://doi.org/10.1080/13561820.2019.1636007.

Social Care Institute for Excellence, 2018. Integrated care research and practice. Author, London. Online. Available: www.scie.org.uk/integrated-care/research-practice.

South Island Alliance, 2021. Calderdale Framework. Author, Christchurch.

Smith, T., Fowler-Davis, S., Nancarrow, S., et al, 2018. Leadership in interprofessional health and social care teams: A literature review. J. Healthc. Leadersh., 31 (4), 452–467. Online. Available: https://doi.org/10.1108/LHS-06-2016-0026.

Stadick, J.L., 2020. The relationship between interprofessional education and health care professional's attitudes towards teamwork and interprofessional collaborative competencies. J. Interprof. Educ. Pract., 19 100320, 1–7. Online. Available: https://doi.org/10.1016/j.xjep.2020.100320.

State of Victoria, 2021. Royal Commission into Victoria's Mental Health System, final report, summary and recommendations, Parl Paper No. 202, Session 2018–21. Author, Melbourne.

Sustainable Health Review, 2019. Sustainable Health Review: Final report to the Western Australian Government. Department of Health, Western Australia, Perth.

Sutarsa, N., Banfield, M., Passioura, J., et al, 2021. Spatial inequities of mental health nurses in rural and remote Australia. Int. J. Ment. Health Nurs., 30, 167–176. Online. Available: http://doi.org/10.1111/inm.12769.

Szafran, O., Kennett, S.L., Bel, N.R., et al, 2019. Interprofessional collaboration in diabetes care: Perceptions of family physicians practicing in or not in a primary health care team. BMC Fam. Pract., 20, 44. Online. Available: https://doi.org/10.1186/s12875-019-0932-9.

Taylor, J., O'Hara, L., Talbot, L., et al, 2021. Promoting health. The primary health care approach, seventh ed., Elsevier, Chatswood.

Tiller, E., Fildes, J., Hall, S., et al, 2020. Youth Survey Report 2020. Mission Australia, Sydney.

Tori, K., 2021. Nurse practitioners. In: Guzys, D., Brown, R., Halcomb, E., Whitehead, D. (Eds), An introduction to community and primary health care, third ed., Cambridge University Press, United Kingdom, pp. 421–431.

Well Child Tamariki Ora Review Advisory Rōpū and Steering Group, 2020. Well Child Tamariki Ora review report. Online. Available: www.health.govt.nz/publication/well-child-tamariki-ora-review-report.

Western Australian Office of the Chief Psychiatrist, 2021. Authorised mental health practitioners. Government of Western Australia, Perth.

Wightman, L., Hutton, A., Grant, J., 2021. Child and family health nurses' role in the care of infants and children: A scoping review. J. Child Health Care, 1–13. Online. Available: https://doi.org/10.1177/13674935211026123.

Wilkinson-Stokes, M., 2021. A taxonomy of Australian and New Zealand paramedic clinical roles. Australas. J. Paramedicine, 18, 1–20. Online. Available: https://doi.org/10.33151/ajp.18.880.

World Health Organization (WHO), n.d. The health of Indigenous peoples. WHO, Geneva.

World Health Organization (WHO), 2018. Continuity and coordination of care: A practice brief to support implementation of the WHO Framework on integrated people-centred health services. WHO, Geneva. Online. Available: http://apps.who.int/iris/bitstream/hand le/10665/274628/9789241514033-eng.pdf?ua=1.

World Health Organization (WHO), 2020. Nursing and midwifery. WHO, Geneva.

World Health Organization (WHO), 2021. Health promoting schools. WHO, Geneva.

World Health Organization (WHO), Regional Office for Europe, 2021. Maternal and newborn health. WHO, Copenhagen.

Wranik, W.D., Price, S., Haydt, S.M., et al, 2019. Implications of interprofessional primary care team characteristics for health services and patient health outcomes: A systematic review with narrative synthesis. Health Policy 123, 550–563.

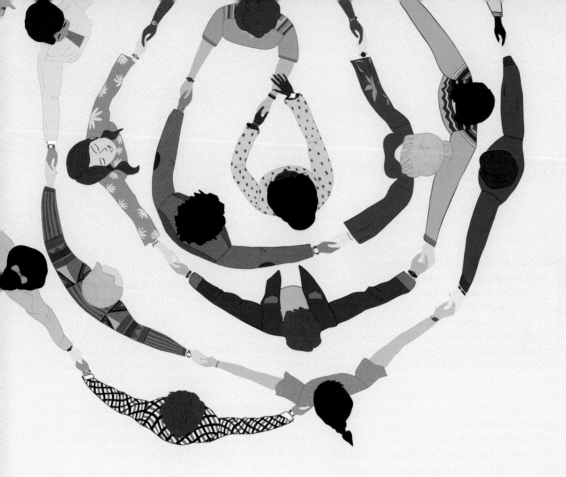

Section 3

Health and wellness throughout the lifespan

Introduction to the section

This section reflects the importance of promoting health and wellness at each stage along the life course from birth to death. Chapter 7 focuses on the contemporary family and healthy children. Because the family is so important to both individual and community health, we provide a detailed section to guide your learning, covering the rapid social, technological and workplace changes that are influencing family life and couple relationships across the transitions of partnering, marriage and, in some cases, marital separation. We also discuss the unique circumstances of some families living in our communities, including migrant and refugee families, families coping with illness or disability and rural families. We also discuss the impact of COVID-19 on family functioning. The second part of Chapter 7 focuses on child health. Child health is commonly understood as the most significant indicator of how families, neighbourhoods, communities and nations are able to provide health-enhancing conditions for daily living. We consider the burgeoning body of research into biological embeddedness, the role of environmental stimuli and the social determinants of child health and how these contribute to raising healthy children.

Chapter 8 traverses life from adolescence through to older age, focusing on three stages along life's journey: adolescence, adulthood and older adulthood. The health status of adolescents in any community provides a barometer of a community's progress in creating and supporting a healthy start to life, and creating a template for the future. At this crucial stage, a large segment of the population is launched from childhood to adulthood, from dependence to independence. How adolescents deal with the various challenges and negotiate the many transitions of a few delicate years often heralds how well they will cope with the transitions of adult life.

Healthy adulthood reflects the culmination of socially and environmentally supported choices for health and wellness made by individuals at earlier stages of their development. Adulthood is also the time when many chronic diseases emerge and when the risks of ill health or injury are acute. For younger adults, particularly parents, social and occupational pressures loom large and our discussion extends to issues related to formal and informal work and family life.

The final section of the chapter examines the features of healthy ageing. Managing chronic conditions is of major concern in this part of life's pathway, and we revisit some of the main strategies for helping people shape their lifestyles and their communities to promote healthy ageing. A social perspective of ageing is outlined, including the need to attend to older people's numerous transitions: those related to family members joining or leaving the family home, retirement, loss and the adjustments of widowhood.

Our two families, the Smiths and the Masons, also feature in both chapters, as the case study unfolds with a different focus for each, ranging from the family to the children, adolescents, adults and older family members. As you read through the chapters, we encourage you again to think about the big issues, some of which we mention at the end of each chapter, and reflect on practice and its evidence base.

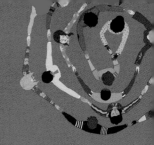

CHAPTER 7
The early years

Introduction

Few people would challenge the notion that the family is the most important influence on the health of a society. The family is where individuals are nurtured and guided to adopt and adapt beliefs, behaviours, values and attitudes that will help their members become healthy and competent citizens of wider worlds. There are many influences on health and development that arise from the interactions between families and communities. Some of the most important of these are habits of mind and action that emerge from a child's early experience in the family.

Daily interactions between family members create opportunities for inherent traits and predispositions to be shaped into positive or negative behaviours in relation to health and wellbeing.

These become habitual and refined as they are reinforced and nurtured, and as family members interact with others external to the family. Families play an important role in nurturing their children along their developmental pathways. This has a reciprocal effect on parents or caregivers as each interaction provides not only an opportunity for parental dialogue, but also renewed consideration of the way adult family members are relating to one another. In this era of increasing cross-border migration, there are also many lessons to be learned about the distinctiveness of these family interactions in families with different cultural traditions.

Adult family members make lifestyle choices, and this can be crucial to a child's decision-making in relation to healthy lifestyles. Children's choices are cultivated by what is observed and modelled within the family, and how family health is entrenched in

OBJECTIVES

By the end of this chapter you will be able to:

1 discuss local, national and global influences on families and children in a range of settings

2 describe the major risk and protective factors influencing families and children in contemporary society

3 describe the impact of preconceptual and antenatal care on children's health and developmental pathways

4 using a primary health care and social determinants framework, develop community goals and strategies for sustaining child and family health and wellbeing within a range of family structures.

the social conditions and relationships beyond the family. In this respect, families play a significant gatekeeping role as the main link between individuals and their environments. Because families themselves are dynamic, their roles change in various ways and this has implications for family health and wellbeing. As individual family members change and develop in their encounters of daily life, the family as an entity also changes to adapt to the outside world, which affects its ability to provide a supportive environment for adult members and children. Each opportunity to adapt and change can be used to share strengths and challenges, and to teach children the skills to be self-regulating and competent, to create and sustain health and wellbeing as they negotiate the critical stages along the pathways to adulthood.

In a contemporary world where change is both rapid and constant, the way family members interact with their environments determines the extent to which the family can provide support, protection, encouragement and direction to each of its members. Families that are able to provide a firm grounding for all their members to deal with outside stressors can foster understanding, tolerance and social cohesion within the family and community. Alternatively, a lack of strong family bonds to shelter or safeguard family members from adverse influences can have harmful effects on family members and the wider community.

One of the greatest indicators of health and wellness in a community is the extent to which it invests in and nurtures its children. As we outline in this chapter, our knowledge of the factors that contribute to child health is growing at a rapid rate, and there is widespread understanding that the most important avenue to good health in any community is supporting a healthy start to life. This includes support for parents from the time they begin to plan a family, through conception, childbirth and parenting. Community life is crucial to good parenting and it requires commitment at all levels of society to develop community structures and processes that will be helpful to parents and others who interact with children.

This chapter examines the importance of primary health care practice for families and children in the early years. Our social determinants of health (SDH) perspective addresses the multiple,

reciprocal, positive and negative influences on family life and how these may change over time. Towards that end, this chapter explores families and children in the context of today's societies, how they are changed by contemporary life and the role of nurses and other health practitioners in helping them achieve and sustain health and wellbeing. Part 1 of this chapter explores healthy families and their role in supporting, protecting, encouraging and directing family members. Part 2 focuses on children and those factors that influence healthy children to grow and thrive in the context of their family and today's communities.

Part 1: Healthy families
WHAT ARE FAMILIES?

When we think of family, some of us think of the protective envelope that provides a refuge from the stresses and strains of contemporary society. Others see family as a combat zone, a kind of repository for the collective problems of both the inside and the outside world. Most people hold a view of family that lies somewhere between these two extremes.

> ### KEY POINT
>
> **What is ... the family?**
>
> A protective gatekeeper between individual family members and their culture, and wider society. Family is the most important influence on the health of a society.

Defining the family is important for several reasons. These include some of the most important social and structural determinants of health, such as the socio-legal family environment. Socio-legal arrangements dictate which members have access to children's school records, who is eligible for reproductive assistance and who is legally responsible for children's health decisions. The concept of family is difficult to define as the meaning varies considerably within community and population groups. For statistical and reporting purposes, the Australian Bureau of Statistics (ABS) describes family as being:

> Two related people who live in the same household. This includes all families such as couples with and without children, including same-sex couples, couples with dependants, single mothers or fathers with children, and siblings living together. At least one person in the family has to be 15 years or over.

(ABS 2020)

Similarly, Statistics New Zealand (2021a) defines a family as including 'sole parents, couples with and without children, and people living alone'. Both countries have comparable family types, with the most common form being a couple with children (opposite-sex and same-sex couples), followed by couples without children and one parent with children. There is an increasing number of families reliant on grandparents to provide childcare or family support due to economic and social necessity and underpinned by cultural and social values (Ee et al 2020).

Across Australia and New Zealand, most children live with one or both of their parents. However, due to adverse SDH such as parental substance abuse, mental or physical illness and family violence, some parents are unable to provide safe care for their children. Temporary or ongoing out-of-home care is arranged, with grandparents being a major source of these arrangements. In Australia, the 2016 census revealed more than 35 200 children aged 0 to 12 years had grandparents as their primary caregivers (Australian Institute of Health and Welfare [AIHW] 2019a, AIHW 2020a).

Social and cultural structures influence how people relate to each other within families. For example, the kinship system within Aboriginal communities involves both biological parents and other family members having defined social structure roles within families. Extended family members assume diverse roles, particularly in relation to raising children. It is important for health professionals to have an understanding of a child's extended kinship structure, along with knowledge of their primary carer. Inclusion of Aboriginal and Torres Strait Islander health workers, liaison and peer support workers in discussions with parents and caregivers will assist with appropriate understandings of family structures and responsibilities (Hartz 2018).

In Australian and New Zealand Indigenous groups, 'family' is pre-eminent. Australian Indigenous groups have variable languages with which to describe their families and the notion of family connectedness; however, government agencies describe all Australian Aboriginal and non-Aboriginal families as 'family' using common terminology. In Australia, working with Aboriginal family groups is inclusive of Aboriginal people, such as child and family health workers, who are from the same group as the group they work with, or those who are known to be accepted by the families. These Aboriginal health workers may be part of mainstream government services, community-controlled Aboriginal health services or non-government organisations and are educated in family therapy, research and policy development as well as having local cultural knowledge. Examples of services employing such health workers include the Bouverie Centre in Victoria (Bouverie Centre 2021) and the Yorgum Aboriginal Family Counselling Service in Western Australia (Yorgum Healing Services 2021). The Bouverie Centre works in conjunction with participating Aboriginal community cooperatives, child and family services and La Trobe University. Yorgum Healing Services is an Aboriginal community-controlled family counselling service that provides specialist assessment and counselling and links family members, including Aboriginal grandmother groups, to those who require their services.

In New Zealand, Māori families are known as whānau. Whānau is an extended family group comprising three to four generations. Traditionally, whānau were made up of 20 to 30 people and were generally self-sufficient in everything except for matters of defence where they called on hapū (subtribe) and iwi (tribe) for support. Whānau cared for their older members (kaumatua and kuia) and their tamariki (children) collectively; where a child lost a parent or the family was too large to support a child, the child became known as whangāi and was cared for by the larger whānau, and this is still common practice today (New

Zealand Government 2019). For Māori, whānau is what they say it is. The collective nature of whānau is important to understand in relation to family policy in New Zealand and will be discussed later in the chapter.

These descriptions highlight a focus on family function rather than structure, where family can be seen as a continuing system of interrelationships. Changes in population demographics and societal recognition of alternative family patterns have influenced contemporary structures of families across Australia and New Zealand. Increasing diversity through migration, higher proportions of older family members through longer life expectancy, reduced numbers of children within families and increasing acceptance of same-sex relationships and single parent households are significantly changing interactions within families and their linking to their communities (Brown & Jeon 2021).

increasingly involved with care of their children, with a higher proportion of women actively engaged in the workforce. As such, children are progressively more reliant on a wider range of carers both within and external to the family unit (Brown & Jeon 2021, Coles et al, 2018). Australian research has shown that shared-care arrangements for children with a non-resident parent is becoming increasingly prevalent, with a concurrent decline in the proportion of children having no contact with a non-resident parent (Wilkins et al 2020).

There has been a recent trend for young adults to return to their parental home which has been particularly influenced by unemployment and housing shortages during the COVID-19 pandemic, resulting in changes in family economic and social dynamics (Fry et al, 2021). Additionally, more older adults are retiring later in life, with women having a more noticeable move away from early retirement than their male counterparts (Wilkins et al 2020).

KEY POINT

'Relational' view of family and diversity

- Families connect and shape one another's lives through variations in biological, legal and socially constructed relationships.
- Shared values and beliefs within and between families may vary, reflecting diversity in family functioning (Brown & Jeon 2021, p. 88).

FAMILY DEVELOPMENTAL PATHWAYS

Developmental theorists suggest that families and their members go through various life stages influenced by biological and psychosocial factors. This biopsychosocial approach demonstrates the transitions during adulthood where long-term relationships are made and caring responsibilities during parenthood are needed (Orenstein & Lewis 2020). With these stages embedded within diverse contemporary family structures and societies, there is a wide range of roles within families. Fathers are

Where to find out more on ...

Contemporary family structures

- Families Then & Now: Households and families: https://aifs.gov.au/publications/households-and-families.

FAMILY FUNCTIONS

Although there is considerable diversity among families, in most cases communities situate the family at the centre of social life, thereby being a conduit through which society transmits to individuals its social and cultural norms, roles and responsibilities. It also acts as a communicative structure from within, providing a scaffold for interactions, with the goal of bonding individuals into a cohesive whole with shared attitudes, values and opinions. When this goal is achieved, the family is able to give voice to needs and preferences, which has the potential to inform societal policies and processes that can strengthen the community.

According to their developmental stage, members make decisions affecting access to healthcare and social services, prevention of illness, preservation of the natural and built environment, the cultivation of knowledge and strategies to manage the social determinants of their health and wellbeing. These are the essential elements of a healthy society. However, family life can also exert a negative influence on these decisions, constraining individuals and circumstances, precipitating illness, failing to protect its members from harm or endangering their physical, psychosocial or cultural environments. Families are therefore the pivot point around which societies revolve.

Families have a vital role in developing nurturing environments around children's learning and wellbeing. The ability of children to develop responsive relationships within the family helps to promote secure attachments, emotional security and trust. These personal attributes contribute to positive brain development which, in turn, develops confidence with relationships external to the family and lifelong social skills, peer interactions and resilience (Center on the Developing Child 2021a).

The family functions just listed represent an ideal. When families are able to provide these caring functions and encourage protective functions such as family and community values and linkages, there is a greater likelihood of positive health and wellbeing. This promotes the development of social cohesion and social capital (Taylor et al 2021). For Indigenous families in Australia and New Zealand, family and kinship are central to their functioning and sense of community, with shared roles of responsibility and consideration for family members. Social and emotional wellbeing is closely linked to family, community, culture, spirituality and connectedness to country (Ward 2018).

Families have changed dramatically in the 21st century in form, function and relationships. In this era of globalisation and mass migration, most societies, especially in wealthier countries, are composed of more culturally and linguistically diverse (CALD) families than in the past. Sexual minority groups such as same-sex mothers and fathers are becoming increasingly recognised within communities; however, there is limited data relating to their unique challenges (Perales et al 2020). While the demographic profiles of families have altered, they remain a significantly important source of our closest relationships within a wide range of family structures (Qu 2020).

Nationally and internationally, the world of work has also transformed family roles and function considerably, as have changing attitudes and policies affecting areas such as parental leave, care of children and schooling (Brown & Jeon 2021). As an example, in both Australia and New Zealand, grandparents are called upon to provide informal, short- and long-term childcare. This is often at great personal cost given that many are themselves engaged in part-time employment and some have carer responsibilities for a spouse or older family member. Assuming custody of grandchildren, either formally or unofficially, can give way to feelings of grief or loss, disappearance of parenting abilities of their own children, as well as financial difficulties for child-rearing costs. Most grandparents readily accept the responsibility and reciprocity of their grandchildren, recognising the importance and value of the role, but they may also have fewer opportunities for maintaining their own physical and psychosocial support. Despite the pressures, the pleasures and rewards of maintaining connections with grandchildren are appreciated by the grandparents (RCN 2022). Childcare and the many ways it affects contemporary family life and work choices remains a major issue for social policy planners and healthcare practitioners supporting parents and their wider families.

Common changes in the formation and stability of families are relationship dissolution and re-partnering where fresh approaches to cohesive relationships are needed. Changing SDH, such as societal values, information technologies and social networking, education, availability of health services, secure housing and pandemics, create opportunities and challenges for families and parents, influencing their relationships and structures (AIHW 2020a). These have considerable financial and family functioning ramifications requiring support from a range of health practitioners. Box 7.1 outlines contemporary trends affecting family life, health and wellbeing.

In the context of these changes, the challenge for health practitioners is to explore ways of promoting and supporting family choices, enabling and enhancing health for all family members.

BOX 7.1

TRENDS AFFECTING FAMILY LIFE, HEALTH AND WELLBEING

- Most parents are both employed, often working long hours.
- Maternal employment is at an all-time high.
- Fathers take 1 to 4 weeks' leave after birth.
- Many jobs have been casualised, leaving parents with job insecurity.
- Casual pay rates are being reduced for weekend work.
- Many parents are underemployed.
- Some parents work from home.
- Many parents are expected to be electronically contactable for work 7 days a week.
- Women tend to work part-time, increasing hours as their children grow.
- Single mothers have low employment rates.
- Many children are in childcare by the first year of life.
- Grandparents are undertaking considerable childcare.
- Parents may have long absences from home with fly-in-fly-out/drive-in-drive-out employment or deployment with armed services.

Promoting family health is, at times, a daunting challenge given that it occurs in the face of constant change, but it is also fascinating, providing us with constantly evolving understandings of how families define themselves and how they manage their lives and health across a variety of situations.

As we have seen, family systems are continuously developing. Family functioning is dynamic and impacted by changing relationships and SDH. Family nursing scholars have tended to define family and family function according to three basic theoretical perspectives. The first is structural functional theory, where families are identified by how they are organised and what practices they undertake to address family needs and promote family health (Kitchen 2016). Another approach to defining the family is within developmental theory, which views families in terms of a sequence of life cycle stages, each with developmental tasks such as establishing a marriage, child rearing, children leaving home and retirement (Rago 2016). The third and most influential theoretical tradition is seen within the rubric of family systems theory, where the family is seen as an entity in itself, consisting of subsystems (of siblings, for example). Current and multigenerational reciprocity in functioning between subsystems (family members) and interactions between members and the family's environment affect the family as a whole (Center for Family Systems Theory of Western New York, Inc 2021). It is also important to take a socio-ecological approach to assessing and reporting on children and families. This enables exploration of immediate influences on the family unit in addition to direct and indirect effects of communities, societies and environments (AIHW 2020a).

These theoretical approaches can all be used to define the family as a basis for assessing and categorising family needs; however, each carries a presumption of understanding that may not be congruent with the primary health care philosophy and socio-ecological framework for health. The various theories and assessment tools may not consider the relational enquiry approach where intrapersonal, interpersonal and contextual factors affecting families are considered, which will limit a holistic understanding of their needs (Younas 2020). Due to adaptive interactions, family forms have unique structures, roles and challenges impacting on their function and connections to community (AIHW 2020a, Brown & Jeon 2021, Qu 2020). Because of this variability, the relational view of families is more appropriate in a primary health care context. The family as a relational entity is inclusive of the family's perspectives, choices, internal interactions and interactions with the external world in the face of changes and challenges.

Assessing a family on the basis of a set of guidelines or behavioural norms also sends a message that there are normative criteria and expectations for interactions and behaviours. This can be disempowering for families who experience historical, social or cultural disadvantage. A more authentic approach to working with families is first to discover and explore background issues affecting the family, and then work in partnership to encourage their participation in identifying any changes they seek to make or options for care (Hartz 2018). We have discussed family assessment frameworks such as the Calgary Family Assessment Model (Wright & Leahey 2013, Shajani & Snell 2019) and Friedman's Family Assessment Tool (Friedman et al 2003) and care planning in Chapters 5 and 6. These emphasised the partnership approach to working with families which is underpinned by the way health practitioners define family and family function, and work with them to facilitate their self-perceived health and wellness.

Where to find out more on ...

Support for non-parent carers

- www.servicesaustralia.gov.au/individuals/subjects/support-non-parent-carers

Parental leave support to help parents to take time off to parent a newborn or recently adopted child

- www.servicesaustralia.gov.au/about-paid-parental-leave-scheme?context=23121

Being a grandparent carer

- http://raisingchildren.net.au/articles/grownups_grandparent_carer_nutshell.html

---

CONTEMPORARY ISSUES WITHIN DISTINCTIVE FAMILIES

As discussed in Chapter 3, there are distinctive and special populations within global, national and local communities. In this next section of the chapter, we will explore family function and approaches to health and wellbeing for families within these communities.

Rural and remote families

Families living in rural and remote areas experience greater life satisfaction than those living in urban areas (Wilkins et al 2020). However, they are also impacted by a range of adverse SDH. A variety of stressors that are unique to life and work in rural and remote areas result in higher levels of mental health illnesses for individuals and families, and there are challenges to the availability of professional support for both diagnosed and undiagnosed conditions. Accessibility to the health workforce is disproportionate to these increasing requirements for primary mental health care services. Consequently, self-harm and suicide are more prevalent (National Rural Health Alliance [NRHA] 2021).

Poverty through lower incomes or deprivation due to inflated costs of accessing essential goods and services is highest for families in Australian rural and remote areas, with greater unemployment and under-employment and higher costs of living being contributing factors. Disadvantages in educational opportunities contribute to poorer employment prospects and lower incomes (AIHW 2018). Families who are especially vulnerable include those headed by sole parents and households dependent on social security incomes (AIHW 2020a).

On average, Australians living in rural and remote areas have shorter lives, higher levels of disease and injury and poorer access to and use of health services, compared with people living in metropolitan areas. Poorer health outcomes in rural and remote areas may be due to multiple factors including lifestyle differences and a level of disadvantage related to education and employment opportunities, as well as access to health services. There is a disproportionate number of people living in rural and remote areas with chronic illnesses and disabilities, sustaining injuries and having less equitable access to and use of primary health care services. Management of these conditions is complex due to reduced health infrastructure, geographical distances and costs affecting access to and use of health services (AIHW 2019b).

Community health nurses and other health practitioners working with families in rural and remote areas have practice challenges related to distances from services and the support of their colleagues. Their understanding of families' needs, priorities, assets and values will guide partnership and interdisciplinary approaches to relevant plans of care that take into account the effect of relevant SDH. However, care needs to be taken with community expectations of rural health nurses' availability at all times, including social situations. Ad hoc and opportunistic clinical contacts need to be carefully managed. Additionally, there is increased pressure on nurses in small communities to maintain client confidentiality (Guzys 2021).

Refugee and migrant families

In Australia and New Zealand, the last few decades have seen a steady growth of migrants from Asian countries and the subcontinent, the United Kingdom and other European countries, as well as cross-migration between the two countries. Refugee families also contribute to the multicultural vibrancy of the family and society in both countries in spite of the difficulties many of these groups experience in the resettlement processes. At a societal level, migration from poor to wealthy countries can create tensions, particularly if public opinion debates focus on the strain on the host country's resources from waves of migration. At the same time, there is widespread discussion over how to meet work skill shortages. Obviously, the two issues need to be resolved in the same arena, but the challenge remains for health and social service planners to identify how migrant and refugee people can be educated and employed in the areas of greatest need without disempowering them, or denigrating their lifestyles.

Some families experience a conflict of competing cultures and new family structures, as young family members straddle traditional family values and new ways of thinking. Their challenges include being accepted into the mainstream culture and difficulties with language that affect education and employment, and changes in family roles, including gendered division of housework and decision-making. Unemployment and casual work contracts can place further stress on family functioning (Ayika et al 2018).

Support from community health practitioners is a major influence on ongoing patterns of family development and the family's ability to connect with networks in the wider community. Working with refugee and migrant families can be challenging, with clinical practice recognising and incorporating the SDH and a trauma-informed framework. Working from a primary health care perspective can ensure that there is accessible, equitable and empowering healthcare that encourages health literacy and self-determination (Desmyth et al 2021). Engaging with migrant and refugee families in a community context needs to be focused on promoting inclusiveness, family cohesion and the transmission of strengths, needs and preferences along their variable developmental pathways and transitions. We explore issues of refugee and migrant health further in Chapter 9.

KEY POINT

Migration to a new country can create new opportunities for families but can also be one of the most stressful periods in a family's life course.

The transition to a new country is complex for all family members and affects family functioning in both subtle and overt ways. There is a high risk of pre-migration trauma and disadvantage leading to significant physical and psychosocial health vulnerabilities. Disadvantage during recent COVID-19 restrictions has also been highlighted due to health and social support predominantly being available online with significantly less face-to-face support. Limited language competencies and health literacy, compounded by reduced accessibility to the internet, have resulted in digital exclusion (Desmyth et al 2021).

Where to find out more on ...

Communicating with migrant and refugee communities during COVID-19: Learnings for the future

- www.refugeehealthnetworkqld.org.au/wp-content/uploads/2021/02/Report-Communications-during-COVID-19-FINAL.pdf

Working with young people from refugee and migrant backgrounds: Applying the National Youth Settlement Framework in mainstream services (webinar)

- https://aifs.gov.au/cfca/webinars/working-young-people-refugee-and-migrant-backgrounds

Fly-in fly-out families

Although each style of employment poses challenges to family life, the increase in the fly-in fly-out (FIFO) (also known as drive-in drive-out) employment pattern has had a major impact on families. FIFO families are likely to be functioning well, but there are potential negative impacts of this lifestyle on parents and children. Some families experience stress with adjusting their everyday routines on the return of the workers, such as renegotiating domestic and parenting roles and responsibilities. Concerns have also been raised by FIFO workers and their partners on the consequences of these disruptive work practices on their children's developmental health and wellbeing (Gardner et al 2018).

An Australian study investigating the mental health impacts of FIFO work arrangements has highlighted both positive and challenging aspects. Partners acknowledged development of their practical abilities, independence and emotional flexibility. However, there were burdens with needing to cope with all the parenting and family demands while their partners were away, during which time separation loneliness was felt by both partners and children. Communication was identified strongly as a relationship challenge by all family members, with recommendations for regular and quality communication with workers and their families while they were away to accommodate family routines (Centre for Transformative Work Design 2018). Community health nurses and other health practitioners need to work in partnership with this unique population to design and implement flexible primary health care approaches to enhance family health and wellbeing, with a particular focus on parenting issues.

Where to find out more on ...

The effects of FIFO workforce practices on families (webinar)

- https://aifs.gov.au/cfca/events/effects-fly-fly-out-fifo-workforce-practices-families-australia

Violence in the family

One of the greatest risks to the health and wellbeing of families is violence among family members; the infliction of abuse by one family member against another. There are various forms of family violence, including child-to-parent violence, elder abuse, intrafamilial abuse or intimate partner violence, the last of which is the most frequent form of violence in the family. Intimate partner violence is perpetrated by partners or ex-partners who engage in coercive intimidation, manipulation and exertion of power that may consist of physical, sexual and psychosocial violence and financial exploitation. Women and children are disproportionately impacted by family violence because perpetrators are more likely to be men than women. Periods of increased risk are during pregnancy and family separation, with children being affected directly or through witnessing violence against their mother (New Zealand Ministry for Women [NZMFW] 2021). For many women, the cycle of daily disempowering conditions becomes the norm for their lives in the ordinary interactions of marriage or partnership. Family violence can also be perpetrated against men and same-sex partners, involving a range of physical and psychosocial impacts.

Across a wide scope of sociocultural and economic environments, witnessing and experiencing family violence, particularly intimate partner violence, has a profound effect on children's lifelong emotional, social, behavioural and cognitive developmental health (NZMFW 2021, World Health Organization [WHO] 2021a). In some families, there is a co-occurrence of family violence and child abuse (Coulter & Mercado-Crespo 2015), which increases the risk of later victimisation in childhood, adolescence and adulthood (NZMFW 2021). Box 7.2 describes some of the many forms of family violence.

Aboriginal women in Australia and Māori women in New Zealand experience more family violence than non-Indigenous peoples (AIHW 2021a, NZMFW 2021). Within the discussion of family violence, it needs to be highlighted that the experiences of Indigenous women are complex and include a combination of factors related to colonisation history, racism and marginalisation as well as social and economic vulnerability (AIHW 2021b).

The onset and prevalence of family violence against women has increased during recent COVID-19

BOX 7.2

· ·

FORMS OF FAMILY VIOLENCE

· ·

- Physical abuse
- Sexual abuse
- Emotional or psychological abuse
- Verbal abuse
- Spiritual abuse
- Stalking and intimidation
- Social abuse and geographic isolation
- Financial abuse
- Abuse of animals

Source: On the Line, 2021. Types of domestic and family violence. On the Line, Footscray.

Family and domestic violence is more prevalent in rural and remote areas, underpinned by risk factors such as social and geographical isolation, lack of transport, limited support services, poverty and greater availability of firearms. System-level barriers also exist such as lack of agreements among available services (Youngson et al 2021). We explore intimate partner violence in more detail in Chapter 9.

Where to find out more on ...

Health impacts of domestic and family violence across urban, rural and remote areas:

- www.aihw.gov.au/reports/australias-health/health-impacts-family-domestic-and-sexual-violence

pandemic lockdowns, with safety concerns being a consideration when seeking help (Boxall et al 2020). The special issues of migrant and refugee families are also a consideration, where women in particular are vulnerable to physical and sexual violence, in addition to financial abuse, social isolation and coercion related to insecurity of their immigration status. An interdisciplinary approach is needed to help clients address assimilation into new communities, using trauma-informed care to facilitate culturally safe models of care. Of note, encouraging refugee and migrant clients to engage with communities and develop leadership roles has the potential to guide culturally appropriate programs which underpin primary health care approaches to prevention of family violence (El-Murr 2018).

Where to find out more on ...

Rates of violence in Australia

- www.ourwatch.org.au/quick-facts/

Data summaries of family violence in New Zealand:

- www.nzfvc.org.nz/family-violence-statistics/at-a-glance

There are several practice points for community health nurses and other practitioners engaged with families experiencing family violence. Effective, non-judgmental and confidential communication is essential, with interactions often having to be outside the family home. How to undertake an assessment of family violence is challenging as is accessing evidence-based pathways to guide practitioners in helping families. Early detection and intervention by community health practitioners has strong potential for preventing family violence; however, difficulties such as lack of service collaboration, risk assessments being underrated and complexity of client issues can be challenging (Youngson et al 2021). Identifying factors that could mediate the relationship between family structure and family violence need to be explored sensitively and integrated into strategy planning in partnership with family members. It is important that a primary health care approach is used, with a range of interdisciplinary agencies, to facilitate appropriate, realistic, culturally relevant and sustainable outcomes.

POINT TO PONDER

What visible behaviours might you see in a child health clinic in encountering a mother and child who are victims of intimate partner abuse?

GOALS FOR HEALTHY FAMILIES

A comprehensive primary health care approach can meet the needs of families at multiple contact points throughout life. Policies and practices supporting universal and targeted health and wellbeing support can be undertaken by a range of interdisciplinary practitioners such as child, adolescent and family health nurses, nurse practitioners, midwives, social services' support practitioners and general practitioners. Evidence-based frameworks such as the Ottawa Charter provide a guide for their work in the community, enhancing their skills and advocacy for the health and wellbeing of families and communities (Taylor et al 2021). Bronfenbrenner (1986) highlighted the interactions, linkages and impacts between families and other settings such as the community, social networks and work environments, in addition to public policies which provide a secure base for families and communities. In turn, the intrafamilial processes such as love and acceptance offer dependable settings for children for their developmental health and wellbeing. From our earlier chapters, you will recall global factors impacting on governments and communities, such as the influence of conflict and migration. Figure 7.1 shows the different influences of these on family and child health and wellbeing.

As primary health care practitioners, it is imperative that we develop strategies for assisting families that are linked to the wider social and cultural context of their lives. In working with families, contemporary skills and services need to be developed from a base of research evidence to inform accessible, adequate and appropriate care. We need to orient our research strategies to strength-based approaches, considering what works, and to provide exemplars of good and best practice in family care. To this body of evidence we should add our practice-based arguments for preventive care, which is visionary, culturally appropriate and relevant to each family's environment, taking into account impacts of current and historical SDH. Caring, as the fundamental essence of practitioner practice, mandates our involvement in social and political processes. This guides us towards working in an intersectoral way as facilitating partners

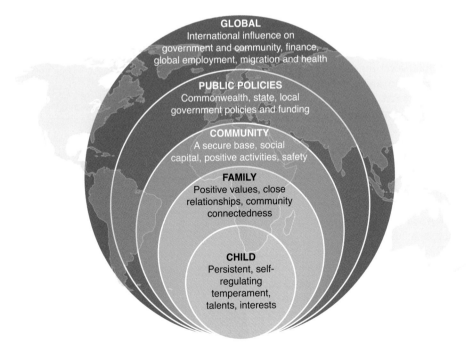

Figure 7.1 Child, family, community, societal and global assets and protective factors

with families to secure accessible, equitable and empowering health and wellbeing.

Part 2: Healthy children
BIOLOGICAL EMBEDDING AND GENETICS

Healthy children can be defined on the basis of a wide variety of indicators, some of which change throughout childhood. Being born healthy to a family with adequate resources and supports gives a child a head start, whereas coming into an environment of social disadvantage or experiencing ill health or disability compromises a child's chance of achieving health and wellbeing over the life course (Moore 2021). The traditional debate on the influences of nature (genetics) and nurture (environment) on an individual's growth and development has been advanced and understood in more depth through the study of epigenetics, where the influence of a person's behaviours and their physical and psychosocial environments on their gene expression can be explored. A child's health depends on a combination of antenatal, postnatal and early years biology, family and environments that provide opportunities to lead a healthy, nurtured and well-nourished lifestyle with a minimum of stress. Biological and social processes that change the way genes are expressed with subsequent variations in cellular-level functioning are termed epigenetic changes. These are associated with long-term health consequences for children, with early harmful psychosocial environments and adverse childhood experiences (such as low socioeconomic status, racism, excessive adversity and adverse parenting) having the potential to cause epigenetic change (Box 7.3). However, epigenetic changes are not necessarily permanent. Modification is possible through alterations to health activities, social activities and environmental circumstances (CDC 2020a, Shonkoff et al 2021).

Child and adult stress is an ongoing, adaptive process of interaction with physical and psychosocial environments, developing adaptive responses for immediate situations and learning to anticipate for future challenges. Stress responsiveness has a critical interaction with brain development, with increasing recognition of the

---

BOX 7.3

POTENTIAL OUTCOMES OF ADVERSE CHILDHOOD EXPERIENCES

- Unsafe health activities and practices
- Chronic diseases
- Fewer opportunities to develop capacities to participate in life activities
- Teen pregnancies
- Premature death

Source: Centers for Disease Control and Prevention (CDC), 2020b. Preventing adverse childhood experiences. Atlanta, GA, US Department of Health & Human Services.

---

impact of chronic stress on brain health leading to the concept of allostasis and allostatic load/overload (McEwen & Akil 2020). Toxic stress is a concern for lifetime effects on a child's physical, mental and social health, with greater likelihood of developmental delays. This response occurs when there is frequent, sustained and protracted adversity without family protective systems in place (Center on the Developing Child 2021b).

KEY POINTS

- Epigenetics is the study of how behaviours and environment can cause changes affecting gene expression, thereby altering cell function (CDC 2020a).

- Epigenetics is the mechanism for biological embedding (Aristizabal et al 2020).

- Allostasis is the process of adapting to predictable and unpredictable stress, with the production of mediators such as cortisol maintaining stability (McEwen 2000, McEwen & Akil 2020, p. 12).

- Allostatic load refers to the 'wear and tear' of the physiological systems responsible for managing our stress response, leading to dysregulation of these systems (Whelan et al 2021, p. 1).

Epigenetics is the mechanism through which the changes to genetic expression are biologically embedded in altered physiology across body systems, thereby influencing long-term physical and psychosocial health outcomes (CDC 2020a). Biological embedding usually refers to experiences with negative influences on long-term and intergenerational health trajectories, which needs to be taken into account by community health practitioners when planning interventions and strategies. Working in partnership with families and communities to reduce the risk of biologically embedding toxic stress in the early years is crucial for enabling positive lifelong health and wellbeing outcomes. Primary health care approaches are important in developing family-centred policies and strategies to individualise each child and family's coping and resilience, in order to develop positive foundations for lifelong development (Shonkoff et al 2021).

Where to find out more on ...

Epigenetics and health:

• www.cdc.gov/genomics/disease/ epigenetics.htm

Positive, tolerable and toxic stress responses, including a video:

• https://developingchild.harvard.edu/science/ key-concepts/toxic-stress/

PRECONCEPTUAL AND ANTENATAL CARE

As identified, epigenetic influences on gene expression can occur with associated biological embedding during the antenatal period. This highlights the need for healthy and nurturing physical and psychosocial environments during the preconceptual period in order to optimally enhance growth and development during pregnancy. Community-based preconception care facilitates biomedical, behavioural and social

health interventions for women and families prior to conception. In partnership, women, men and interdisciplinary community health practitioners can develop modifiable and non-modifiable strategies to reduce the risk of an unwanted and unhealthy pregnancy. Enhancing opportunities for healthy lifestyles encourages sound fetal growth, especially during the sensitive periods of development (Dorney & Black 2018). Prevention discussions prior to pregnancy may include uptake of vaccinations, use of folic acid and iodine supplementation, maintenance of healthy weight, nutrition and exercise, assessment of psychosocial health and cessation of tobacco, alcohol, illegal drugs and over-the-counter medications. Notably, fetal alcohol spectrum disorder (FASD), caused by maternal alcohol use, is a preventable condition resulting in lifelong developmental and behavioural conditions (Hartz 2018). The importance of healthy environments, particularly avoidance of TORCH infections, needs to be promoted (Royal Australian College of General Practitioners [RACGP] 2018):

- Toxoplasmosis
- Other, such as syphilis, varicella and mumps and listeriosis
- Rubella
- Cytomegalovirus
- Herpes simplex.

Community health nurses and other health practitioners have an important role in developing primary health care approaches to preconception care in partnership with families. These strategies need to recognise SDH that impact on health inequities, health literacy and clients' readiness for lifestyle changes.

Where to find out more on ...

Preconception care: Maximising the gains for maternal and child health

• www.who.int/maternal_child_adolescent/ documents/preconception_care_policy_ brief.pdf?ua=1

Antenatal care by a community health practitioner from the earliest stages of pregnancy can help pregnant women and their partners identify the need for lifestyle changes and ways of sustaining those changes throughout the pregnancy and beyond the birth of the child. It also provides an opportunity to help parents create the emotional foundations for the child's life; one of the most important elements of early parenting. High levels of stress and anxiety in the mother can cause epigenetic influences on the function of the fetal–placental unit, compromising fetal growth and causing a risk of preterm birth or low birth weight. Further potential developmental difficulties in the antenatal period include fetal arousal and physiological changes which are suspected to delay maturation of fetal neurological development, in addition to structural brain changes with associated adverse effects on the development of the brain. These issues further affect postnatal growth and development of children through infant temperament difficulties and compromised physical, emotional and behavioural development (Shonkoff et al 2021). There are also adverse impacts on the quality of parenting as antenatal stress is a strong predictor of postnatal anxiety and depression and reduced maternal attachment to their children. Knowledge of this early neurological development of the fetus, along with our understanding of the effects of stress on neural development during the critical periods, underlines the importance of community health practitioners working in partnership with women and their partners to develop health-promoting activities that are meaningful, realistic and culturally appropriate for their individual circumstances (Munns 2021, Shonkoff et al 2021).

KEY POINT

Antenatal care provides an opportunity for parents to create the emotional foundations for a child's life and to initiate lifestyle changes.

Maternal attendance at regular antenatal care in the first trimester of pregnancy is associated with improved maternal health and fewer medical interventions later in the pregnancy, which support good child health and wellbeing outcomes. It is important for community health practitioners such as nurses and midwives to identify and engage with vulnerable women and their partners as they are less likely to present to antenatal services. Women living in low socioeconomic areas, Indigenous women and adolescents have particular issues with attendance (AIHW 2021a). We need to consider the SDH impacting on mother's abilities to obtain antenatal care and apply a primary health care approach when facilitating care, such as provision of culturally appropriate services which are accessible and affordable with gender-specific healthcare practitioners.

Where to find out more on ...

The Australian Nurse–Family Partnership Program

This program utilises the skills of home-visiting nurses and family partnership worker/Aboriginal community workers to work with Aboriginal families during pregnancy to 2 years of age (www.anfpp.com.au). This is an adapted program from the evidence-based Nurse–Family Partnership model developed by David Olds in the United States. See Chapter 10 for further discussion on the research into early nurse home-visiting programs.

Antenatal visits can act as a platform for planning and empowerment for parents through trusting relationships with health practitioners that will help women develop the skills for decision-making on birthing. Preparation includes gathering information about preferred place of birth and the choice of birth attendant or birth companion. A contemporary model of birthing care is midwife-led continuity of care, where a known and trusted midwife or small group of known midwives provide stable antenatal, intrapartum and postnatal services. This is the most common type of maternity care in New Zealand. Health promotion activities such as promotion of breastfeeding and safe sleeping for babies can also be undertaken (Red Nose 2021, Starship Foundation 2019, WHO 2018). The challenge for community health nurses, midwives and social support practitioners is to support parents, their families and communities in the antenatal period in order to establish safe physical and psychosocial environments for a healthy start to life and lifelong health trajectories.

RESILIENCE AND CRITICAL PATHWAYS TO CHILD HEALTH

From all the research into early parenting and development, we know that the health of children reflects: the social determinants that impact on their world; the national policy environment that encourages or discourages the expression of their culture; their genetic make-up, and that of their parents; their ability to access early, high-quality education; the family's socioeconomic status, including their place of residence; their access to and preferences for health services; family harmony, the extent to which healthy behaviours are modelled in the family and community; and features of the physical environment. There are three critical pathways that summarise steps towards achieving health for children.

KEY POINT

Critical step 1 towards healthy children: the health and wellbeing of women.

The first critical step on the pathway to healthy children is to focus on the health and wellbeing of women and this begins with educating women throughout the world. Women's education and empowerment have significant effects on their socioeconomic capability, and that of their children and communities. Equally important is their ability to be involved in decisions benefiting themselves and their families, which has links with recognising gender equality and prevention of gender-based violence (Mundkur et al 2020).

KEY POINT

Critical step 2 towards healthy children: linking child, family and community to build resilience.

A second critical pathway overlaps the first, in that health promotion activities should reorientate health services to empower families and communities, thereby encouraging self-help and social support to enhance resilience (WHO 2021b). A socio-ecological view of child health includes attention to the characteristics of the child, family and community, ensuring adaptation to challenges and development of resilience is supported by positive relationships such as close caregiver attachment and effective parenting with emotional security and sensitive caregiving (Masten & Barnes 2018). An interesting resource to help develop resilience is 'The Worry Book' (van der Hart & Waller 2011), where children, adolescents and adults are encouraged to reflect on their processes of worrying, removing the focus from their actual problems.

Children also need to be seen from very early in life as learners. Their learning and development in the early years is integral to their wellbeing, from play in the family, to childcare, preschool and beyond. Developmentally appropriate learning is important for children not only for their educational attainment, but also to facilitate social skills such as interpersonal communication and positive self-esteem (AIHW 2020a). Supporting early, high-quality childcare and education are therefore important policy initiatives.

KEY POINT

Critical step 3 towards healthy children: early childhood education, high-quality childcare.

Good-quality early childhood education is one of the most important government policy initiatives in relation to child development, education and productivity. It has universal positive impacts on all children, with the benefits including higher levels of workforce participation by parents and carers and improved literacy and numeracy for children, leading to higher educational achievement across all schooling. There is also a range of social benefits that includes less contact by children, adolescents and adults with the justice system and reductions in the rates of adverse smoking and obesity and associated healthcare costs (PricewaterhouseCoopers 2019).

Overall, the goals for child health are to address the major health issues for their wellbeing in today's society, including adequate societal investment in the early years, supportive communities that protect and enable child and family health, health literacy for parents and their children and continuing evolution of the evidence base for child and family health. The most optimal circumstance for a healthy child is to be born into a child-friendly, healthy and safe family and community. To support parents in this endeavour, community health nurses need to assist families in key developmental areas with activities such as:

- maintaining culturally appropriate support for parents, children and their communities (AIHW 2021b), with particular reference to Australian Aboriginal and New Zealand Māori families
- encouraging exclusive breastfeeding for 6 months within their circumstances and environment (WHO 2021c)
- promoting safe, stable physical and psychosocial development (CDC 2020b)
- promoting developmentally appropriate strategies for infant sleeping (New Zealand Ministry of Health [NZMOH] 2021a)
- prevention of injuries and accidents (Kidsafe WA 2021)
- promotion of up-to-date immunisation for children, parents and caregivers (CDC 2019)
- promoting food security, particularly for vulnerable population groups (United Nations 2021).

To achieve positive child health in any community, all known risk factors and factors that develop children's resilience and capacity to cope with their environments must be acknowledged and incorporated into a community's goals and targets for prevention, protection and health promotion. Resilience is centred on complex interrelationships between risk (adversity) and protective factors. Adverse physical and psychosocial environments can lead to harmful outcomes such as substance abuse. However, supportive relationships for children from family, schools, relatives, friends and community have been shown to reduce the impact of negative influences. International research has identified six policy areas to moderate barriers to risk factors impacting on healthy child development and wellbeing, and to enhance protective factors through opportunities and resources, thereby fostering the development of resilience:

- empowering vulnerable families
- policies strengthening children's emotional and social skills
- child protection policies
- policies improving educational outcomes
- policies improving health outcomes
- policies reducing children's poverty and material deprivation (OECD 2019, p. 12).

Developmentally appropriate literature for children and youth is available to help them address concerns and worries that may be so concerning they lead to poor resilience, with online strategies to help engage as primary health care prevention or secondary early intervention support.

Where to find out more on ...

An information booklet for children and youth to support their mental health and wellbeing:

- https://enliven.org.au/wp-content/uploads/2020/06/GP-Practice_Booklet_mental_health_FINAL.pdf

Contacts and websites to engage and support children and youth:

- www.beyondblue.org.au/who-does-it-affect/young-people/helpful-contacts-and-websites

Information for children and young people:

- www.ccyp.wa.gov.au/info-for-children-and-young-people/

BOX 7.4

PRACTICE PROFILE: SCHOOL NURSE

Hi. My name is Alison and I am a community health nurse working in the high school setting.

What the role entails:

The role is based on a comprehensive social model of care. This role includes traditional aspects of general nursing care including: basic emergency care to ill and injured students; direct hands-on care to students and staff for subacute minor conditions; immunisation; health screening for vision, hearing and weight; and the management of chronic health conditions. High school nurses spend a large amount of time with students, teachers and parents to address student mental health problems. Seventy five per cent of the day usually involves assessment and care for adolescents who seek help for physiological and psychosocial reasons. The students may present with a somatic complaint related to mental health problems that include anxiety and depression. During a typical day, I will provide information and support to students in the classroom and on a one-on-one basis on topics such as sexual health, healthy eating, smoking prevention and cessation and the prevention of sexually transmitted infections. I will also provide information to the parents and teachers on topics including adolescent development, asthma, medication and anaphylaxis management, infectious diseases, immunisations and asthma. I work within the health-promoting school framework and this involves working with internal and external allied health providers.

How I came to be in the role:

I have a genuine interest in adolescent development and wanted to work in a challenging position where I could make a difference. I completed a Graduate Diploma in Community Health and following this I undertook further qualifications in school health. In the beginning I worked in district schools assessing primary school children. Following this, I accepted the challenge to develop further skills and knowledge about adolescent development.

What I find most interesting about the role:

The role is complex and interesting because each student and family's needs are different. I find it most rewarding to support adolescents who seek help and to promote adolescent mental health care.

Advice for anyone wanting to become a high school nurse:

Enhance your skills and knowledge about adolescent development by undertaking tertiary studies in this specialty area. A good starting point is to undertake a graduate certificate in community health, specialising in child and adolescent health. Be prepared to critically analyse situations and have well-developed communication skills that are required to assist with students, parents and teachers who present with sensitive problems. As this is a highly sought-after position and the process is fiercely competitive, undertake sound research on the application process and seek help through a mentor to achieve your goal to work in this area of specialty.

Partnerships between community health practitioners such as nurses and midwives enable a comprehensive primary health care approach to health and wellbeing strategies for families, children and youth (see Box 7.4). The periods of preconception, antenatal, postnatal and the early years are considered crucial times for engagement with families with significant opportunities available to develop relevant, empowering and sustainable support strategies with potential for current and lifelong affirmative outcomes.

CHILDREN IN CARE

Vulnerable children who are removed temporarily or permanently from their families of origin are entering care at a younger age. They are staying in their care arrangements for longer periods and are at risk of adverse developmental physical and psychosocial outcomes. Due to unique SDH, Aboriginal children in Australia have an over representation in care (AIHW 2019c, CAHS 2021, WADoC 2018).

All Australian states and territories have a legislated government child protection agency that has legal control for children in care and ensures each child has a care plan identifying their health and wellbeing needs. Community child and school health nurses are required to forward reports of assessment outcomes to the relevant agency and liaise with the child and carer, case managers and other support professionals when undertaking strategies relating to assessment outcomes (CAHS 2021). Communication, working in partnership and organisational abilities are important for nurses working with children in care.

In New Zealand, Māori children are similarly overrepresented in care with 69% of children aged 0 to 3 months in care identifying as Māori although Māori comprise only 16.5% of the population (Children's Commissioner 2020). Further, the inequity between Māori and non-Māori is increasing with decisions to remove Māori infants often made prior to birth (Children's Commissioner 2020).

OBESITY

As children grow, the compound effects of the SDH become more evident, and this is particularly concerning in relation to the global 'obesity epidemic' (Box 7.5). Overweight and obesity are influenced by SDH which can impact positively or provide challenges to individuals in Australia and New Zealand when addressing this major public health issue. Individual factors such as genetics and physiology, in addition to health inequalities and environmental and societal factors, contribute to the current high prevalence for children and their families. There is evidence of a social gradient effect, which means that children who are disadvantaged

---

BOX 7.5

WHY IS THERE AN OBESITY EPIDEMIC?

- Genetic predisposition
- Excess maternal weight gain
- Social disadvantage, poverty
- Poor nutrition (high salt, sugar diets)
- Poor oral health
- Fast food outlets in neighbourhoods
- Trend towards 'eating out'
- Unscheduled meal times
- Inadequate physical activity
- No parks, walkable/safe/playable spaces
- Poor parental role-modelling
- Education, knowledge, skills
- Too much 'screen time'
- Lack of school support

---

socially, economically and geographically are at increased risk of becoming overweight. There is an association between SDH such as food security, the built environment and residence in outer regional and rural areas (AIHW 2021c).

Obesity is as much a problem for Australian and New Zealand children as it is throughout the world, which is a concern given that obesity is a risk factor for heart disease, type 2 diabetes and some types of cancer (AIHW 2021c). In a 2019/20 survey in New Zealand, approximately 9.4% of children aged 2 to 14 years were classified as obese. Māori and Pacific children are also more likely to be obese than other New Zealanders, with Pacific children (29.1%) being twice as likely to be obese as Māori (13.2%) (NZMOH 2021b). In 2014/15, around 25% of Australian children aged five to 17 years were overweight or obese (ABS 2018).

Researchers and community health practitioners are collaborating to examine evidence-based management for overweight and obesity in children. Family-, child- and community-centred strategies include taxation on high-sugar food and beverages, regulation of food marketing campaigns and nutrition warning labels (Obesity Evidence

Hub 2021a,b,c). The role of the community child and school health nurse is paramount in health education, health promotion, growth monitoring, family assessment and referrals for children and their families. Working in partnership with parents enables them to understand their child's growth and development. Current recommendations are for nurses to focus on children's functions rather than discussing weight directly, as some parents may regard highlighting of weight issues as criticism of their parenting. Undertaking body mass index (BMI) assessment in child and school settings allows nurses to identify children with growth that is not within healthy parameters. Once assessments have been made to exclude growth faltering, supportive positive lifestyle changes can be made with a focus on healthy nutritional and exercise behaviours for the whole family (CAHS 2018).

Where to find out more on ...

Australia's physical activity and exercise guidelines:

- www.health.gov.au/health-topics/physical-activity-and-exercise/physical-activity-and-exercise-guidelines-for-all-australians?utm_source=health.gov.au&utm_medium=callout-auto-custom&utm_campaign=digital_transformation

New Zealand's physical activity guidelines:

- www.health.govt.nz/our-work/preventative-health-wellness/physical-activity

It is tempting to blame parents for child overweight and obesity problems, but there is a web of social and environmental factors that have created obesogenic environments, many of which affect parents, children and communities. Therefore, solutions have to be aimed at the broader circumstances that create unhealthy lifestyles for the entire family and communities.

CHILD POVERTY

The health of the world's children is of concern to everyone who claims global citizenship. Most children in the world are cared for and loved, but many other children and their families suffer from poverty. Those living in impoverished circumstances with few resources to mitigate risks are most vulnerable to ill health (AIHW 2020b). Poverty is an adverse SDH affecting health inequities and acting as a stressor on brain development both antenatally and in the early years. As we have discussed, these epigenetic influences have long-term consequences to health and wellbeing. Child poverty is also associated with toxic stress, poor educational achievement and social exclusion, with immediate and long-term psychosocial outcomes such as unemployment, homelessness and a wide range of negative physical and psychological outcomes that restrict lifelong potential and capacity building (Shonkoff et al 2021).

In New Zealand and Australia, many children and their families are living in poverty, with Māori, Pacific peoples and Aboriginal and Torres Strait Islander people being overrepresented. In 2018/19, 14.9% of New Zealand children between 0 and 17 years were classified as living in poverty, with approximately 23% of Māori children and 28.6% of Pacific children affected (Statistics New Zealand 2021b, Child Poverty Action Group 2021). Australian statistics reflect an increase in child poverty from 16.4% in 2014 to 16.9% in 2017, which equates to one in six children. The effects of the COVID-19 pandemic have placed many more families and children at risk of falling below the poverty line (Davidson et al 2020).

Of note is public discourse related to family poverty. Health behaviours that are challenged by adverse SDH can be interpreted by others through the narratives of discrimination, which put forward ideas that poorer health and social outcomes relate to biology, family or individual weaknesses. This leads to an urgent imperative for community health nurses to promote interdisciplinary support for action to address health messaging and health literacy and promote equity policies and practice (Berentson-Shaw 2018). (See Fig 7.2.)

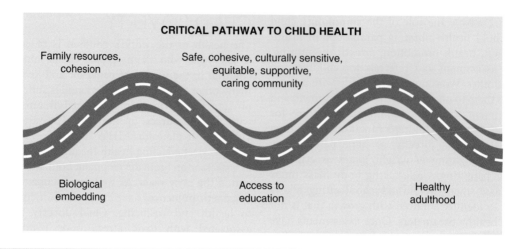

Figure 7.2 Critical pathway to child health and wellbeing

GOALS FOR HEALTHY CHILDREN

A partnership approach between community health practitioners and children, their families and communities is needed to achieve optimal and sustainable child health and wellbeing. A particular focus is on parental support to enhance their role in providing healthy physical, social and emotional environments for their children. Fetal development and the early years are windows of opportunity for cognitive, physical and social-emotional growth along with primary health care interventions that offer opportunities for positive development with lifelong benefits (Shonkoff et al 2021).

Conclusion

Reflecting back on Figure 7.1, we can see how children are nested within and influenced by protective factors from families, communities, public policies and global factors. A child's health depends on the combination of biology, family and the extended environments that provide opportunities to lead healthy, nurtured and well-nourished lifestyles with a minimum of stress. Community health practitioners, particularly child and school health nurses and midwives, can provide a base of expertise using primary health care principles to advocate against social and structural inequalities affecting the health and wellbeing of children, families and their communities. Understanding the impacts and interactions between families, communities, public policies and global factors allows nurses, midwives and other practitioners to guide opportunities for accessible and culturally appropriate support, particularly during periods of social disruption such as pandemics. Taking into account both enhancing and adverse SDH, they are able to undertake interdisciplinary approaches within their practice and work collaboratively with children, parents and communities to encourage health literacy and their participation in health decisions that will sustain lifelong wellbeing. We have split the following reflective and case study sections in two, focusing on families in the first section and children in the second.

Reflecting on the Big Issues for families

- Family life is multidimensional and consists of the family system, sibling subsystems and extended kinship networks.

- Family health and wellbeing is a product of individual and family interactions and the way family members interact with the external world, including the immediate community and society.

- The primary goal for empowering family members is to work in partnership with them to undertake collaborative planning to help them develop individual, family and community capacity and choices for family health and wellbeing.

- It is important for nurses and other health practitioners to be aware of family issues such as marital

separation, family violence, family caregiving, work–life issues and the intersection of gender, culture and family histories in causing family change.

- The environments within which families interact are influenced by SDH such as transport, housing, social support, pandemic disruptions and racism which impact on their ability to maintain their health and wellbeing. Urban, rural and remote families experience different levels of vulnerability.

- Nursing interventions should be based on research evidence as well as careful assessment of the family and the circumstances and events surrounding them.

CASE STUDY 7a

Family life for the Smiths and Masons

Returning to our families, we see that Rebecca and Huia attended child health clinics in their respective communities for their children's annual check-ups. As Rebecca outlined relatively minor child health issues, the nurse conducted an in-depth assessment of some of the special family issues facing the family—in particular those related to FIFO work, the father–child relationships, father role identity, the marital relationship, couples' counselling, the need for extended family support or appropriate substitute support systems. These are sensitive issues, so communication strategies were foremost in the nurse's approach when working with Rebecca.

Huia and Jason have both been able to attend their clinic appointment due to extended clinic hours for working

parents. The well child/Tamariki Ora nurse performing Jake's 4-year-old before-school check had some helpful suggestions for parenting strategies and the couple plans to implement some of these strategies, work together as a team and be consistent in their parenting.

In the mining community the occupational health nurse conducted a company-endorsed interactive family training session for all workers, where issues were addressed relating to housing, transportation, community support for transient families and mining management support for families.

Reflective questions: How would I use this knowledge in practice?

1 Prepare a genogram and ecomap of the Smith and Mason families.

2 What family goals would you establish for each family to ensure health and wellbeing for all family members?

3 How would you approach family assessment if you were conducting a home visit?

4 Would you alert the school nurse of any problems with the family? Why or why not?

5 What actions would you take if family violence was disclosed during the family interview with either of the mothers?

6 During the interactive sessions with the miners, how would you address family relationship issues and conflict resolution?

7 What resources would you use to ensure you had access to current research evidence for your actions?

Reflecting on the Big Issues for children

- The most important investment governments can make is in supporting child and family health.
- The SDH have a profound impact on the health and wellbeing of children and families.
- One of the most significant threats to child health is poverty.
- Healthy pregnancy and antenatal care establish a platform for good health and development in childhood.
- Exclusive breastfeeding for 6 months is the ideal for nourishing infants.
- Family lifestyle and parenting practices have a profound impact on child health.
- Community healthcare practice should be evidence based and connected to child and family outcomes.

CASE STUDY 7b

Child health for the Smith and Mason families

With Colin absent from the home so much, Rebecca is left to cope with the children's issues, especially Gemma's eczema, which she thinks may be linked to stress as well as an unknown allergy. She is also concerned about Emily's difficulties at school and hesitates to involve Colin too much in her approach to seeking help for her. The school nurse has been to see Rebecca about Emily to try to help her work out some behavioural strategies to help her.

In Pakakura Jake has been admitted to hospital again for an acute asthma attack, which has meant that Huia has had to take time off work and arrange for someone else to care for the other children as Jason is away. Huia's job is under threat because of her frequent absences due to Jake's asthma.

Reflective questions: How would I use this knowledge in practice?

1 What are the main priorities you would identify in a first home visit with Rebecca or Huia?

2 How would you assess the Smith and Mason household environments for risks and protective factors for their children?

3 How would your knowledge of Jason and Colin's employment and Huia's role as a teacher change your approach to assessing their needs and that of their children?

4 Which support services in Huia and Rebecca's home communities would be most likely to provide support for their needs and that of their family?

5 What are the most visible effects of the SDH on both families?

6 Explain how you would ensure that both families had sufficient health literacy for their parenting responsibilities.

7 Describe three aspects of their school or recreational setting that would be crucial to providing family support. For each, explain the importance of the setting in promoting child health and its link to primary health care principles.

References

Aristizabal, M.J., Anreiter, I., Halldorsdottir, T., et al, 2020. Biological embedding of experience: A primer on epigenetics, 117 (38), 23261–23269. https://doi.org/10.1073/pnas.1820838116.

Australian Bureau of Statistics (ABS), 2020. Labour force status of families. ABS, Canberra.

Australian Bureau of Statistics (ABS), 2018. National health survey: First results. ABS, Canberra.

Australian Institute of Health and Welfare (AIHW), 2018. Australia's health 2018. Australia's health series no. 16. AUS 221. AIHW, Canberra.

Australian Institute of Health and Welfare (AIHW), 2019a. Child protection Australia: 2017–18. Child welfare series no. 70. Cat. no. CWS 65. AIHW, Canberra.

Australian Institute of Health and Welfare (AIHW), 2019b. Rural and remote health. Cat. no. PHE 255. AIHW, Canberra.

Australian Institute of Health and Welfare (AIHW), 2019c. Child protection Australia 2017–18. AIHW, Canberra.

Australian Institute of Health and Welfare (AIHW), 2020a. Australia's children. Cat. no. CWS 69. AIHW, Canberra.

Australian Institute of Health and Welfare (AIHW), 2020b. Australia's health 2020. AIHW, Canberra.

Australian Institute of Health and Welfare (AIHW), 2021a. Australia's mothers and babies. AIHW, Canberra.

Australian Institute of Health and Welfare (AIHW), 2021b. Australia's welfare 2021. AIHW, Canberra.

Australian Institute of Health and Welfare (AIHW), 2021c. Inequalities in overweight and obesity and the social determinants of health. Cat. no. PHE 278. AIHW, Canberra.

Ayika, D., Dune, T., Firdaus, R., et al, 2018. A qualitative exploration of post migration family dynamics and intergenerational relationships. SAGE Open October-December, 1–10. Online. Available: http://doi.org/10.1177/2158244018811752.

Berentson-Shaw, J., 2018. Telling a new story about 'child poverty' in New Zealand. The Workshop and The Policy Observatory, Auckland.

Bouverie Centre, 2021. Help for families. Grow as a family and as individuals. La Trobe University, Brunswick. Online. Available: www.bouverie.org.au.

Brown, N., Jeon, Y-H., 2021. Partnering in care. In: Crisp, J., Douglas, C., Rebeiro, G., Waters, D. (Eds), Potter and Perry's fundamentals of nursing, sixth ed. Elsevier, Chatswood, pp. 84–97.

Boxall, H., Morgan, A., Brown, R., 2020. The prevalence of domestic violence among women during the COVID-19 pandemic. Statistical Bulletin no. 28. Australian Institute of Criminology, Canberra.

Bronfenbrenner, U., 1986. Ecology of the family as a context for human development: Research perspectives. Dev. Psychol., 22 (6), 723–742.

Center on the Developing Child, 2021a. Serve and return. Harvard University, Cambridge, MA.

Center on the Developing Child, 2021b. Toxic stress. Harvard University, Cambridge, MA.

Centers for Disease Control and Prevention (CDC), 2019. Pregnancy and vaccination. US Department of Health & Human Services, Atlanta.

Centers for Disease Control and Prevention (CDC), 2020a. What is epigenetics? US Department of Health & Human Services, Atlanta.

Centers for Disease Control and Prevention (CDC), 2020b. Preventing adverse childhood experiences. US Department of Health & Human Services, Atlanta.

Center for Family Systems Theory of Western New York, Inc., 2021. History of family systems theory. Author, Buffalo.

Centre for Transformative Work Design, 2018. Impact of FIFO work arrangements on the mental health and wellbeing of FIFO workers. Western Australia Mental Health Commission, Perth.

Child and Adolescent Health Service (CAHS), 2018. Community health clinical nursing manual: Guideline. Overweight and obesity. Government of Western Australia, Department of Health, Perth.

Child and Adolescent Health Service (CAHS), 2021. Children in care—conducting an assessment. Government of Western Australia, Department of Health, Perth.

Child Poverty Action Group, 2021. Latest child poverty figures. Author, Auckland.

Children's Commissioner, 2020. Statistical snapshot: Pēpi Māori 0–3 months and the care and protection system (January issue). Online. Available: www.occ.org.nz/assets/Uploads/20200116-OCC-StatisticalSnapshot.pdf.

Coles, L., Hewitt, B., Martin, B., 2018. Contemporary fatherhood: Social, demographic and attitudinal factors associated with involved fathering and long work hours. J. Sociol., 54 (4), 591–609.

Coulter, M.L., Mercado-Crespo, M.C., 2015. Co-occurrence of intimate partner violence and child maltreatment: Service providers' perceptions. J. Fam. Viol., 30, 255–262.

Davidson, P., Bradbury, B., Wong, M., 2020. Poverty in Australia 2020: Part 2, Who is affected? ACOSS/UNSW Poverty and Inequality Partnership Report No. 4. ACOSS, Sydney.

Desmyth, K., Eagar, S., Jones, M., et al, 2021. Refugee health nursing. J. Adv. Nurs., 77 (10), e30–e32. Online. Available: https://doi.org/10.1111/jan.14910.

Dorney, E., Black, K.I., 2018. Preconception care. Aust. J. Gen. Pract., 47 (7), 424–429. Online. Available: http://doi.org/10.31128/AJGP-02-18-4485.

Ee, N., Maccora, J., Hosking, D., et al, 2020. Australian grandparents care. National Seniors, Canberra.

El-Murr, A., 2018. Intimate partner violence in Australian refugee communities. Scoping review of issues and service responses. CFCA paper no. 50. Child Family Community Australia, Southbank.

Friedman, M.M., Bowden, V.R., Jones, E.G., 2003. Family nursing: Research, theory & practice. Prentice Hall, Upper Saddle River.

Fry, R., Passel, J.S., Cohn, D., 2021. A majority of young adults in the US live with their parents for the first time since the Great Depression. Pew Research Center, Washington, DC.

Gardner, B., Alfrey, K-L., Vandelanotte, C., et al, 2018. Mental health and wellbeing concerns of fly-in fly-out workers and their partners in Australia: A qualitative study. BMJ Open, 8, e019516. Online. Available: http://doi.org/10.1136/bmjopen-2017-019516.

Guzys, D., 2021. Rural health nursing. In: Guzys, D., Brown, R., Halcomb, E., Whitehead, D. (Eds), An introduction to community and primary health care, third ed. Cambridge University Press, United Kingdom, pp. 253–263.

Hartz, D., 2018. Indigenous child health. In: Guzys, D., Brown, R., Halcomb, E., Whitehead, D. (Eds), An introduction to community and primary health care, third ed. Cambridge University Press, United Kingdom, pp. 212–230.

Kidsafe Western Australia, 2021. Kidsafe WA. Author, West Leederville.

Kitchen, D.P., 2016. Structural functional theory. The Wiley Blackwell Encyclopedia of Family Studies (Online). Online. Available: http://doi.org/10.1002/9781119085621.wbefs273.

Masten, A.S., Barnes, A.J., 2018. Resilience in children: Developmental perspectives. Children, 5 (7), 1–16. Online. Available: http://doi.org/10.3390/children5070098.

McEwen, B.S., 2000. Allostasis and allostatic load: Implications for neuropsychopharmacology. Neuropsychopharmacology, 22, 108 –124.

McEwen, B.S., Akil, H., 2020. Revisiting the stress concept: Implications for affective disorders. J. Neurosci., 40 (1), 12–21.

Moore, T.G., 2021. Core care conditions for children and families: Implications for integrated child and family services. Prepared for Social Ventures Australia. Parkville, Victoria: Centre for Community Child Health, Murdoch Children's Research Institute, The Royal Children's Hospital, Melbourne. Online. Available: https://doi.org/10.25374/MCRI.14593878.

Mundkur, A., Nguyen, L., Fitzgerald, I., et al, 2020. Working paper. Linking women's economic empowerment, eliminating gender-based violence and enabling sexual and reproductive health and rights. UNFPA & Care, Thailand & Australia.

Munns, A., 2021. Community midwifery: A primary health care approach to Aboriginal antenatal care. Aust. J. Prim. Health, 27, 57–61. Online. Available: https://doi.org/10.1071/PY20105.

National Rural Health Alliance (NRHA), 2021. Mental health in rural and remote Australia. Fact sheet. NRHA, Canberra.

New Zealand Government, 2019. Te Ara. The Encyclopedia of New Zealand. Tribal organisation. Manatū´ Taonga Ministry of Culture and Heritage, Wellington.

New Zealand Ministry for Women (NZMFW), 2021. What is violence against women? NZMFW, Wellington.

New Zealand Ministry of Health (NZMOH), 2021a. Safe sleep. NZMOH, Wellington.

New Zealand Ministry of Health (NZMOH), 2021b. Obesity statistics. NZMOH, Wellington.

Obesity Evidence Hub, 2021a. Case for a tax on sugar-sweetened beverages (SSBs) in Australia. Cancer Council, Victoria.

Obesity Evidence Hub, 2021b. Marketing unhealthy food and drinks to children: Global framework. Cancer Council, Victoria.

Obesity Evidence Hub, 2021c. Next prevention: Nutrient warning labels. Cancer Council, Victoria.

OECD, 2019. Changing the odds for vulnerable children: Building opportunities and resilience, OECD Publishing, Paris. Online. Available: https://doi.org/10.1787/a2e8796c-en.

On the Line, 2021. Types of domestic and family violence. On the Line, Footscray.

Orenstein, G.A., Lewis, L., 2020. Erikson's stages of psychosocial development. Stat Pearls Publishing, Treasure Island.

Perales, F., Reeves, L.S., Plage, S., et al, 2020. The family lives of Australian lesbian, gay and bisexual people: A review of the literature and a research agenda. Sex. Res. Social Policy, 17, 43–60. Online. Available: https://doi.org/10.1007/s13178-018-0367-4.

PricewaterhouseCoopers, 2019. A smart investment for a smarter Australia: Economic analysis of universal early childhood education in the year before school in Australia. PWC, Sydney.

Qu, L., 2021. Households and families. Australian Institute of Family Studies, Melbourne.

Rago, M., 2016. Family development theory. The Wiley Blackwell Encyclopedia of Family Studies. Online. Available: http://doi.org/10.1002/9781119085621.wbefs359.

Raising Children Network (RCN), 2022. Being a grandparent carer. Raising Children Network (Australia) Limited, Melbourne.

Royal Australian College of General Practitioners (RACGP), 2018. Guidelines for preventive activities in general practice, ninth ed., updated. RACGP, East Melbourne.

Red Nose, 2021. Safe sleeping. Author, Docklands.

Shajani, Z., Snell, D., 2019. Wright and Leahey's nurses and families: A guide to family assessment and intervention, seventh ed. F.A. Davis, Philadelphia.

Shonkoff, J.D., Slopen, N., Williams, D.R., 2021. Early childhood adversity, toxic stress and the impacts of racism on the foundations of health. Annu. Rev. Public Health, 42, 115–134.

Starship Foundation, 2019. Infant safe sleeping in Starship. Starship Foundation, Auckland.

Statistics New Zealand, 2021a. Family. New Zealand Government, Wellington.

Statistics New Zealand, 2021b. Child poverty statistics: Year ended June 2020—corrected. New Zealand Government, Wellington.

Taylor, J., O'Hara, L., Talbot, L., et al, 2021. Promoting health. The primary health care approach, sixth ed. Elsevier, Chatswood.

United Nations, 2021. Global issues. Food. UN, Geneva.

van der Hart, W., Waller, R., 2011. The worry book. InterVarsity Press (IVP), Illinois.

Ward R., 2018. Cultural understandings of Aboriginal suicide from a social and emotional wellbeing perspective. In: Best, O., Fredericks, B. (Eds) Yatdjuligin. Aboriginal and Torres Strait Islander nursing and midwifery care, second ed. Cambridge, Port Melbourne, pp. 192–211.

Western Australia Department of Communities (WADoC), 2018. Annual Report 2017–18. WADoC, Perth.

Whelan, E., O'Shea, J., Hunt, E., et al, 2021. Evaluating measures of allostatic load in adolescents: A systematic review. Psychoneuroendocrinology, 131 (105324), 1–9. Online. Available: https://doi.org/10.1016/j.psyneuen.2021.105324.

Wilkins, R., Botha, F., Vera-Toscano, E., Wooden, M., 2020. The Household, Income and Labour Dynamics in Australia Survey: Selected findings from Waves 1 to 18. Melbourne Institute of Applied Economic and Social Research, University of Melbourne, Melbourne.

World Health Organization (WHO), 2018. WHO recommendations on antenatal care for a positive pregnancy experience: Summary. WHO, Geneva.

World Health Organization (WHO), 2021a. Violence against children. WHO, Geneva.

World Health Organization (WHO), 2021b. Health promotion. WHO, Geneva.

World Health Organization (WHO), 2021c. Breastfeeding. WHO, Geneva.

Wright, L.M., Leahey, M., 2013. Nurses and families: A guide to family assessment and intervention, sixth ed. F.A. Davis, Philadelphia, PA.

Yorgum Healing Services, 2021. Link up. Author, East Perth. Online. Available: https://yorgum.org.au/services/#stolen-generations.

Younas A., 2020. Relational inquiry approach for developing deeper awareness of patient suffering. Nurs. Ethics, 27 (4), 935–945. Online. Available: https://doi.org/10.1177/0969733020912523.

Youngson, N., Saxton, M., Jaffe, P.G., et al, 2021. Challenges in risk assessment with rural domestic violence victims: Implications for practice. J. Fam. Violence, 36, 537–550. Online. Available: https://doi.org/10.1007/s10896-021-00248-7.

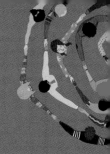

Transitions to adulthood and beyond

Introduction

Life comprises a series of transitions from before birth through to death. Many people manage these transitions with ease, using each phase of life as a building block to the next. But for some people, each phase presents challenges that at times may seem insurmountable. Supporting people to manage these transitions through life in a way that promotes health and wellbeing, achieves equity and builds and sustains resilience is an important role for the health practitioner. In Chapter 7 we examined the importance of primary health care practice with children and families in the early years and in Chapter 8 we expand this to explore the experiences of adolescents, adults and older adults as they transition through life. During adolescence, social determinants outside the family home become a greater influence on health and wellbeing than in childhood. Peers, media, education and early workplace experiences become prominent. As the individual transitions from adolescence to adulthood and on to older adulthood, community and structural determinants continue to remain influential, employment becomes a major influence in adulthood, with family growing in importance as one ages (Patton et al 2017). Figure 8.1 captures the changing proximal social determinants of health across the life course and provides the basis for exploring these life transitions throughout the chapter. This developmental approach enables us to consider the importance of promoting health and wellness at each stage along the life course from before birth to death. It is important to be mindful that although development is generally linear, biological, social and cultural factors such as intergenerational relationships will influence individual and family

OBJECTIVES

By the end of this chapter you will be able to:

1 identify the main factors contributing to healthy adolescence

2 explain the primary influences on health and wellness in adulthood

3 discuss the critical pathways to healthy ageing

4 explore the role of technology in supporting transitions across the life course

5 using a primary health care and social determinants framework, develop community goals and strategies for sustaining adolescent, adult and older adult health and wellbeing within a range of family structures.

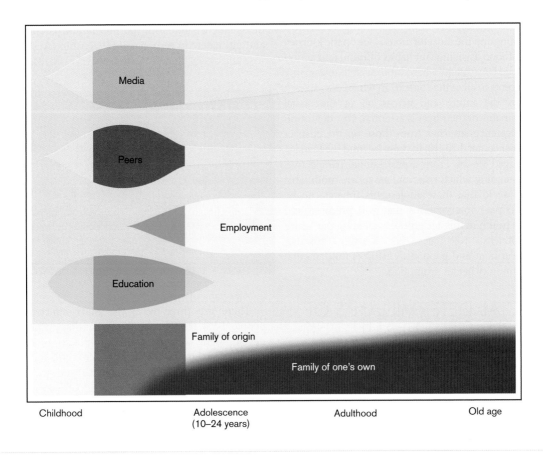

Figure 8.1 Changing proximal social determinants of health across the life course

Source: Patton, G.C. et al, 2017. Our future: A Lancet commission on adolescent health and wellbeing. The Lancet, 387 (10036).

pathways through life. We have avoided a focus on the specifics surrounding health status of each group but provide pointers for where you can access the most up-to-date information on this for each population group. Throughout the chapter we outline some of the fundamental principles of working across the life course.

Part 1: Healthy adolescence

CONTEXT

Adolescents—that is, young people in their teenage years—play a vital role in community life, contributing energy and vibrancy to the population through the spirit of youth and a promise for the future. In most cases, adolescents are in good health and their health and wellbeing is focused on school and the developmental tasks and transitions of adolescence. Although decisions made during adolescence can also affect our wellbeing in the long term (Weiss & Ferrand 2019), it is the social sphere within which adolescents interact that is predominant. It is the pivot around which their lives and their identity revolves. Although the adolescent journey is sometimes described as fraught with confusion, conflict and risk, an alternative view sees adolescents 'at promise' instead of 'at risk', and we address the pathway from risk to promise and, ultimately, to resilience. Adolescence is the most dramatic, the most interesting and the most tortuous stage on the journey to adulthood as significant habits of mind and action are formed. A strengths-based approach to supporting adolescents in all of the contexts in which they stretch towards the future and across all of the social determinants of their lives is essential. Our definition of adolescence stretches from those on the cusp of adolescence, aged 10–13, to those beyond the teenage years, aged 19–24. From a professional perspective, understanding which risks and assets are modifiable in the world that these adolescents inhabit can be used to plan interventions that will promote and sustain health in this age group. Evaluating the health practitioner's role in the journey towards empowerment and good citizenship is fundamental to community health promotion.

SOCIAL DETERMINANTS OF ADOLESCENT HEALTH, RISK-TAKING, RESILIENCE AND DECISION-MAKING

The social ecology of adolescent development can be seen as a matrix of interrelated factors that influence adolescents' health and wellbeing. As with other population groups, the social determinants of their lives present strengths, weaknesses, opportunities and threats. The main strength of adolescents is that most tend to be physically well. The weaknesses or risks inherent in adolescent life generally revolve around the fact that, because they are in the formative stages of development, most adolescents are not yet able to take control of their lives or health-related decisions. But the strongest determinants of adolescent health are not these individual factors, but the structural determinants that provide them with education, employment and the equitable living conditions that will allow them to develop their full potential in adult life (Azzopardi et al 2019). To provide a capacity-building transition to adulthood, opportunities to participate in education and the workforce must also be accompanied by safe and supportive families, schools, peers and communities. These are the structural conditions within which young people are exposed to strengths or compromises to health during transitions through school, from education to work, from family dependence to

independence, autonomy, partnering and parenthood, and ultimately to responsible citizenship (Australian Institute of Health and Welfare [AIHW] 2018).

KEY POINT

Adolescent transitions include:
- primary to secondary school to higher education
- education to workforce
- family to self-responsibility for health
- family living to autonomy, partnering, parenthood
- growing towards responsible citizenship.

There are three ways the SDH affect young people. First, the 'latent effects' that determine early development occur when a child's biological mechanisms are preset in utero. Second, there are experiences that determine health and wellbeing over the life trajectory, called the 'pathway effects'. Third, there are 'cumulative effects' from the advantages or disadvantages that a person experiences from exposure to unfavourable environments over time (Raphael 2019). Years ago the prevailing view was that the young brain was fully developed in childhood, yet research evidence now shows that the brain architecture of both children and adolescents is malleable, and social, emotional and neural development takes place until the early twenties (Yahfoufi et al 2020). Understanding this second 'sensitive period' in a young person's development has important implications for health promotion, in that some of the negative effects of structural factors in the early years, such as poverty, unemployment, racism, poor housing, cultural or gender-based inequities or anti-social behaviours at school, can be modified in adolescence, predominantly by strong family and community support including well-designed health interventions in schools (Bundy et al 2018, Dahl et al 2018, DeMichelis 2016, World Health Organization & UNICEF 2021). As health professionals, this leads us to renewed optimism for the success of family- and school-based interventions that will help young people navigate their transitions successfully. School-based nurses have a particularly important role to play in advocating to address inequities and improving access to healthcare for young people (Jones et al 2021).

Contemporary health promotion strategies are also informed by understanding the distinctions between early, middle and late adolescence. Early adolescence involves entering puberty, beginning the process of sexual maturation and shifting focus from family to friends. Early adolescents (age 13–14) ask 'Am I normal?' Middle adolescence sees physical development continue, with increasing reliance on friends and peer groups. This stage is accompanied by the risk of adopting peer-influenced behaviours such as experimenting with drugs and alcohol. Middle adolescents (15–16) ask, 'Who am I?' In late adolescence, physical changes have levelled off and cognitive development continues, with adult thinking becoming closer to maturity (Patton et al 2017). Late adolescents (age 17–18) ask, 'What is my place in the world?' Understanding the subtle differences between the various stages helps frame adult interactions with adolescents in slightly different ways.

KEY POINT

Stages of adolescence

- Early—puberty, sexual maturation, friendships
- Middle—physical development, reliance on friends, peer groups
- Late—cognitive development, adult thinking

Adolescence has traditionally been a period characterised by risk-taking behaviours (including alcohol and drug use, unprotected sex, smoking and taking part in extreme activities), as young people explore and push their boundaries and seek to understand their place in society. Box 8.1 lists some of the risks and challenges facing young people in Australia and New Zealand. But these activities are subscribed to by adults at least as frequently and in some cases more frequently than adolescents (Kloep et al 2016). By characterising adolescents as 'at risk'

BOX 8.1

RISKS AND CHALLENGES FACING YOUNG PEOPLE

- Alcohol use
- Substance use
- Mental health issues
- Suicide
- Smoking
- Unprotected sex
- Bullying including cyber-bullying
- Overweight and obesity
- Lack of exercise
- Poor nutrition
- Eating disorders
- Injuries

---

and spending substantial resources on finding out why adolescents may engage in risky behaviours, we paint a highly negative picture of adolescents and potentially lose the opportunity to investigate why people of any age take risks, and understand the potential of young people (Kloep et al 2016). By understanding the potential of young people and what makes them resilient, we can then develop strategies that will help support young people as they transition to adulthood.

In this book, we draw on Masten and Barnes' (2018, p. 2) definition of resilience which they broadly define as the capacity of a system (including individuals, families, economies, ecosystems and organisations) to adapt successfully to challenges that may threaten the function, survival or future development of that system. Masten and Barnes' definition is intended to be scalable across system levels and across disciplines. This definition of resilience fits with our socio-ecological approach to community health that draws on the interactions between individuals, families, communities, society and the global environment to achieve wellness. During adolescence, when a myriad of developmental challenges take place, a young person must successfully adapt to these or be at risk of a range of psychopathologies (Zinn et al 2020). Of great interest to researchers is how young people who face significant early life adversity still manage to experience positive outcomes. Factors such as a positive relationship with a competent adult, having good learning and problem-solving skills, having positive relationships with peers and family, having self-efficacy and positive self-identity including an understanding of one's 'prospective' or future self, coping skills, engagement in a well-functioning school, connections with well-functioning communities and areas of identified competence all contribute to resilience in young people (Masten & Barnes 2018, Zinn et al 2020). We can support this development of resilience, and strengthen young people's coping mechanisms, by helping them to build strong interpersonal, cultural, institutional, social and political relationships (DeMichelis 2016). Strong, positive relationships and role models will help guide young people to find their place in society and assist them in identifying and managing risks and challenges to their health and wellbeing (Patton et al 2017).

Where to find out more on ...

Adolescent health

- Adolescent health status in New Zealand: www.youth19.ac.nz
- The latest statistics on youth health in Australia: www.aihw.gov.au/reports/australias-health/health-of-young-people
- Global information on youth health: www.who.int/topics/adolescent_health/en/ and www.geastudy.org/
- The Global Strategy for Women's, Children's and Adolescents' Health 2016–2030: www.who.int/life-course/partners/global-strategy/globalstrategyreport2016-2030-lowres.pdf?ua=1&ua=1
- Training courses for health professionals working with young people (including free online courses): www.wharaurau.org.nz
- Resources for health professionals and young people: www.rch.org.au/cah

ASSESSING THE NEEDS OF YOUNG PEOPLE

The major health goals for adolescents include mental and emotional health and maturity, good physical health and safety, academic engagement, minimisation of conditions that create risks to health and wellbeing, sustainable lifestyle habits in healthy environments, adolescent-appropriate nursing and health services, creating enabling environments and empowering structures and processes for successive generations. Addressing these goals can help adolescents move from risk to promise and all are embedded in the ecological framework outlined in Figure 8.2 (adapted from Blum et al 2012).

It is important to remember that in an ecological model, what happens to a child or adolescent at each developmental stage is influenced by what happened in each earlier stage, meaning that interventions should be different for different populations and determined by the differing types of risks and protective factors that have been present in the life of the child or adolescent (Tomlinson et al 2021). Work by Patton and colleagues (2017) shows a simplified version of the ecological model to capture more clearly how development across the lifespan from preconception to adulthood impacts on adolescent health needs, risks and problems, how actions are required to address these at the structural, community and health service levels and how these factors lead into adulthood and onto the next generation. (See Figure 8.3.) Box 8.2 describes examples of the types of life course interventions and policies that will help achieve the goals for adolescent health.

One of the most important things the health practitioner can do when working with adolescents is to develop the attitudes, knowledge and skills that foster engagement with young people while maintaining engagement and interaction with the family (Patton et al 2017). The single most important predictor of resilience in children and young people is access to at least one stable, caring and supportive relationship with an adult in their life (National Scientific Council on the Developing

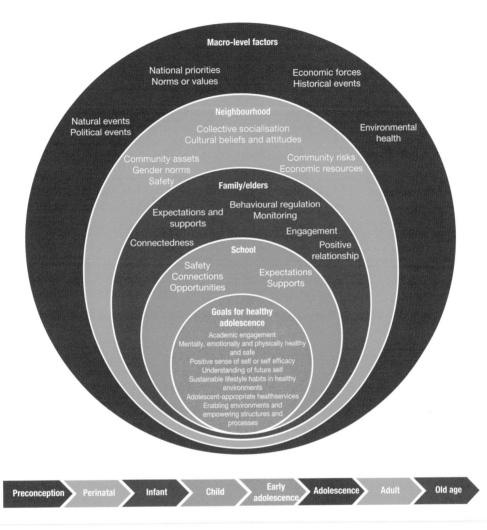

Figure 8.2 The ecological framework for adolescent health

Source: Reprinted with permission from Elsevier. Adapted from Blum, R. et al., 2012. Adolescent health in the 21st century. The Lancet, 379 (9826).

Child 2015). Health practitioners need to consider the ways they can work across sectors to support and enable young people to engage with their parents or caregivers, with their communities through partnership with adults, in training and mentorship, and in creating new structures and processes that facilitate young people's involvement in decision-making (Patton et al 2017, World Health Organization & UNICEF 2021). Digital media and technology provide exponential opportunities for engagement and service delivery that matches young people's needs and digital savvy. Young people not only use technology, they are dependent on it. It is up to us as health practitioners to identify and use these opportunities to develop new models of care based around these

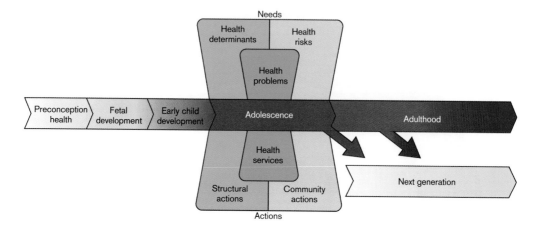

Figure 8.3 Conceptual framework for defining health needs and actions in adolescents and young adults

Source: Patton, G.C. et al, 2017. Our future: A Lancet commission on adolescent health and wellbeing. The Lancet, 387 (10036), 2431.

BOX 8.2

....

EXAMPLES OF LIFE COURSE INTERVENTIONS AND POLICIES THAT WILL HELP ACHIEVE GOALS FOR ADOLESCENT HEALTH

....

Biological and psychosocial interventions

- Antenatal, childbirth and postnatal care
- Nutrition
- Responsive care
- Vaccination
- Management of childhood illness
- Physical activity
- Adolescent-friendly sexual and reproductive health services
- Adolescent and caregiver mental health
- Care for developmental delays, disorders and disabilities
- Injury and suicide prevention

Supportive policies

- Minimum wage
- Universal healthcare
- Maternity protection
- Food safety and labelling

- Affordable childcare
- Universal access to education
- Sexual and reproductive rights
- Road safety regulations
- Tobacco and alcohol taxation and regulation
- Family-friendly workplace policies
- Social protection schemes

Supportive physical environment

- Clean water
- Adequate sanitation
- Clean air
- Clean energy
- Environments free from toxins
- Secure places for recreation
- Safe roads
- Smoke-free public places
- Child friendly urban design

Source: Adapted from Tomlinson, M., Hunt, X., Daelmans, B., Rollins, N., Ross, D., Oberklaid, F., 2021. Optimising child and adolescent health and development through an integrated ecological life course approach. BMJ (Online), 372, m4784. Online. Available: https://doi.org/10.1136/bmj.m4784.

technologies. Talking and working with young people in a way that enables us to co-design these new models will ensure we draw on their expertise of what they need as well as facilitate young people's need to build social capital through engagement with their communities, peers and health providers. Examples such as SPARX and SPARX-R (www.sparx.org.nz) that use online gaming and cognitive behavioural therapy to help adolescents experiencing mild to moderate depression show how effective this approach can be (Fleming, Stasiak, et al 2019, Malatest International 2016). Co-design is important though as the SPARX researchers found when they trialled the tool with young offenders. This group did not engage with the program in the way expected, highlighting that what may be effective in one setting and with one group of adolescents may not be as well received in a different setting (Fleming, Gillham, et al 2019).

Good assessment is the key to understanding young people and provides an opportunity to intervene where needed—particularly with young people who are engaged in risky behaviour or who may be experiencing mental health issues. For example, the risk of suicide among young people experiencing depression is high and it is important to recognise the warning signs of an impending suicide attempt. Box 8.3 ('Jessica's story') has a link to a video featuring a young Australian named 'Jessica', aged 19, and follows her non-fatal attempt to take her own life and the factors leading up to this. The video is an enactment but provides a realistic example of the experiences of young people that can lead to suicidal ideation and attempt. Pathways to self-harm are outlined in Figure 8.4. Lesbian, gay, bisexual, transgender/transsexual, queer, intersex, asexual, takatāpui, fa'afafine (LGBTQIA+) young people are at particular risk of bullying, verbal and physical abuse and challenges to their self-esteem due to their sexual orientation (Eisenberg et al 2019). For these reasons, particular attention must be paid to supporting young people who may identify as LGBTQIA+ or be questioning. We will explore this area further in Chapter 9.

Where to find out more on ...

Information and support for LGBTQIA+ and questioning young people

- Australia: https://minus18.org.au
- New Zealand (Rainbow Youth): www.ry.org.nz

Undertaking a HEEADSSS (Home, Education/Employment, Eating, Activities, Drugs and Alcohol, Sexuality, Suicide and Depression, Safety) assessment, whether digitally or face-to-face, is one of the first steps in working with young people (Ho et al 2019, Klein et al 2014, Smith & McGuinness 2017). Appendix C includes a copy of the HEEADSSS tool. The assessment gathers information on the most common influences on an adolescent's life at home, at school and in other social environments. The tool can help nurses and other health practitioners gain a multidimensional, yet individual, perspective of adolescent life. The assessment data can be used to foster closer engagement with their world, identify strengths, and ultimately, strategies to help protect and nurture them through uncharted pathways. Assessment can also be collaborative, aimed at helping inform a whole-of-community approach. Teachers, administrators, parents, community members and others can encourage constructive opportunities and validate the adolescent's ability for decision-making.

BOX 8.3

....

JESSICA'S STORY

....

Suicide—Jessica's story
www.youtube.com/watch?v=WdC3nhxA66U

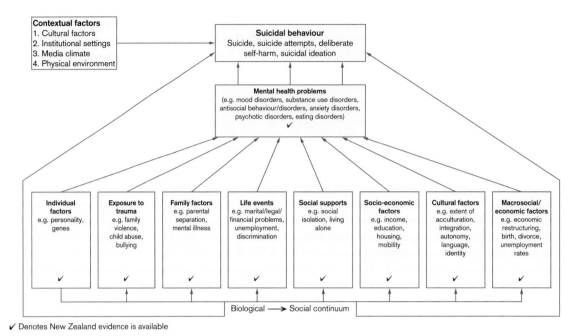

✔ Denotes New Zealand evidence is available

Figure 8.4 Pathways to self-harm

Source: Ministry of Health, 2015. Suicide Prevention Toolkit for District Health Boards (February issue). Ministry of Health, Wellington. Online. Available: www.health.govt.nz/system/files/documents/publications/suicide-prevention-toolkit-for-dhbs-feb15_3-v3.pdf.

Two of the most important environments influencing adolescent health are the school and social environment. Schools play a privileged and strategic role in the development of adolescent identity and competence and in helping young people make positive choices for healthy behaviours (Boen et al 2020, Bundy et al 2018, McCluskey 2015). School-based health services provide interventions designed specifically for young people, providing a safe, supportive and accessible environment for young people to seek help. With the right time, professional development, clinic access and support, school nurses can have substantial input into improving mental and physical health care for young people

and play an important role in public health advocacy to address equity and the social determinants of health (Jones et al 2021, McCluskey 2015). In particular, team-based school-based health services where school pastoral care staff and health professionals work together are associated with better mental health among students who use them (Denny et al 2019). Unfortunately, the variable distribution and role of school nurses in both Australia and New Zealand means some young people continue to miss out. Advocating for enhanced school and locality-based youth health services—particularly in rural, remote and socio-economically deprived areas—is an important role for all health practitioners.

Where to find out more on ...

Youth health and school services

- Information on youth health (New Zealand): www.youth19.ac.nz
- School health services (Western Australia): http://healthywa.wa.gov.au/Articles/S_T/School-health-services
- New Zealand school nurses: www.nzschoolnurses.org.nz
- National School Nursing Professional Practice Standards (Australia): http://anmf.org.au/pages/school-nursing-standards
- WHO's Helping adolescents thrive toolkit: www.who.int/publications/i/item/9789240025554

BOX 8.4

....

GOALS FOR ADOLESCENT HEALTH

....

The major health goals for adolescents include:

- mental and emotional health and maturity
- good physical health and safety
- academic engagement
- minimisation of conditions that create risks to health and wellbeing
- sustainable lifestyle habits in healthy environments
- adolescent-appropriate nursing and health services
- creating enabling environments and empowering structures and processes for successive generations.

Nurses and other health practitioners can support parents and caregivers by providing a bridge between home, school and the community. Although the primary community for most adolescents is the school, the family environment and family support behaviours are critical in helping adolescents through behaviour changes and identity formation, especially in relation to alcohol and substance use, sexual identity and coping with bullying (Bundy et al 2018, Patton et al 2017, World Health Organization & UNICEF 2021). Because many parents and caregivers do not have time to be closely engaged with the school or social environment, it is important that teachers, nurses and other health and support practitioners take advantage of every encounter, to assess how they are coping with parenting, to keep the channels of communication open and to maintain non-judgmental support and a positive attitude. This can be approached by communicating understanding of the complexity of adolescent issues, and of the importance of building family resilience and a strong sense of place. Resilient children and young people surrounded by resilient families have a greater chance of escaping social and economic disadvantage, lower risks of psychological problems as an adult and smoother transitions along the life course (Patton

et al 2017, United Nations 2016, Zinn et al 2020). Goals for adolescent health are found in Box 8.4.

Part 2: Healthy adulthood

CONTEXT

Adulthood is the time of a person's life when the intersecting influences of biology, the environment and lifestyle are most apparent. The years between age 20 to around 50 are concerned with finding one's place in the family, work environment and society, and reconciling the needs of various roles and expectations. By the time people have become adults, their innate predispositions combine with their past and current lifestyles and a variety of life circumstances to establish relatively stable patterns for the future. For most, the prospect for a long life free of the burden of illness and disability is good. However, other people achieve less than optimal health because of genetic predisposition, the social determinants of their childhood or current circumstances. Fortunately for most adults in

Australia and New Zealand, the environment provides considerable potential for overcoming vulnerability to ill health and achieving high levels of health and wellbeing. Unlike some other parts of the world, most people in this part of the world have access to nutritious food, clean air and water, good housing, education and employment possibilities, scientific and technological expertise, relatively low levels of community violence and accessible and appropriate healthcare and social support services.

Adult health and wellbeing also reflect the culmination of the policy environments that have circumscribed people's lives and constrained or facilitated their choices for health and lifestyles. These include a wide range of policies; for example, those governing taxes on alcohol or tobacco, or workplace policies permitting sick leave when workers are ill, or family leave when children need to be cared for. Besides these influences, health in adult life is also a product of family structure, ethnicity, education, employment and place of residence. How an individual has learned to cope with any of these influences, as well as historical illness, injury, disabling conditions or various stressors may be indicative of whether they are able to cope with unexpected events in adult life. Stress and coping are therefore central elements in sustaining health in adult life. Coping strategies also indicate how well an adult is able to continue on the pathway to older age.

The environments surrounding adult life are critical factors in determining their health. This is particularly evident in the effects of the social environment on health and quality of life. A growing body of research linking health to socioeconomic disparities, cultural and economic factors sets the stage for greater knowledge of adult health than was available in the past. Some aspects of the environment are a cause for urgent concern, with the health effects of climate change and other global changes having a major effect on the way we live our lives in the 21st century. Contemporary lifestyles are also influenced by new developments in research and technology. Unique programs of research are forging ahead in informing health promotion and disease treatments, particularly since the mapping of the human genome and the development of stem cell therapies to respond to errant genes and their expression in the human body. This 'translational' body of research knowledge is an important part of the toolkit for guiding adults towards better health.

Where to find out more on ...

Information on causes of death and disability in adulthood

- Australian Institute of Health and Welfare: www.aihw.gov.au/reports-data/health-conditions-disability-deaths
- New Zealand Ministry of Health: www.health.govt.nz/nz-health-statistics/health-statistics-and-data-sets/health-new-zealanders-data-and-stats

Priorities for health interventions are based on data indicating the major causes of morbidity and mortality. Long-term or chronic conditions such as type 2 diabetes or cardiovascular disease are the most urgent concern for Australian and New Zealand adults. The global picture of health is similar and shows that chronic diseases are now the most significant cause of mortality worldwide, causing 70% of deaths (World Health Organization [WHO] 2020d). Many of these are linked to modifiable lifestyle factors such as exercise and nutrition. Addressing risk factors for chronic disease such as smoking, inactivity, obesity and overweight, and poor diet are an important focus for health practitioners.

For people who are obese or who have been diagnosed with chronic illnesses, nutrition counselling is often a first step in making lifestyle improvements. Advice needs to be tailored to individual needs, as a one-size-fits-all prescription for healthy eating may present barriers for certain individuals. Many people live in circumstances that prevent them from adopting healthy lifestyle practices that may be appropriate for someone else. Some of these circumstances that act as barriers to change include pregnancy, living in a situation where they have little personal support or are subjected to ridicule from family members or close friends or having co-morbidities. Any of the chronic conditions may change a person's appetite and attitude to food as well as their access to preferred products. Some diabetics, for example, have difficulty with the constant food vigilance that can be involved in managing their condition. They may feel uncomfortable eating with others, or have variable treatment regimens. Many people live alone and those with chronic disease, limited finances, functional difficulties or who suffer from loneliness, anxiety or depression may simply fail to take the time to prepare appropriate meals. Ensuring healthy foods are readily available in the neighbourhood is also essential for enabling those needing to make dietary changes to do so. Healthy foods need to be affordable and accessible and it may be necessary to lobby locally and nationally to make this happen. Ensuring local health authorities have effective food security policies to support the sustainable development goal of zero hunger is as important in Australia and New Zealand as it is in other countries. In New Zealand, 19% of children and 14% of the entire population live in severely to moderately food-insecure households (Comeau et al 2020, Ministry of Health 2019). In Australia, food insecurity is estimated to affect between 4% and 13% of the population and between 22% and 32% of the Indigenous population (Bowden 2020).

Encouraging schools and hospitals to sell only healthy foods in vending machines and supporting supermarkets to replace sugar-laden foods at the checkout with fruits and healthy snacks are simple steps that can be easily taken. Sugar has now been identified as one of the most dangerous food items for health and the WHO has been encouraging governments to take steps to encourage manufacturers to reduce the sugar content of their food and improve labelling for consumers since 2014. The WHO guidelines on sugar intake for children and adults recommend reducing free sugar intake throughout the life course and reducing this intake to less than 10% of total energy intake (WHO 2015). Health practitioners can check to ensure their government is following this advice and support efforts to improve nutrition labelling and decreases in sugar content. These interventions help address the obesogenic environment—that is, those environments that are more likely to promote weight gain and obesity. Interventions that focus on the whole family may be effective in supporting people to make changes to their diet (Funaki-Tahifote et al 2016, Morgan et al 2020).

KEY POINT

Nutrition counselling needs to be tailored to meet individual needs. Cultural imperatives, the social context of eating and motivation influence the ability of individuals to make the dietary changes they need to maintain good health.

Social, cultural and environmental factors are important in promoting lifestyle changes, especially those intended to increase exercise and other activities. Organised physical activities at the neighbourhood level can provide opportunities to develop supportive social networks as well as helping manage chronic conditions, or preventing further deterioration once a person has experienced an acute episode such as a cardiac event. The environmental determinants for healthy lifestyles include safe walkways, cycleways and well-lit streets to allow working people to exercise and socialise after working hours and choose healthy options for commuting to work. Intersectoral planning by engineering, transportation, recreation, health and education professionals can help make neighbourhoods conducive to activities. Structured group exercise programs tend to create a feeling of wellbeing that can enhance value, belongingness and attachment to others, which builds social capital. At a personal level, exercise: improves muscular and cardiorespiratory fitness; improves bone and functional health; reduces the risk of hypertension, cardiovascular disease, stroke, diabetes, cancer and depression; and reduces the risk of falls (WHO 2018b, 2020c). For this reason, 'sweat' has been called the natural antidepressant.

The relationship between health and place is an important element of the social context that creates lifestyle risks. Urban living has risks from crime, neighbourhood violence, various air, water and food pollutants, motor vehicles and a proliferation of fast-food outlets. However, compared to urban dwellers, people living in regional or rural areas, many of whom are Indigenous, are at significantly higher risk of chronic illness and mental health issues (particularly depression) due to geographical isolation, lack of support, poor access to primary care services, low levels of health literacy and high rates of smoking and alcohol consumption (AIHW 2019, Jones et al 2020).

> ### Where to find out more on …
>
> **Rural and remote health**
>
> - Australia Government: www.aihw.gov.au/reports/rural-health/rural-remote-health/contents/rural-health
> - New Zealand Government: www.health.govt.nz/our-work/populations/rural-health
> - Rural Health Alliance Aotearoa New Zealand: https://rhaanz.org.nz

Health promotion strategies that revolve around health literacy and empowering people to take control over their lifestyles are important, but these are often hampered by a lack of access to resources. Unlike urban dwellers many rural people do not have opportunities for group sports or other activities, and many regional towns and rural areas do not have access to green parks, exercise playgrounds for children or safe walking trails close to schools. When they need assistance, there are few specialists available to treat chronic illnesses or to offer them preventative programs. In addition to supportive services and programs, the 'digital divide' between those with and without access to internet information can worsen inequities by preventing the level of education enjoyed by people in the city.

In Australia, nurses are the most commonly found health practitioner in rural and remote communities, providing a broad range of services including acute healthcare, health promotion and community development activities (McCullough et al 2021). Often these nurses come to communities with significant acute care experience but little in the way of primary

health care knowledge or expertise (McCullough et al 2021, Muirhead & Birks 2019). To this end, they frequently find themselves struggling to reconcile the cultural mores of Indigenous populations with the Western biomedical requirements of contracts that require patient compliance (McCullough et al 2021). Developing partnerships with community members, collaborating at a community health service level and ensuring educational pathways for rural and remote nurses including how primary health care principles can be incorporated into nursing practice are all essential for ensuring the care provided in rural and remote communities meets the needs of those living there (McCullough et al 2021, Muirhead & Birks 2019). Primary health care approaches to nursing practice can be embedded in all settings from the bedside to the most remote community. Chapter 3 discussed this in detail.

WORK

Work is one of the main activities of adults and, where working conditions and culture are conducive, is generally good for health and wellbeing (Australasian Faculty of Occupational & Environmental Medicine 2019). Work contributes to individual autonomy, personal development, empowerment and feelings of satisfaction in the ability to support one's family and to help others (Bickenbach 2019). Work also contributes to mental wellbeing and improved quality of life (Reichard et al 2019). Conversely, long-term work absence, work disability, unemployment, unsafe working environments and workplace incivility can have a negative impact on health and wellbeing, contributing to stress, inequalities and poor outcomes (Bickenbach 2019).

Workplace stressors affect members of cultural and socioeconomic groups differently, but in general, workplace stress is becoming more prevalent across all categories of workers. This is linked to changing social conditions. Life in the twenty-first century has become fast-paced for many adults, with resounding effects on the family, the workplace and society. For example, labour market policies in some places have resulted in growing numbers of people in 'precarious' work. Precarious work is characterised by a fundamental uncertainty in conditions, duration and pay, and may include work described as seasonal, casual, seasonal contracting or zero hours contracts (Jonsson et al 2021, Rosenberg 2018). Precarious work is linked to poor health with clear associations between precarious work and self-rated poor general and mental health (Jonsson et al 2021). Questions about how to stem the flow of people into precarious employment and the subsequent impact of that on individuals' lives and their families are important to consider and the answers will frequently lie in the policies of government. But understanding the lived experience of the 'precariat' and understanding the reality of what it is like to struggle daily to make ends meet is everybody's business. Ensuring people in these circumstances lead dignified lives and have access to appropriate services and support to achieve this are goals of primary health care practice.

The 'busyness' of lifestyles and changes in workplace demands, such as precarious work, fly-in fly-out (FIFO) jobs, high workloads and employer expectations regarding digital media and the ability to be able to access work 'anywhere, anytime', are major sources of stress (Ilić Petković & Nikolić 2020). There are clear links between stress and physical and psychosocial outcomes with those experiencing stress in the workplace at greater risk of depression, cardiovascular disease, diabetes and musculoskeletal issues (Ilić Petković & Nikolić 2020, Somers & Casal 2021). Workplace policies themselves can add to or alleviate stress. Some, but not all, countries have flexible workplace policies, where employees can negotiate work hours that are more suitable to their lifestyle. Whether this is working around children and family or for personal satisfaction, flexibility can help improve work–life balance. However, when flexibility in the workplace results in precarious work or a lack of income security, workers hesitate to take sick leave, even in the face of severe illness or injury. This creates additional stress, especially with the threat that the worker may be dismissed without explanation or financial compensation, which affects the entire family. The COVID-19 pandemic put the spotlight on access to sick leave in both Australia and New Zealand with many arguing current sick leave provisions were insufficient to enable workers to take required sick leave following testing for or diagnosis of the virus (Speers 2020). New Zealand went as far as changing the law to increase sick leave provisions

from 5 to 10 days per annum (Ministry of Business, Innovation and Employment 2021). Many large resource sector companies employ nurses and other health practitioners to work on improving and managing health and safety on site which includes providing support for workers who may be experiencing depression, stress and anxiety as a result of their working circumstances. These practitioners can also support workers to access appropriate leave entitlements. However, despite the implementation of new and extensive health and safety laws in both Australia and New Zealand, health and safety at work remains problematic in both countries.

Health and safety at work

Health and safety at work are essential for ensuring all workers come home safely. Between 60% and 70% of the population in both Australia (www.abs.gov.au/ausstats/abs@.nsf/mf/6202.0) and New Zealand (www.stats.govt.nz/information-releases/labour-market-statistics-march-2021-quarter) are employed, meaning health and safety in the workplace can be considered a major risk to most adults' health and wellbeing. Illness and injury at work has the potential for long-term disability, which can affect not only the worker, but also their family and community. Workplace events also cause losses in worker productivity which, in cases where a worker does not have job security, can exacerbate socioeconomic disadvantage. Accidents and injuries also incur costs to businesses and the healthcare system. Workplace accidents are highly variable, depending on the type of work and the workplace culture, particularly in terms of safety and support. Musculoskeletal injuries are the most common work-related injuries. Another prevalent work-related injury is hearing loss, caused by excessive noise in the workplace. In some cases, workplace injuries are linked to individual worker characteristics as well as to the work environment, including the worker's commitment to health and safety. For example, the consumption of alcohol or substances, either during or before work, can interfere with jobs that require the operation of machinery or intense concentration. Other factors affecting health and safety in the workplace include the type of work undertaken, the pressures placed on workers to meet productivity targets and exposure to hazardous substances or safety risks. Productivity pressures can cause biological, physical or psychosocial risks or a combination of these.

Where to find out more on ...

Workplace health and safety

- Australia: www.safeworkaustralia.gov.au
- New Zealand: www.worksafe.govt.nz

For this reason, primary prevention activities include a hazard or risk assessment in the workplace. This begins with an ergonomic assessment of the workplace and the working conditions. Ergonomic assessment involves examining the engineering aspects of the relationship between the worker and their work environment. Ergonomic hazards are those that induce fatigue, boredom or glare, or tasks that must be conducted in an abnormal position. Examples include work that causes vibration, repetitive motion, poor workstation–worker fit and lifting heavy loads. Biological hazards can include exposure to bacteria, moulds, insects, viruses or infectious co-workers. Chemical hazards can include exposure to dangerous liquids, gases, dust, vapour or fumes. Physical hazards include extremes of temperature, noise, radiation, poor lighting, lifting or exposure to unprotected machinery. Nurses, for example, are at risk of musculoskeletal injuries, obesity and overweight and cardiovascular disease due to the physical nature of their work and the shift work required (Pessoa Pousa & de Lucca 2021, Stimpfel 2020). During the Covid-19 pandemic, in response to government directives, workplaces responded rapidly to implement changes. These changes were ultimately designed to alter human behaviour and suppress the pandemic. Mask wearing, social distancing and working from home, while designed to keep people safe, have also impacted on people's physical, mental and social health (Plant & Fendley 2021). Managers who are responsible for supporting health and safety need ongoing support to address these workplace health and safety risks (Sigahi et al 2021).

THE SANDWICH GENERATION

Through the middle stages of adulthood, a combination of unique stressors can prove challenging. Juggling work, caring for children and, increasingly, caring for older parents can test the resilience of many, particularly women, who are more likely to take on these multiple roles. Called the 'sandwich generation', these women (and some men) contribute more than 1500 hours per year each of unpaid family care (Deloitte Access Economics 2015, Grimmond 2014, Kia Piki Ake Welfare Expert Advisory Group 2019). Informal caregiving is recognised as a chronic stressor, creating physical and psychological strain over extended periods of time and family caregivers can earn up to 10% less than non-caregivers despite similar occupational backgrounds, largely attributable to working part-time (Kia Piki Ake Welfare Expert Advisory Group 2019). Ultimately, many give up work to care full-time, further affecting their finances (Spann et al 2020). The COVID-19 pandemic has had a particularly significant impact on female caregivers with multiple pathways to disadvantage. These include higher risk of contracting the disease due to their caregiving roles, loss of work due to the disestablishment of many part-time and informal roles frequently taken on by women, and increased unpaid domestic work due to the closure of schools and businesses forcing family members to stay home to provide care (Ayittey et al 2020). Despite negative outcomes for sandwich carers, there are benefits. These include the emotional and relational rewards associated with caring for loved family members (Evans et al 2019). Being aware of these multiple stressors on the adult enables nurses and other health professionals to put in place appropriate strategies and interventions to support healthy adulthood.

GOALS FOR HEALTHY ADULTHOOD

The best approach for adult health is community participation in all matters concerning health and wellbeing, irrespective of whether the objective is to overcome risks or enhance the quality of people's lives. The most pertinent issues in planning for healthy adulthood are social: to overcome inequity and inequality. The focus of today's health promotion agenda for adults should be to address the SDH, to reduce risk, to improve the quality of work and family life, to prevent and better manage chronic diseases, including mental health, and to respond capably to current and future threats including both infectious diseases and threats to the environment. To address these issues requires public awareness of the seriousness of each, and dissemination of accurate information that will be both instructive and supportive. The focus should remain on communities in creating and maintaining health to decrease the incidence of chronic diseases, develop safer workplaces, living spaces and societies and provide greater opportunities for people to achieve better physical, mental, spiritual, environmental and culturally safe health. Box 8.5 outlines a set of specific recommendations that help guide nurses and other health practitioners in their work with adults. It is important to take an ecological approach and consider the needs of each individual in the context of their community and society as well as the impact of global issues on their circumstances. Achieving a healthy adulthood enables the individual to manage the transition to healthy ageing with ease.

Part 3: Healthy ageing
CONTEXT

The central challenge for healthy ageing lies in creating the conditions for people to age with optimal health and wellbeing and a good quality of life. But what is ageing? In the twenty-first century, social commentators quip that 40 is the new 20, and 60 the new 40. Does this make 80 the new 60, and, if so, what does that mean for the way we nurture health and wellbeing along the latter stages of life's pathway? We know that the quality of ageing depends on the cumulative effects of social determinants in the earlier years. But there are also developmental changes that occur in the years from 65 to 90 and beyond, and these have not often attracted the attention of healthcare planners. Instead, planning has tended to revolve around population trends towards disease states, and how to prevent, treat and

---

BOX 8.5

....

GOALS FOR ADULT HEALTH

....

The major goals for adult health include:

- ensuring an appropriate balance between comprehensive and selective primary health care, particularly in addressing chronic conditions for disadvantaged populations
- providing political support for health in all policies
- integrating primary, secondary and tertiary intervention for adult health in the workplace and community
- adopting a life course approach for the prevention of chronic conditions
- promoting an ecological risk-reduction approach by focusing on the environments for good health
- using intersectoral collaboration to address physical and mental health issues comprehensively
- ensuring cultural safety in all interactions
- designing health promotion strategies that are empowering, with people and families as partners at the centre of care
- using health resources efficiently and effectively, eliminating boundaries between professionals
- using the World Health Organization's Ottawa Charter as a guideline for health promotion
- considering the career needs of adults as they plan for retirement.

---

palliate these. This 'illness' rather than 'wellness' focus is disempowering for older people, especially for those trying to cope with the cumulative effects of lifelong disadvantage. Community-based actions to support and enhance healthy ageing should revolve around health promotion; improving the social, physical, economic and policy environments within which older people can enjoy good health into their later years and engage in healthy lifestyles.

Communities for healthy ageing need to acknowledge the extent to which older persons contribute to the social, cultural and geographical life of the community. People over the age of 65 are vital to childcare and other aspects of family life, particularly for their grown children who may be living in busy, dual-earner families. Many older persons are also carers for family members with disabling conditions. Importantly, older citizens are also a viable economic force. Some continue in the workplace longer than their forebears, bringing wisdom to a wide range of industries, including healthcare. As people remain in the workforce longer, employers will need to accommodate any declines in older workers' capacity, including work content or physical loading, stressful work environments and the psychosocial elements of good work practices. They will also need to ensure there is a culture that supports worker interaction and social engagement. Vulnerable groups among older generations in need of supportive environments include the migrant population, the rural population, the economically disadvantaged and those attempting to fulfil casual employment positions. Strategies for mentoring young workers can have maximum value for both the mentors and the mentees, as older people are encouraged to pass on their experience to those who need to develop knowledge and skills.

Older adults also have the potential to dominate shifts in the economy through their spending, investments and service requirements. They are a political force through the sheer weight of numbers, capable of swaying the policy climate for health, the environment and their grandchildren's educational future. In some communities, older people help calm the social climate through their understanding, and by having a more emotionally balanced perspective that comes with the patience of ageing. Others' lives may be destitute and lonely. The combination is unique for every person and experienced differently, depending on social and environmental supports. First and foremost among the goals for healthy ageing is empowerment, to nurture older citizens' participation in community life and in their healthcare decisions.

HEALTH IN OLDER AGE

Many people over the age of 65 in Australia and New Zealand lead healthy and productive lives, some thriving in ways they could not during their middle years, when their life circumstances prevented them from achieving a balance between work, recreation and family responsibilities. A large number of older people are also unwell, suffering from chronic diseases or long-term conditions that limit their mobility or sense of wellbeing. But these two groups are not polar opposites. There are numerous older people whose health lies between the extremes of high-level wellness and immobility. The challenge for nurses and other health practitioners working with older persons is to see each person in terms of individual strengths and needs, and in the context of the environments that support or constrain their health and wellbeing. This includes understanding their individual journey, and what it has meant for the way they experience health. Although the lives of many have been affected by conflict, including the First and Second World Wars (1914–1918 and 1939–1945) and the Korean and Vietnam wars of the 1950s to 1970s, the current generation of older people born in Australia and New Zealand now live in relative peace and harmony. But some have also been beleaguered by the global financial crises of the 1980s and 2008–2009 that eroded their retirement income, causing uncertainty about the future. Conflicts and disrupted living circumstances have also affected the earlier years of many immigrants and refugees who are ageing in both countries. Ageing is also proving difficult for LGBTQIA+ elders, some of whom have suffered the cumulative strains of lifelong discrimination which continues into aged and residential care facilities (Zanetos & Skipper 2020). The older years are also challenging for Indigenous people who may live in remote areas with few services or supports.

Where to find out more on ...

The health of older people

- Australia: www.aihw.gov.au/ageing
- New Zealand: www.health.govt.nz/our-work/life-stages/health-older-people and www.health.govt.nz/our-work/life-stages/health-older-people/lilacs-nz-research-programme

Those in rural and remote areas need special attention. For those ageing at home in rural and remote areas, community services are often absent, leaving them at a disadvantage. The shrinking of the rural sector is an issue that has caused many older rural people considerable stress. Age-friendly community networks, especially for the large proportion of women caring for family members and their caregivers, can help rural people remain connected and feeling valued until the end of life. Older people in rural areas believe maintaining social connections and remaining optimistic are key to helping them age in place (Anderson et al 2020, Hancock et al 2019). Often, though, it is their chronic and long-term conditions that contribute to older people making the move from their rural homes to cities, to be closer to health services. Away from their familiar space and sense of independence, many experience the crowding and financial stress of cities for the first time, during and after retirement. Many of these people have led self-reliant and independent lives, yet find their preferences subsumed within lifestyles unfamiliar to them. Nurses and other health practitioners working with older people in the community need to be vigilant to ensure that rural voices are heard, and that policies include strategies for action with a focus on the specific needs of elders.

Today, society is gradually becoming aware of the need to value older people as instrumental to sustaining community capacity. Older people themselves are also more inclined to consider the potential of modifying their environments and engaging in robust personal behaviours for healthier lives. These include healthy nutrition, physical exercise, low-risk personal habits and coping styles and a general refocusing on what can enrich, rather than compromise, their health and happiness in the later years. Healthy lifestyles among older people are visible in communities that provide environmental supports, such as the beach communities on Queensland's Gold Coast, which attract a large number of retirees. The local Gold Coast Council has established walking trails alongside the beaches, with exercise stations approximately every 10 metres. The stations are equipped with weather-resistant gym equipment that is shared by young and old people alike on a daily basis. The equipment represents a small investment in the health and fitness of citizens that might otherwise be precluded from exercising because of a lack of transportation or finances. Free Tai Chi sessions on the beach offered courtesy of Gold Coast Council's 'Active and Healthy Gold Coast' strategy are another way in which the council demonstrates its commitment to health and wellbeing (see Fig 8.5).

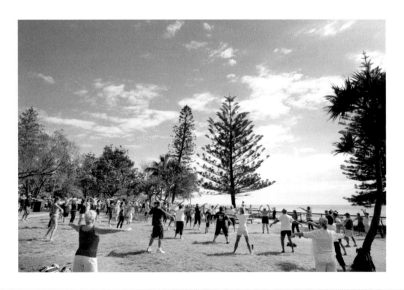

Figure 8.5 Free Tai-Chi classes on the Gold Coast

AGEIST ATTITUDES

Despite today's older adults having grown up in an era of experimentation, dramatic social change and relative prosperity, they are still subject to ageist attitudes, behaviours and stereotypes from those younger than themselves. Ageism is a type of discrimination against older adults on the basis of misconceptions about their characteristics, attitudes, abilities and capacity. The most obvious example of ageism is the global state of alarm at population ageing with some describing older persons as a 'demographic time bomb' or as universally and exclusively needy, dependent and frail (Desjardins 2017, Milne 2019). Ageism can result in older adults being over- or under-treated in our healthcare systems, can limit their ability to find work, contributes to the provision of poor healthcare and can shorten life (Saif-Ur-Rahman et al 2021, Shpakou et al 2021). In many cases, where ageism is present, there is little consideration of personality characteristics, or personal responses to provocation, pain, disability or recent life events. Instead, the older adult's concerns are often stereotyped as if they were typical of the entire demographic group. Making assumptions about the experiences of older people is risky. The video and website found in Box 8.6 show the results of research with women over 60 and their diverse experiences of intimacy. The work shows that preconceived ideas surrounding intimacy and older women are often not true. Initiatives such as the co-location of kindergartens with aged care facilities and other intergenerational activities can help remove the stigma of ageing and may be particularly helpful for those with dementia (Janke et al 2019).

BOX 8.6

....

STILL DOING IT

....

- Video: www.youtube.com/watch?v=NVgcdULvtX0
- Website: www.stilldoingit.com

RETIREMENT

Some policy experts have argued that retirement is a risk factor for illness or frailty, while others have mounted a counterargument—that leaving the stress of the workplace and assuming a healthier lifestyle during retirement has major health benefits. Some older workers prefer to remain in the workforce (although often cut down on hours) as a way of remaining connected with their colleagues and their self-identity. Older nurses, for example, may struggle with some of the physical challenges of nursing, but have developed substantial resilience in order to manage these challenges and continue to work often into their seventies (Clendon & Walker 2016). Others stay for financial reasons. During the retirement or semi-retirement phase of life, increased leisure time provides opportunities for closer social engagement than during a person's working life. Social engagement helps maintain emotional closeness, or social intimacy, as well as instrumental assistance, which is usually seen in having greater social support for times when it is needed. Social engagement in older age is considered a key component of healthy ageing with substantial health benefits for the individual and the wider community (Hancock et al 2019). Participating in social activities tends to help people feel they have maintained mastery over their life; that they continue to accomplish things despite any constraints associated with ageing such as functional impairments, widowhood or lack of family support. Encouraging social engagement is an important goal for nurses and other health practitioners who work with older adults.

One of the greatest community assets in many cities and communities today is the vast array of volunteer networks that often provide a critical link to social life and social services. These networks often comprise numerous people having reached older age themselves. Their guidance is often invaluable in helping others make the transitions from rural to urban, home to community or residential care, or to services and facilities they need. Volunteering is one of the most rewarding activities for older adults, as it helps build a strong sense of control. Often volunteers have a deep understanding of older adults' problems from first-hand experience, and they often recognise the type of information or assistance that is needed. They may also have the time and patience to listen when it is most needed, especially for people who may be suffering from depression or other mental illness. Volunteers also develop a sense of self-esteem through their actions, especially knowing the extent to which their input is valued.

One of the most vital movements of current times is the response to widespread recognition of the need for lifelong learning, through courses such as those in the University of the Third Age (U3A). Older students are often willing to share life experiences, integrating their insights into course material. Older people also approach learning in unique ways, using new knowledge to forestall deterioration of their cognitive abilities, eager to build linkages between old and new knowledge. Studying and learning helps build cultural bridges, linking personal and public perspectives, blending emotional insights with enhanced awareness of the world. The advent of the internet has also provided some older persons with a thirst for even more knowledge, and different ways of exploring the world. Organisations such as SeniorNet (www.seniornet.co.nz) provide opportunities for older people to learn internet skills at a pace that is appropriate to their needs.

One way to promote connectedness within the ageing community is to reinforce the value of religious institutions, where this is appropriate to community members. Relocation to a different environment may cause older adults enormous stress if they are unable to retrieve the familiarity of the church, temple or synagogue or those who provide religious support. Our role as health advocates should include assessing older community members' needs for communication and spiritual worship. This may involve arranging transportation, social networks of lay people with similar religious affiliations or visits by members of the church, especially for older adults who are incapacitated and cannot meet the obligations of their faith.

CHALLENGES IN OLDER AGE

Although many people age well, as noted earlier, many will also face challenges that warrant further attention here. In addition to the cumulative effects of long-term conditions such as cardiac disease and diabetes, dementia is one of the major causes of disability and dependency among older adults worldwide (WHO 2020a). The numbers of people with dementia in Australia and New Zealand are expected to rise primarily due to continued growth and ageing of the population in both countries (AIHW 2020, BPAC 2020). 'Dementia' is considered an umbrella term that includes a number of conditions that affect the function of the brain. Approximately two-thirds of people with dementia have Alzheimer's disease (WHO 2020a). People with dementia and their carers can adopt strategies to help manage the disease, minimise losses and reduce isolation (Livingston et al 2020). These strategies may include facilitating participation of the person with dementia in activities and helping them to maintain their sense of identity (Livingston et al 2020, Read et al 2021). Carers themselves may be under tremendous stress as they experience changes in their own role as they care for their family member (Livingston et al 2020, Read et al 2021). Nurses and other health practitioners have an important role in supporting people with dementia and their families by providing information and advice, non-judgmental support and referral for further assessment and intervention where needed (BPAC 2020).

> ## Where to find out more on ...
>
> ### Dementia and Alzheimer's disease
>
> - Australia: www.dementia.org.au and www.alz.org/au/dementia-alzheimers-australia.asp
> - New Zealand: www.alzheimers.org.nz and https://dementia.nz/

Older people with dementia may also be at particular risk of elder abuse (Collins et al 2020). The United Nations and the WHO define elder abuse as 'a single, or repeated act, or lack of appropriate action, occurring within any relationship where there is an expectation of trust which causes harm or distress to an older person' (WHO 2020b).

Elder abuse includes physical, psychological and sexual abuse, financial exploitation and neglect (Collins et al 2020, WHO 2020b). It is estimated that between 2% and 14% of older Australians and New Zealanders experience abuse every year (Collins et al 2020, Office for Senior Citizens 2015). Elder abuse has significant ramifications for the individual and for communities. People experiencing elder abuse suffer significant psychological distress, may die earlier, are more likely to use health services and be hospitalised and have poorer mental health and depression (Collins et al 2020, WHO 2020b). Nurses and other health practitioners have an important role to play in identifying and preventing elder abuse and supporting those who have experienced it. Many older people are reluctant to report abuse (Dow et al 2020). Because of this, holistic assessment of the older person should include screening for elder abuse. However, a recent Australian study found a range of limitations to many current assessment tools (Brijnath et al 2020). The authors suggested that any tool must be concise, easy to use, take into account the older person's health and social context and provide a referral pathway if elder abuse is suspected (Brijnath et al 2020). The authors also recognised the value of co-designing a screening tool and to this end set about designing the Australian Elder Abuse Screening Instrument (AuSI) in collaboration with health practitioners (Gahan et al 2019). The tool is available at www.nari.net.au/Handlers/Download.ashx?IDMF=b793ff77-d3ff-4440-91df-bd883a1ba86d. In addition, using the McMurray community assessment framework will help nurses and other health practitioners identify key community resources to support people identified as experiencing or at risk of elder abuse.

Prevention approaches to elder abuse can be classified into two broad themes: changing values and attitudes among the broader community and among professionals and individuals who have contact with older people; and addressing the risk factors for elder abuse (Kaspiew et al 2016). Evidence to support effective approaches to preventing elder abuse is limited. The WHO (2020b) suggest the following approaches show some promise:

- providing caregiver support before and after abuse occurs

- providing school-based intergeneration programs to decrease negative attitudes and stereotypes towards older people
- increasing professional awareness of the problem.

A multifaceted approach to addressing elder abuse will be the most effective with nurses having a role at each level from individual identification to supporting families where abuse is a risk, and to community-wide interventions to encourage greater knowledge and understanding of the strengths and value of older people in the community.

Frailty is also gaining recognition as contributing to morbidity and early mortality among older adults. Frailty (sometimes called frailty syndrome) is multidimensional and is characterised by the presence of three or more phenotypes: unintentional weight loss, self-reported fatigue, weakness, low level of physical activity and slowness (Barbosa da Silva et al 2020, Papadopoulou et al 2021). Not captured in the phenotype model is the contribution of social or environmental factors to the progression of frailty, both of which should be included in an assessment to ensure a comprehensive understanding of a person's situation (Freer 2020). Frailty is also a component of geriatric syndrome which includes urinary incontinence, falls, delirium and pressure ulcers. Geriatric syndrome may be a better predictor of death than the presence or number of certain diseases in older people (WHO 2018a). The use of a validated tool such as the Clinical Frailty Scale can help in determining the frailty status of an individual and was used during the COVID-19 pandemic to assist in making clinical decisions such as allocating scarce resources (Rockwood & Theou 2020). Figure 8.6 shows the Clinical Frailty Scale. Of note is the ability to prevent many of the common components of ageing, underlining the importance of comprehensive primary health care approaches to supporting people to age well.

Dementia and frailty combined with other common long-term conditions present among older people means many are taking multiple medications in order to manage their health. As a result, polypharmacy is a significant issue among older people in Australia and New Zealand. Older people on multiple medications are more prone to drug-related complications due to the complex medicine regimens they may be required to adhere to and the

CLINICAL FRAILTY SCALE

1 VERY FIT People who are robust, active, energetic and motivated. They tend to exercise regularly and are among the fittest for their age.

2 FIT People who have **no active disease symptoms** but are less fit than category 1. Often, they exercise or are very **active occasionally**, e.g., seasonally.

3 MANAGING WELL People whose **medical problems are well controlled**, even if occasionally symptomatic, but often are **not regularly active** beyond routine walking.

4 LIVING WITH VERY MILD FRAILTY Previously "vulnerable," this category marks early transition from complete independence. While **not dependent** on others for daily help, often **symptoms limit activities**. A common complaint is being "slowed up" and/or being tired during the day.

5 LIVING WITH MILD FRAILTY People who often have **more evident slowing**, and need help with **high order instrumental activities of daily living** (finances, transportation, heavy housework). Typically, mild frailty progressively impairs shopping and walking outside alone, meal preparation, medications and begins to restrict light housework.

6 LIVING WITH MODERATE FRAILTY People who need help with **all outside activities and with keeping house**. Inside, they often have problems with stairs and need **help with bathing** and might need minimal assistance (cuing, standby) with dressing.

7 LIVING WITH SEVERE FRAILTY **Completely dependent for personal care**, from whatever cause (physical or cognitive). Even so, they seem stable and not at high risk of dying (within ~6 months).

8 LIVING WITH VERY SEVERE FRAILTY Completely dependent for personal care and approaching end of life. Typically, they could not recover even from a minor illness.

9 TERMINALLY ILL Approaching the end of life. This category applies to people with a **life expectancy <6 months**, who are **not otherwise living with severe frailty**. (Many terminally ill people can still exercise until very close to death.)

SCORING FRAILTY IN PEOPLE WITH DEMENTIA

The degree of frailty generally corresponds to the degree of dementia. Common **symptoms in mild dementia** include forgetting the details of a recent event, though still remembering the event itself, repeating the same question/story and social withdrawal.

In **moderate dementia**, recent memory is very impaired, even though they seemingly can remember their past life events well. They can do personal care with prompting.

In **severe dementia**, they cannot do personal care without help.

In **very severe dementia** they are often bedfast. Many are virtually mute.

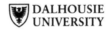 **DALHOUSIE UNIVERSITY**

Figure 8.6 Clinical Frailty Scale

physiological changes associated with ageing. Adverse events and interactions associated with this polypharmacy can lead to a greater risk of falls, fractures, confusion, incontinence, constipation and other issues that can cause distress. These events can also lead to admission to hospital or residential care facilities (Stevenson et al 2020). Stevenson and colleagues (2020) advocate for medication-related harm to be considered a component of geriatric syndrome—separate in itself to the other elements listed earlier. Nurses and other health practitioners, such as pharmacists, have an important role in ensuring older people are managing their medicines well, providing education and support in the home or clinic. Identifying where polypharmacy may put an older person at risk and putting in place appropriate strategies to manage this, including regular medicine reviews, referral and reconciliation, is important. Often older people may also be taking over-the-counter medicines or complementary and alternative medicines and may be reluctant to share this with their health practitioner. Careful assessment can help identify where this may be occurring and allow preventative strategies to be put in place early.

Where to find out more on …

Information on medication safety

- Health Quality & Safety Commission New Zealand: www.hqsc.govt.nz/our-programmes/medication-safety
- Australian Commission on Safety and Quality in Health Care: www.safetyandquality.gov.au/our-work/medication-safety

---

SUPPORTING TRANSITIONS TO AND WITHIN OLDER ADULTHOOD

Building personal health capacity in the later years should be multidimensional, addressing psychosocial health issues and health literacy, as well as any risks related to disability or poor general health. Effective pain management strategies can support older people to overcome the impact of pain on their lives and develop the resiliency needed to age well. One of the most useful resources is a website developed in Western Australia to help people understand and manage pain: Pain*Health* (http://painhealth.csse.uwa.edu.au). The website explains different types of pain, provides various personal stories of pain and outlines ways of coping with pain through techniques such as mindfulness and goal setting as well as medication management.

Mental health services for older people continue to be sporadic, especially in regional and rural areas, and community nurses with specific training in mental health remain one of the best sources of assistance for families trying to manage dementia-related behaviours. The Mental Health Nurse Incentive Program in Australia, which facilitates credentialled mental health nurses to work in primary health care and provide direct care to those experiencing mental illness, has been shown to be a cost-effective and beneficial program for recipients, nurses and other clinicians (Happell & Platania-Phung 2019). These nurses are also an ideal support

for family members trying to manage their own anxieties related to caregiving.

Another important role for nurses working in home and community care is to help older people manage chronic conditions and prevent deteriorating health. Integrated care focused on improving coordination for those with chronic and complex conditions has been shown to enhance care, improve coordination of services and be valued by patients and providers (McMurray et al 2021). Shared care records are a cornerstone to success in these types of programs but often a lack of integrated e-record creates barriers to the longevity of coordinated care activities (McMurray et al 2021). The interdisciplinary approach associated with integrated care programs should extend across the continuum of care, to include acute care episodes and palliative care, involving the older person and family members as partners in care with specialist support where required from palliative care professionals.

Nurses and/or nurse practitioners are also among the most frequent visitors to long-term care homes, and in this capacity they can help promote continuity between services and caregivers and decrease hospital admissions (Craswell et al 2020, Hullick et al 2021, Kwa et al 2021). These nurses play an important dual role in helping create awareness of the range of issues that may be challenging in care, as well as encouraging evidence-based practice and the translation of new information into practice changes such as person-centred care. The videos found in Box 8.7 showcase how nurses, clinical nurse specialists and nurse practitioners are working together to improve their care for older people. Research into the types of skills required of nurses working with

---

BOX 8.7

· ·

NURSES IN LONG-TERM CARE HOMES

· ·

- www.youtube.com/watch?v=NFzAGoQJ8Ys
- www.youtube.com/watch?v=346cAbTSe3c

older people in residential care settings shows that they need advanced assessment skills, the ability to manage complex care, and a focus on primary health care and keeping people well (Davis 2016, Phelan 2016). In fact, during the COVID-19 pandemic in Australia, the chance of an aged and residential care facility resident contracting the disease decreased substantially for every registered nurse employed (Kiejda 2020). Nursing plans should also be mindful of people's sense of place. Older adults living in residential care settings are, in essence, at 'home'. Nurses can help others in the aged care setting work within a primary health care approach that includes social inclusion, connectedness, cultural safety, person-centred care, health literacy and appropriate use of technology to tailor plans to people's multidimensional needs.

Another aspect of service provision demanding attention is the need to tailor services to the needs of different community groups of older citizens. Older adults are not a homogeneous group, nor do they represent a common culture, or common experiences of illness or disability. It is therefore important to assess people's individual needs before assigning them to one type of care. Care facilities are already being redesigned to accommodate various subgroups within residential and semi-residential care, and this is a step in the right direction. Home to residential care will probably be the most problematic transition for the oldest old, and current initiatives for 'ageing in place' need to be customised to individual preferences and needs (Mayo et al 2021). Understandings of ageing generally are important. Older people value physical comfort, but place equal, if not greater, importance on social integration, their ongoing contribution to society, security, autonomy and enjoyment (Hancock et al 2019). However, it is important to remember that ageing in place in the community will work for some, but not all people, and services should accommodate a range of preferences and choices where possible.

THE FUTURE

The most significant societal-level challenge for the next decades will be how to best care for the over-85 age group, which is the fastest growing group globally (United Nations 2019). Population ageing will require adjustments in pension and income security schemes to support the ageing population. Healthcare systems will also have to accommodate changing needs. Acute care hospitals will be populated by a large proportion of the oldest old, many of whom will experience multiple health problems. With shortened hospital stays, nurses practising in the community have already begun to provide the bulk of care across extended periods of time for a wide range of acuity. In the near future, evolving technologies and therapeutic techniques will transform home care. Nurses will be part of the rapidly developing models of care that will see treatments customised to individual needs. Their roles will be central to caring for the communities where ageing takes place, supporting health-promoting behaviours, advocating for environmental supports for lifestyle modifications and helping people navigate the myriad services available. Many older people are embracing technologies, and these can be used to optimise care. Many older people are internet savvy, some using social networking to stay in touch with family members, and others using it to search for services or supports. Developing internet literacy can help people remain in their homes safely, access groceries and other services and prevent deterioration in their health. For example, there are electronic devices now with motion and vibration sensors that can detect falls. Other mobile devices connect health practitioners with older people living alone to collect information about their medical condition or alert authorities when they have a problem. Technological devices can also monitor sleep, toileting and urinary tract infections. The wide range of technological developments that we see now and will continue to see in the future must be implemented with equity in mind. Not all people have access to the internet and many older people struggle with technology, particularly among the oldest old. New technology must be implemented in a way that does not contribute to increasing the 'digital divide' and must be universally accessible to all, not just those who can afford it.

Goals for healthy ageing

Involving older persons as partners in health is crucial to developing age-appropriate healthcare systems and healthy ageing. Older persons consume more healthcare than any other demographic group. They carry the major burden of chronic diseases and have the greatest use of primary care services. But they also contribute to the overall care of the population, especially for those with disabilities. This unpaid work should warrant a greater voice in healthcare planning, and some older persons do participate in this type of planning. But, far too often, older people are excluded from participating in meaningful ways for service improvements. As a numerically dominant group they should be given greater opportunities to influence models of healthcare, based on their experiences and needs. This will become even more important in future, with the development of personalised therapies from genomics and molecular biology on the horizon. Box 8.8 outlines our goals for healthy ageing.

BOX 8.8

. . . .

GOALS FOR HEALTHY AGEING

. . . .

- Access, equity, empowerment and cultural safety
- Physical, emotional and spiritual health
- Intersectoral collaboration for services and resources based on individual needs and strengths
- A balance between independent living and adequate service provision based on appropriate technologies
- Acknowledgment of the relationship between health and place
- A place to feel safe and comfortable in living a dignified life
- Adequate financial and healthcare resources to sustain the latter stages of life irrespective of geographic location
- Policies to promote social inclusion and social engagement

Conclusion

Taking a life course approach to this and the previous chapter has enabled us to consider the key influences on health from pre-pregnancy through childhood, adolescence, adulthood and on to older adulthood. Supporting people to manage transitions through life is an important goal for nurses and other health practitioners working in primary health care settings. Understanding the challenges to health as well as those factors that strengthen people's response to challenges enable us to develop appropriate interventions. Next we reflect on the big issues identified in this chapter before returning to the Smith and Mason families to consider the challenges of dealing with current and future adolescent issues to maintain family health and harmony, issues related to the health of the adults in the Smith and Mason families and issues related to ageing.

Reflecting on the Big Issues

- Through each transition from adolescence to adulthood to older adulthood, every person's experience will be individual and each will have differing health and wellness needs.

- Adolescents are generally healthy but often have psychosocial issues that create risks to their health.

- Adolescents can be seen as 'at promise' as well as 'at risk'.

- From a socio-ecological perspective, home, school and the social environment are closely connected in adolescents' lives.

- Adult health is socially determined and needs to be seen in the context of a person's life course development.

- Adult health can be compromised by unhealthy behaviours.

- The physical environment has a major influence on health behaviours, suggesting an important relationship between health and place.

- Equity is a major factor in adult health, with chronic illnesses experienced more intensely by those who are disadvantaged.

- As most adults spend the majority of their time in the workplace, the health of both worker and workplace is a major focus for intervention.

- The work–home life nexus can create major stress, especially for women trying to lead a balanced life.

- Workplace relationships can be a source of psychological ill health.

- Older people are often the subject of stereotypical age discrimination in the workplace, in social life and in healthcare.

- Older people need to be valued for their wisdom, calmness and ability to see life in perspective.

- An older person's health and wellbeing is the product of cumulative experiences, indicating the need for a life course approach in evaluating health and wellness.

- Older people undertake a disproportionate amount of family caregiving and community volunteer work.

- The principles of primary health care can be used to ensure that adolescents, adults and older adults have access to health and other services, that their needs are met sensitively and that they develop in equitable life conditions.

CASE STUDY 8a	From preadolescence to adolescence in the Mason and Smith families

Jason and Huia's son John is 12 and on the cusp of adolescence. As parents, Jason and Huia were surprised, alarmed, then sad to learn from his teacher that he has just been diagnosed with a learning disability and is being bullied by his peers as he struggles with reading. After consulting with Huia, John's teacher at the Kura Kaupapa has initiated a referral to the learning and behavioural support teacher who will help provide some strategies for the family to support John.

Healthy adults in the Mason and Smith families

The occupational health nurse has been developing health promotion materials for the miners at Colin's work on a variety of health issues, including heart disease, depression, stress and diabetes. She is finding that the materials provoke some discussion but continues to offer personal assistance to those who don't seem to find the materials helpful.

Rebecca has been developing her health knowledge about her pre-metabolic syndrome and has become quite health literate in the process. Working with the practice nurse to manage her diet and lifestyle, she has brought her blood sugar and weight into a healthy range.

Jason has been finding the health promotion material provided by the occupational health nurse who visits his workplace helpful in managing his blood pressure, but he still struggles with his diet and exercise—particularly with his long commute into the city for work each day.

Huia is worried about losing her job because of Jake's asthma and although the family doesn't need the extra income, she finds the work rewarding and stimulating. She has not shared her concerns with Jason.

Older workers, older Mason and Smith family members

Some of the occupational health nurses are working with older mining managers, many of whom had not expected to continue working after age 65. They are addressing the special needs of the older worker in the context of not only chronic illness management but preventative care and the effect of shiftwork on older workers.

Rebecca's mother has developed breast cancer and is having to travel to the city for chemotherapy. During those weeks of treatment she is staying in Rebecca's home, and this is causing some problems with the young children disturbing her mother's rehabilitation and

adding to the pressure on Rebecca of maintaining family harmony.

Huia's mother has recently had a heart attack and moved into the family home for Huia to look after her, which is normal practice for Māori families. This has created additional pressures on her and now she has become one of the sandwich carers, dealing with both children and parents. Although her mother has tried hard to help around the house, her recent illness hampers her ability to contribute much. Huia has spoken with the Māori nurse practitioner who works in Papakura and she has promised to make a home visit.

Reflective questions: How would I use this knowledge in practice?

1 Explain the main risks of adolescence and how these can be addressed by nurses in a range of settings using a variety of strategies.

2 Using the HEEADSSS assessment (Appendix C), identify some of the needs that you believe would be revealed by an adolescent. Explain how you would promote a sense of community and school connectedness for this person.

3 Explain the health literacy needs of an adolescent, an adult and an older adult. What age-appropriate

strategies would you use to build health literacy in each group?

4 What social, physical and psychological influences have the most important effects on healthy ageing?

5 How does the environment affect older people's risk and potential in relation to falls prevention?

6 How can primary health care principles be used to guide a holistic assessment of the health needs of adolescents, adults and older adults?

References

Anderson, E.M., Larkins, S., Beaney, S., et al, 2020. Coping with ageing in rural Australia. Aust. J. Rural Health, 28 (5), 469–479. Online. Available: https://doi.org/10.1111/ajr.12647.

Australasian Faculty of Occupational & Environmental Medicine, 2019. Employment, poverty and health: A statement of principles (April issue). Online. Available: www.racp.edu.au/docs/default-source/advocacy-library/employment-poverty-and-health-statement-of-principles.pdf?sfvrsn=d084181a_4.

Australian Institute of Health and Welfare (AIHW), 2018. Aboriginal and Torres Strait Islander adolescent and youth health and wellbeing 2018. Online. Available: www.aihw.gov.au/reports/indigenous-australians/atsi-adolescent-youth-health-wellbeing-2018/contents/table-of-contents.

Australian Institute of Health and Welfare (AIHW), 2019. Rural & remote health (January issue). Online. Available: www.aihw.gov.au/getmedia/838d92d0-6d34-4821-b5da-39e4a47a3d80/Rural-remote-health.pdf.aspx?inline=true.

Australian Institute of Health and Welfare (AIHW), 2020. Dementia. Online. Available: www.aihw.gov.au/reports/australias-health/dementia.

Ayittey, F.K., Dhar, B.K., Anani, G., et al, 2020. Gendered burdens and impacts of SARS-CoV-2: A review. Health Care Women Int., 41 (11/12), 1210–1225. Online. Available: https://doi.org/10.1080/07399332.2020.1809664.

Azzopardi, P.S., Hearps, S.J.C., Francis, K.L., et al, 2019. Progress in adolescent health and wellbeing: Tracking 12 headline indicators for 195 countries and territories, 1990–2016. Lancet, 393 North(10176), 1101–1118. Online. Available: https://doi.org/10.1016/S0140-6736(18)32427-9.

Barbosa da Silva, A., Queiroz de Souza, I., da Silva, I.K., et al, 2020. Factors associated with frailty syndrome in

older adults. J. Nutr. Health Aging, 24 (2), 218–222. Online. Available: https://doi.org/10.1007/s12603-020-1310-y.

Bickenbach, J., 2019. A human rights perspective on work participation. In: Bültmann, U., Siegrist, J. (Eds), Handbook of disability, work and health. Springer International Publishing, pp. 1–15. Online. Available: https://doi.org/10.1007/978-3-319-75381-2_17-1.

Blum, R., Bastos, F., Kabiru, C., et al, 2012. Adolescent health in the 21st century. The Lancet, 379 (9826), 1567–1568. Online. Available: https://doi.org/10.1016/S0140-6736(12)60407-3.

Boen, C.E., Kozlowski, K., Tyson, K.D., 2020. 'Toxic' schools? How school exposures during adolescence influence trajectories of health through young adulthood. SSM—Population Health, 11, 100623. https://doi.org/10.1016/j.ssmph.2020.100623

Bowden, M., 2020. Understanding food insecurity in Australia. In: Child Family Community Australia Information Exchange (issue 55). Online. Available: https://aifs.gov.au/cfca/sites/default/files/publication-documents/2009_cfca_understanding_food_insecurity_in_australia.pdf.

BPAC, 2020. Recognising and managing early dementia (February issue). Online. Available: www.bpac.org.nz.

Brijnath, B., Gahan, L., Gaffy, E., et al, 2020. 'Build rapport, otherwise no screening tools in the world are going to help': Frontline service providers' views on current screening tools for elder abuse. Gerontologist, 60 (3), 472–482. Online. Available: https://doi.org/10.1093/geront/gny166.

Bundy, D.A.P., de Silva, N., Horton, S., et al, 2018. Optimizing education outcomes: High-return investments in school health for increased participation and learning. Disease Control Priorities, 8 (Child and Adolescent Health and Development), 265. International Bank for Reconstruction and Development / The World Bank, Washington. Online. Available: http://dcp-3.org/sites/default/files/resources/DCP3 Education Edition_Final.pdf?issu.

Clendon, J., Walker, L., 2016. The juxtaposition of ageing and nursing: The challenges and enablers of continuing to work in the latter stages of a nursing career. J Adv. Nurs., 72 (5), 1065–1074. Online. Available: https://doi.org/10.1111/jan.12896.

Collins, M., Posenelli, S., Cleak, H., et al, 2020. Elder abuse identification by an Australian health service: A five-year, social-work audit. Aust. Soc. Work, 73 (4), 462–476. Online. Available: https://doi.org/10.1080/0312407X.2020.1778050.

Comeau, D. J., Conklin, J., Huang, B., et al, 2020. Assessing the current state of food insecurity in New Zealand. Online. Available: www.rph.org.nz/public-health-topics/nutrition/kai-and-our-community/assessing-the-current-state-of-food-insecurity-in-new-zealand2.pdf.

Craswell, A., Wallis, M., Coates, K., et al, 2020. Enhanced primary care provided by a nurse practitioner candidate to aged care facility residents: A mixed methods study. Collegian, 27 (3), 281–287. Online. Available: https://doi.org/10.1016/j.colegn.2019.08.009.

Dahl, R.E., Allen, N.B., Wilbrecht, L., et al, 2018. Importance of investing in adolescence from a developmental science perspective. Nature (London), 554 (7693), 441–450. Online. Available: https://doi.org/10.1038/nature25770.

Davis, J., 2016. The rhetoric and reality of nursing in aged care: views from the inside. Contemporary Nurse: A Journal for the Australian Nursing Profession, 52 (2–3), p. 191.

Deloitte Access Economics, 2015. The economic value of informal care in Australia in 2015 (June issue). Online. Available: www2.deloitte.com/au/en/pages/economics/articles/economic-value-informal-care-Australia-2015.html.

DeMichelis, C., 2016. Relational resilience: An interdisciplinary perspective. In: DeMichelis, C., Ferrari, M. (Eds), Child and adolescent resilience within medical contexts: Integrating research and practice. Springer International Publishing, pp. 1–10.

Denny, S., Grant, S., Galbreath, R., et al, 2019. An observational study of adolescent health outcomes associated with school-based health service utilization: A causal analysis. Health Serv. Res., 54 (3), 678–688. Online. Available: https://doi.org/10.1111/1475-6773.13136.

Desjardins, J., 2017, June 6. The demographic timebomb: A rapidly aging population. Visual Capitalist. Online. Available: www.visualcapitalist.com/demographic-timebomb-rapidly-aging-population.

Dow, B., Gahan, L., Gaffy, E., et al, 2020. Barriers to disclosing elder abuse and taking action in Australia. J. Fam. Violence, 35 (8), 853–861. Online. Available: https://doi.org/10.1007/s10896-019-00084-w.

Eisenberg, M.E., Gower, A.L., Rider, G.N., et al, 2019. At the intersection of sexual orientation and gender identity: Variations in emotional distress and bullying experience in a large population-based sample of US adolescents. J. LGBT Youth, 16 (3), 235–254. Online. Available: https://doi.org/10.1080/19361653.2019.1567435.

Evans, K.L., Millsteed, J., Richmond, J.E., et al, 2019. The impact of within and between role experiences on role balance outcomes for working sandwich generation women. Scand. J. Occup. Ther., 26 (3), 184–193. Online. Available: https://doi.org/10.1080/11038128.2018.1449888.

Fleming, T.M., Gillham, B., Bavin, L.M., et al, 2019. SPARX-R computerized therapy among adolescents in youth offenders' program: Step-wise cohort study. Internet Interventions: The Application of Information Technology in Mental and Behavioural Health, 18, 100287. Online. Available: https://doi.org/10.1016/j.invent.2019.100287.

Fleming, T. M., Stasiak, K., Moselen, E., et al, 2019. Revising computerized therapy for wider appeal among adolescents: Youth perspectives on a revised version of SPARX. Front. Psychiatry, 10, 802. Online. Available: https://doi.org/10.3389/fpsyt.2019.00802.

Freer, K., 2020. Falling through the cracks: a case study of how a timely integrated approach can reverse frailty. Br. J. Community Nurs., 25 (8), 382–387. Online. Available: https://doi.org/10.12968/bjcn.2020.25.8.382.

Funaki-Tahifote, M., Fung, M., Timaloa, Y., et al, 2016. Better quality and reduced quantity in food/drinks in Pacific settings. Heart Foundation/Pacific Heartbeat, Auckland.

Gahan, L., Gaffy, E., Dow, B., et al, 2019. Advancing methodologies to increase end-user engagement with complex interventions: The case of co-designing the Australian elder abuse screening instrument (AuSI). J. Elder Abuse Negl., 31 (4/5), 325–339. Online. Available: https://doi.org/10.1080/08946566.2019.1682098.

Grimmond, D., 2014. The economic value and impacts of informal care in New Zealand. Infometrics, Wellington.

Hancock, S., Winterton, R., Wilding, C., et al, 2019. Understanding ageing well in Australian rural and regional settings: Applying an age-friendly lens. Aust. J. Rural Health, 27 (4), 298–303. Online. Available: https://doi.org/10.1111/ajr.12497.

Happell, B., Platania-Phung, C., 2019. Review and analysis of the Mental Health Nurse Incentive Program. Aust. Health Rev., 43 (1), 111–119. Online. Available: https://doi.org/10.1071/AH17017.

Ho, J., Fong, C.K., Iskander, A., et al, 2019. Digital psychosocial assessment: An efficient and effective screening tool. J. Paediatr. Child Health, 56, 521–531. Online. Available: https://doi.org/10.1111/jpc.14675.

Hullick, C.J., Hall, A.E., Conway, J.F., et al, 2021. Reducing hospital transfers from aged care facilities: A large-scale stepped wedge evaluation. J. Am. Geriatr. Soc., 69 (1), 201–209. Online. Available: https://doi.org/10.1111/jgs.16890.

Ilić Petković, A., Nikolić, V., 2020. Educational needs of employees in work-related stress management. Work, 65 (3), 661–669. Online. Available: https://doi.org/10.3233/WOR-203120.

Janke, M. C., Purnell, I., Watts, C., et al, 2019. Associations between engagement types, outcome behaviors, and quality of life for adults with dementia participating in intergenerational programs. Therapeutic Recreation Journal, 53 (2), 132–148. Online. Available: https://doi.org/10.18666/TRJ-2019-V53-I2-9647.

Jones, D., Randall, S., White, D., et al, 2021. Embedding public health advocacy into the role of school-based nurses: addressing the health inequities confronted by vulnerable Australian children and adolescent populations. Aust. J. Prim. Health, 27 (2), 67–70. Online. Available: https://doi.org/10.1071/PY20155.

Jones, M., Mills, D., Gray, R., 2020. Expecting the unexpected? Improving rural health in the era of bushfires, novel coronavirus and climate change. Aust. J. Rural Health, 28 (2), 107–109. Online. Available: https://doi.org/10.1111/ajr.12623.

Jonsson, J., Matilla-Santander, N., Kreshpaj, B., et al, 2021. Precarious employment and general, mental and physical health in Stockholm, Sweden: a cross-sectional study. Scand. J. Public Health, 49 (2), 228–236. Online. Available: https://doi.org/10.1177/1403494820956451.

Kaspiew, R., Carson, R., Rhoades, H., 2016. Elder abuse: Understanding issues, frameworks and responses. Online. Available: https://aifs.gov.au/publications/elder-abuse.

Kia Piki Ake Welfare Expert Advisory Group, 2019. Current state: Carers of people with health conditions or disabilities (February issue). Online. Available: www.weag.govt.nz/assets/documents/WEAG-report/background-documents/9513d6b9b0/Carers-of-HCD-010419.pdf.

Kiejda, J., 2020. Nurses are lifesavers for the elderly. Lamp, 77 (5), 8–9. Online. Available: https://thelamp.com.au/specialities/aged-care/nurses-are-lifesavers-for-the-elderly/.

Klein, D., Goldenring, J., Adelman, W., 2014. HEEADSSS 3.0: the psychosocial interview for adolescents updated for a new century fuelled by media. Contemp. Pediatr., 31, 16–28.

Kloep, M., Hendry, L., Taylor, R., et al, 2016. Development from adolescence to early adulthood: A dynamic systemic approach to transitions and transformations. Taylor-Francis e-Books. Online. Available: www.tandfebooks.com/isbn/9781315707952.

Kwa, J.-M., Storer, M., Ma, R., et al, 2021. Integration of inpatient and residential care in-reach service model and hospital resource utilization: A retrospective audit. J. Am. Med. Dir. Assoc., 22 (3), 670–675. Online. Available: https://doi.org/10.1016/j.jamda.2020.07.015.

Livingston, G., Huntley, J., Sommerlad, A., et al, 2020. Dementia prevention, intervention, and care: 2020 report of the Lancet Commission. The Lancet, 396 (10248), 413–446. Online. Available: https://doi.org/10.1016/S0140-6736(20)30367-6.

Malatest International, 2016. Evaluation of SPARX (February issue). Online. Available: www.health.govt.nz/system/files/documents/publications/evaluation-sparx-dec16.pdf.

Masten, A., Barnes, A., 2018. Resilience in children: Developmental perspectives. Children, 5 (7), 98. Online. Available: https://doi.org/10.3390/children5070098.

Mayo, C.D., Kenny, R., Scarapicchia, V., et al, 2021. Aging in place: Challenges of older adults with self-reported cognitive decline. Can. Geriatr. J., 24 (2), 138–143. Online. Available: https://doi.org/10.5770/cgj.24.456.

McCluskey, A.R., 2015. The formative evaluation of a practice framework for nurses working in secondary schools (July issue). Curtin University. Online. Available: https://espace.curtin.edu.au/bitstream/handle/20.500.11937/998/234319_McCluskey 2015.pdf?sequence=2&isAllowed=y.

McCullough, K., Whitehead, L., Bayes, S., et al, 2021. Remote area nursing: best practice or paternalism in action? The importance of consumer perspectives on primary health care nursing practice in remote communities. Aust. J. Prim. Health, 27 (1), 62–66. Online. Available: https://doi.org/10.1071/PY20089.

McMurray, A., Ward, L., Yang, L. (Rachel), et al, 2021. The Gold Coast Integrated Care programme: The perspectives of patients, carers, general practitioners and healthcare staff. Int. J. Integr. Care, 21 (2), 18, 1–15.

Milne, R., 2019, April 3. Demographic time-bomb: Finland sends a warning to Europe. Financial Times. Online. Available: www.ft.com/content/8ebb54bc-5528-11e9-91f9-b6515a54c5b1.

Ministry of Business, Innovation and Employment., 2021. Increasing the minimum sick leave entitlement. Business and Employment. Online. Available: www.mbie.govt.nz/business-and-employment/employment-and-skills/employment-legislation-reviews/increasing-minimum-sick-leave-entitlement/.

Ministry of Health, 2015. Suicide Prevention Toolkit for District Health Boards (February issue). Ministry of Health, Wellington. Online. Available: www.health.govt.nz/system/files/documents/publications/suicide-prevention-toolkit-for-dhbs-feb15_3-v3.pdf.

Ministry of Health, 2019. Household food insecurity among children: New Zealand health survey. Ministry of Health, Wellington. Online. Available: www.health.govt.nz/publication/household-food-insecurity-among-children-new-zealand-health-survey.

Morgan, E.H., Schoonees, A., Sriram, U., et al, 2020. Caregiver involvement in interventions for improving children's dietary intake and physical activity behaviors. Cochrane Database of Syst. Rev., 1. Online. Available: https://doi.org/10.1002/14651858.CD012547.pub2.

Muirhead, S., Birks, M., 2019. Roles of rural and remote registered nurses in Australia: an integrative review. Aust. J. Adv. Nurs., 37 (1), 21–33. Online. Available: www.ajan.com.au/index.php/AJAN/article/view/56.

National Scientific Council on the Developing Child, 2015. Supportive relationships and active skill-building strengthen the foundations of resilience: Working paper 13. Online. Available: http://developingchild.harvard.edu/wp-content/uploads/2015/05/The-Science-of-Resilience.pdf.

Office for Senior Citizens, 2015. Towards gaining a greater understanding of elder abuse and neglect in New Zealand (June issue). Online. Available: https://officeforseniors.govt.nz/assets/documents/our-work/elder-abuse/Elder-abuse-and-neglect-in-New-Zealand-summary-report.pdf.

Papadopoulou, C., Barrie, J., Andrew, M., et al, 2021. Perceptions, practices and educational needs of community nurses to manage frailty. Br. J. Community Nurs., 26 (3), 136–142. Online. Available: https://doi.org/10.12968/bjcn.2021.26.3.136.

Patton, G.C., Sawyer, S.M., Santelli, J.S., et al, 2017. Our future: a Lancet commission on adolescent health and wellbeing. The Lancet, 387 (10036), 2423–2478. Online. Available: https://doi.org/10.1016/S0140-6736(16)00579-1.

Pessoa Pousa, P.C., de Lucca, S.R., 2021. Psychosocial factors in nursing work and occupational risks: a systematic review. Revista Brasileira de Enfermagem, 74, 1–7. Online. Available: https://doi.org/10.1590/0034-7167-2020-0198.

Phelan, A., 2016. Exploring nursing expertise in residential care for older people: A mixed method study. J. Adv. Nurs. 72 (10), p. 2524.

Raphael, D., 2019. Social determinants of health. In: Raphael, D., Bryant, T., Rioux, M. (Eds), Staying alive: Critical perspectives on health, illness, and health care, third ed., Canadian Scholars. pp. 138–170.

Read, S.T., Toye, C., Wynaden, D., 2021. A qualitative exploration of family carer's understandings of people with dementia's expectations for the future. Dementia, 20 (4), 1284–1299. Online. Available: https://doi.org/10.1177/1471301220929543.

Reichard, A., Stransky, M., Brucker, D., et al, 2019. The relationship between employment and health and health care among working-age adults with and without disabilities in the United States. Disabil. Rehabil., 41 (19), 2299–2307. Online. Available: https://doi.org/10.1080/09638288.2018.1465131.

Rosenberg, B., 2018. Precarity in Aotearoa/New Zealand. Kotuitui, 1–4. Online. Available: https://doi.org/10.1080/1177083X.2018.1447491.

Saif-Ur-Rahman, K.M., Mamun, R., Eriksson, E., et al, 2021. Discrimination against the elderly in health-care services: a systematic review. Psychogeriatrics, 21 (3), 418–429. Online. Available: https://doi.org/10.1111/psyg.12670.

Shpakou, A., Klimatckaia, L., Kuzniatsou, A., et al, 2021. Medical care and manifestations of ageism in healthcare institutions: opinion of elderly people. The example of four countries. Fam. Med. Prim. Care Rev., 23 (1), 69–74. Online. Available: https://doi.org/10.5114/fmpcr.2021.103159.

Sigahi, T.F.A.C, Kawasaki, B.C., Bolis, I., et al, 2021. A systematic review on the impacts of COVID-19 on work: Contributions and a path forward from the perspectives of ergonomics and psychodynamics of work. Human Factors and Ergonomics in Manufacturing & Service Industries, 31 (4), 375–388.

Smith, G.L., McGuinness, T.M., 2017. Adolescent psychosocial assessment: The HEEADSSS. J. Psychosoc. Nurs. Ment. Health Serv., 55 (5), 24–27. Online. Available: https://doi.org/10.3928/02793695-20170420-03.

Somers, M.J., Casal, J., 2021. Patterns of coping with work-related stress: A person-centred analysis with text data. Stress. Health, 37 (2), 223–231. Online. Available: https://doi.org/10.1002/smi.2990.

Spann, A., Vicente, J., Allard, C., et al, 2020. Challenges of combining work and unpaid care, and solutions: A scoping review. Health Soc. Care Community, 28 (3), 699–715. Online. Available: https://doi.org/10.1111/hsc.12912.

Speers, D., 2020. A case is mounting for paid pandemic leave. But it won't be a silver bullet. ABC News. August. Online. Available: www.abc.net.au/news/2020-08-02/coronavirus-pandemic-leave-no-silver-bullet-for-economy/12511550.

Stevenson, J.M., Davies, J.G., Martin, F.C., 2020. Medication-related harm: A geriatric syndrome. Age & Ageing, 49 (1), 7–11. Online. Available: https://doi.org/10.1093/ageing/afz121.

Stimpfel, A.W., 2020. Shift work and sleep disruption: Implications for nurses' health. Am. Nurse Today, 15 (11), 23–25. Online. Available: www.myamericannurse.com/wp-content/uploads/2020/09/an11-Shiftwork-1023.pdf.

Tomlinson, M., Hunt, X., Daelmans, B., et al, 2021. Optimising child and adolescent health and development through an integrated ecological life course approach. BMJ (Online), 372, m4784. Online. Available: https://doi.org/10.1136/bmj.m4784.

United Nations, 2016. The global strategy for women's, children's and adolescents' health 2016–2030: Survive, thrive, transform. Online. Available: https://doi.org/10.1017/CBO9781107415324.004.

United Nations, 2019. World population prospects 2019. In: Department of Economic and Social Affairs. World Population Prospects 2019 (Issue 141). United Nations. Online. Available: www.ncbi.nlm.nih.gov/pubmed/12283219.

Weiss, H.A., Ferrand, R.A., 2019. Improving adolescent health: an evidence-based call to action. The Lancet, 393 (10176), pp. 1073–1075. Online. Available: https://doi.org/10.1016/S0140-6736(18)32996-9.

World Health Organization (WHO), 2015. Guideline: Sugars intake for adults and children. World Health Organization 57 (6). WHO, Geneva.

World Health Organization (WHO), 2018a. Ageing and health. WHO, Geneva. Online. Available: www.who.int/news-room/fact-sheets/detail/ageing-and-health.

World Health Organization (WHO), 2018b. Global action plan on physical activity 2018–2030: More active people for a healthier world. https://apps.who.int/iris/bitstream/handle/10665/272722/9789241514187-eng.pdf.

World Health Organization (WHO), 2020a. Dementia. WHO, Geneva. Online. Available: www.who.int/news-room/fact-sheets/detail/dementia.

World Health Organization (WHO), 2020b. Elder abuse. Online. Available: www.who.int/news-room/fact-sheets/detail/elder-abuse.

World Health Organization (WHO), 2020c. Physical activity. Online. Available: www.who.int/news-room/fact-sheets/detail/physical-activity.

World Health Organization (WHO), 2020d. The top ten causes of death. Online. Available: www.who.int/es/news-room/fact-sheets/detail/the-top-10-causes-of-death.

World Health Organization & UNICEF, 2021. Helping Adolescents Thrive Toolkit: Strategies to promote and protect adolescent mental health and reduce self-harm and other risk behaviours. Online. Available: www.who.int/publications/i/item/9789240025554.

Yahfoufi, N., Matar, C., Ismail, N., 2020. Adolescence and aging: impact of adolescence inflammatory stress and microbiota alterations on brain development, aging, and neurodegeneration. Journals of Gerontology Series A: Biological Sciences & Medical Sciences, 75 (7), 1251–1257. Online. Available: https://doi.org/10.1093/gerona/glaa006.

Zanetos, J.M., Skipper, A.W., 2020. The effects of health care policies: LGBTQ aging adults. J. Gerontol. Nurs., 46 (3), 9–13. Online. Available: https://doi.org/10.3928/00989134-20200203-02.

Zinn, M.E., Huntley, E.D., Keating, D.P., 2020. Resilience in adolescence: Prospective Self moderates the association of early life adversity with externalizing problems. J. Adolesc., 81, 61–72. Online. Available: https://doi.org/10.1016/j.adolescence.2020.04.004.

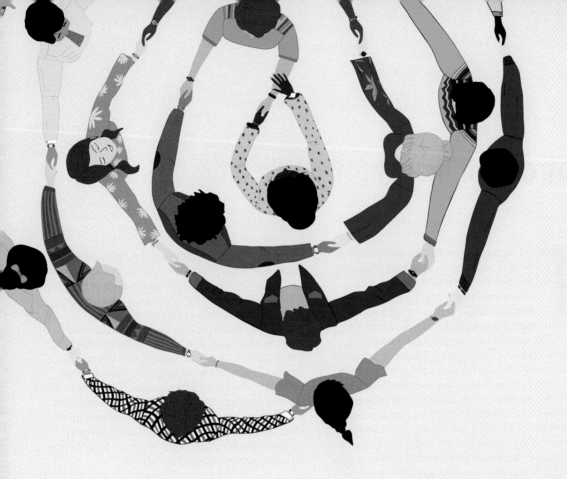

Section 4

Evidence to support primary health care

Introduction to the section

This section begins with an explanation of what is meant by an inclusive community and society, and how these concepts are integral to primary health care. Social inclusion and social exclusion lie at two ends of the same continuum. Along this continuum, people have varying opportunities to achieve health. As mentioned in Chapter 1, social exclusion leaves many members of society without the support and resources they need for health and wellbeing. Social inclusion creates social capital, trust, resilience, norms of reciprocity and cohesion; the essence of a healthy community. These vital elements of community life are important to any discussion of the power relations that exist in society and are our primary focus in Chapter 9. The first part of the chapter focuses on gender before moving onto cultural inclusiveness. Gender is identified as a separate social determinant of health, yet the gender relationships in a family and community may be intensified by the intersection of racial or ethnic issues, family conflict, societal norms of behaviour, migration experiences and gender identity. The chapter unravels the issues inherent in gender, culture and power relationships that impinge on the health and wellbeing of communities and those who live in them before moving on to explore the need for communities to provide the foundations for cultural safety, especially in relation to Indigenous people's health, risk and potential. International reports indicate that there has been some progress in redressing the culturally constructed inequities in societies that have left a legacy of illness, injury and disability among Indigenous people. New initiatives have been developed within the auspices of the World Health Organization's Commission on the Social Determinants of Health, and at a national level, Closing the Gap initiatives in Australia and New Zealand. Yet cultural disadvantage is socially embedded, and the barriers to equality of opportunity and equity of outcomes are well known. Redressing the psychosocial conditions that create disadvantage is a matter of urgency. We therefore focus on Indigenous people's health as a critical element of cultural inclusiveness. Our discussion revolves around the need to share both the risks and the wisdom of each of our nations with one another for mutual benefit and capacity enhancement. The end-point of the chapter is a renewed call to create an ethos of community and social life built on equitable foundations. Perhaps with cross-fertilisation of good ideas, and the cautionary tales of barriers to equity, we can draw into clearer focus strategies for achieving inclusive communities and social justice.

Chapter 10 provides an exploration of research, its major elements and strategies and where we need to fill gaps in our knowledge base for translating evidence into practice. Evidence-based practice is outlined as important to informing community health strategies, but evidence is generated and used in many forms. Everyone working with communities has some level of obligation to be research-minded, and to embrace the trend towards knowledge translation (KT), ensuring research findings are adopted in practice. We have undertaken a major scan of the nursing and midwifery publications over the past several years to develop a sense of what gaps remain in the growing knowledge base for community practice. Reporting on this body of knowledge in Chapter 10 is intended to inspire further participation in research by practitioners as well as students. When research is integral to planning, implementing and evaluating the merits of community-level interventions, we will all be speaking in a language that helps create enthusiasm for change, and incremental development of rational, justified and defensible community health and wellbeing policies and strategies.

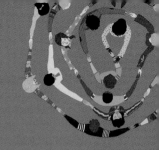

CHAPTER 9
Inclusive communities

Introduction

This chapter focuses on gender, culture and power. Our attention is directed to how gender and culture influence the ways in which people approach and receive healthcare and on how we as health practitioners can work to ensure equity and inclusion for all people. The first part of the chapter focuses on gender and the second on culture.

Attention to gender issues is important for several reasons. Gender is a pivotal social determinant of health (SDH) and instrumental to socioeconomic position (SEP). A person's gender can determine the extent to which they have opportunities to achieve health and wellbeing. People are also assigned relatively different positions in society depending on their gender, particularly in being granted differential education, work opportunities or social support.

Gender influences can be cumulative along the life course. As individuals develop along the critical pathways from birth to older age, gender, like other SDH, shapes not only biology, but experiences and opportunities that become reinforced over time. Because men and women occupy different social positions in the household, workplace and community, they are exposed to different risks and potential. Along the pathways of women's and men's life course, gender differences are apparent at every stage, and this is the case in different countries and contexts. These gender differences interact with other life circumstances to create complex webs of factors affecting health and wellbeing.

Culture provides a different marker for inclusiveness with the most compelling indicator of an inclusive society being the respect conferred on its Indigenous people. Yet, in many countries of the

OBJECTIVES

By the end of this chapter you will be able to:

1 discuss the importance of social inclusion and its relevance to primary health care

2 describe the role of equity in the health of individuals, communities and societies

3 describe the impact of gender influences on health and wellbeing

4 explain the influence of culture on health and social justice

5 define cultural safety as a concept and explain its relevance and importance in the provision of healthcare

6 prioritise a set of goals for primary health care practice when working with diverse communities.

world Indigenous people are treated as outsiders, the 'other' in relation to the dominant culture. This lack of cultural inclusiveness has an enormous impact on their health and wellbeing, and in some cases, determines whether an Indigenous person is able to live a long life in harmony with the natural and spiritual environment, or suffer premature mortality. In many places, cultural exclusiveness divides citizens by race, ethnicity or affiliation, igniting oppressive actions that, at worst, include violent exchanges and civil wars. In other places, cultural exclusion is more subtle and often manifests as unconscious bias expressed in racist attitudes, thinly veiled arrogance and dominant forms of exclusive language. Unconscious bias and previously conscious bias have resulted in the formation of systems, policies and processes that are fundamentally racist and disadvantage people further. Over time, those who are disadvantaged by ethnicity, race or affiliation lose not only opportunities to live vibrant, healthy lives, but their sense of place in the world and in the community. As time goes by, dispossession and hopelessness pervade all aspects of life, and create a self-fulfilling prophecy of vulnerability to ill health and incapacity to change.

The community is an ideal place to address inequities that arise from social and cultural exclusion, particularly in the process of unravelling constraints and facilitating factors involved in developing capacity. Gender and cultural equity and differential access to childhood education, health literacy, prevention, care and economic opportunities are pivotal to community development, community competence and building social capital. Support for equity must therefore begin in the community; otherwise, in this rapidly changing global world, civilisations will grow stagnant. To flourish, societies need to address the way power and social inclusion interact with the SDH, and to seek ways of creating more harmonious, socially just communities.

KEY POINT

The most compelling mark of an inclusive society is the respect conferred on its Indigenous people.

Part 1: Equity, inequality, social exclusion, gender, culture and power

Social exclusion plays an important role in the relationship between many of the SDH and poor health. Socially excluded people are unable to access opportunities to become educated, earn a living, receive social support for their personal needs, live in safe houses and neighbourhoods with a secure food supply and a viable physical environment, raise their children in a non-violent home, cultivate friendships or participate in social and political life.

When people are excluded from full participation in social life, the effects prevent societal development by inhibiting them from reaching their full potential. For example, children living in a jobless household grow up with the risk of becoming socially excluded through a lack of education and other opportunities to change the course of their lives, which can lead to intergenerational poverty. Women confined to physical work from an early age, such as occurs in many developing countries, are socially excluded by virtue of having no opportunities to become educated or to change their status or that of their children. Men working in isolated circumstances may be socially excluded because they have few opportunities to find a partner, raise a family or gain employment in a geographic area with social amenities. Members of sexually diverse minorities such as lesbian, gay, bisexual, transgender/transsexual, queer, intersex, asexual, takatāpui and fa'afafine (LGBTQIA+) groups are at particular risk of social exclusion, and because of the dominance of our Western health and education systems, cultural minorities are often socially excluded from some of the most significant aspects of social life, with profound negative impacts on their health and wellbeing. People with impairments can also be excluded from social participation on the basis of a perceived lack of capabilities. Although social exclusion can arise from a lack of capabilities, it is often the result of a denial of resources, rights, goods and services that are available to the majority of people in society. Clearly, there is a mandate for health and social service practitioners to work towards overcoming social exclusion to promote equity and cohesion in community life. One way in which this can be achieved is by documenting inclusion. The Inclusive Australia Social Inclusion Index focuses on five key aspects of social inclusion:

1 sense of belonging and wellbeing
2 prejudicial attitudes and experiences of discrimination
3 amount and quality of contact with people from minority groups
4 willingness to volunteer in inclusion activities
5 willingness to advocate for social inclusion (Faulkner et al 2019).

The Index covers a wide variety of social inclusion issues in order to capture a 'big picture' view of inclusion in Australia rather than focusing on one particular group as has traditionally been the case (Faulkner et al 2019). The tool enables Australia to track progress and evaluate initiatives designed to improve social inclusiveness and address social exclusion. The latest findings show that Australia still has some way to go to improve inclusion. Nearly one in four Australians had recently experienced a form of major discrimination which in turn was associated with lower wellbeing. Further, although most Australians are not highly prejudiced, 27% still expressed high levels of prejudice against religious and racial minority groups (Faulkner et al 2019).

KEY POINT

Gender, culture, disability or any point of social 'difference' can lead to social exclusion, which is detrimental to health and wellbeing.

Cultural norms can play a major role in social exclusion, particularly in ascribing roles on the basis of gender. Gender differences are grounded in biology, but they are enacted within different social and cultural constructions of roles, norms, behaviours, activities and attributes that are considered appropriate for men and women (Seeta Prabhu & Iyer 2019). Simply put, sex is a biological attribute and gender is a social construct. Gender equality refers to equal opportunities for men and women to enjoy socially valued goods, opportunities, resources and rewards, whereas gender equity recognises and addresses the historical and contemporary disadvantages women face in society that may limit access to these opportunities (Seeta Prabhu & Iyer 2019). Inequitable societies place many women at risk through legal, religious or cultural norms that treat women as productive chattels to care for the household but with little decision-making over their life, health, sexuality and fertility. Even in relatively equitable societies there are differences in the social expectations of masculine and feminine roles, which typically privilege men in the home and workplace (Rees & Wells 2020, Sorrentino et al 2019). The differential expectations and inequalities are manifest in power imbalances created from social pressures to conform to gender roles.

KEY POINT

Gender comprises a set of socio-culturally constructed roles and norms of behaviour for men and women.

Life experiences demonstrate patterns of gendered expectations that have changed little in terms of marriage and family life. Trends in marriage and child-rearing have seen dual-earner families become the norm, with many women choosing to work. However, other women are socially excluded from this mix of work–home lifestyle because of economic circumstances or lack of access to opportunities. Others have greater freedom to choose lifestyles but social norms create pressure on women to nurture, and on men to be breadwinners. Employers also shape understandings of gender by providing greater opportunities to men in the workplace, because of their role as a family provider or on the assumption that men have better management skills. This situation creates job insecurity and lower promotional opportunities for many women, who tend to work flexible schedules to meet home and workplace needs. This became particularly obvious in both Australia and New Zealand during the COVID-19 pandemic where women were more likely to lose their jobs, experienced increased rates of family violence and were frequently required to manage children and work at home (Ayittey et al 2020, Rees & Wells 2020). Factors such as sexism (gender discrimination), the predominance of women in low-paying industries, different working hours and different occupations contribute to a large pay gap between men and women (Boniol et al 2019, Sin et al 2018). The gap in workplace pay and participation between men and women is a significant global problem and achieving gender equality is one of the World Health Organization's (WHO) sustainable development goals. The Australian Government has established the Workplace Gender Equality Agency in an attempt to support organisations and businesses to address the gender pay gap and achieve equality. The gap in pay has substantial long-term impacts on women. As women in the workplace approach retirement, they also discover a gender gap between income and retirement savings, affecting their ability to enjoy retirement to the same degree as their male counterparts. Divorce, widowhood and single parenthood can compound the impact of the gender pay gap (Workplace Equality Agency 2020). A video that describes how the gender pay gap occurs can be found at www.youtube.com/watch?v= gP1aA7GgUvc&t=108s.

Where to find out more on ...

Gender pay gap

- Australia: www.wgea.gov.au
- New Zealand: http://women.govt.nz/work-skills/income/gender-pay-gap

WOMEN'S HEALTH ISSUES

Women's health issues are influenced by many factors: childbirth, gender-linked health conditions including unique reproductive health risks, women's health behaviours and their longevity and social position relative to men. Women's innate constitution gives them an advantage over men in terms of life expectancy, but living longer is a double-edged sword, with older women suffering from chronic diseases for more years of their lives compared with men (Tarricone & Riecher-Rössler 2019). Gender inequality and discrimination results in greater risks from unintended pregnancy, sexually transmitted infections including human immunodeficiency virus (HIV), cervical cancer, malnutrition, lower levels of literacy, interpersonal violence and poorer access to health services (WHO 2021a).

In Australia and New Zealand, leading mortality risks for women are cardiovascular disease, cancer and dementia (Australian Institute of Health and Welfare [AIHW] 2021c, New Zealand Ministry of Health 2019). Gender differences lie in the fact that women's symptoms may be different from those of men's. There are biological differences in areas such as medication regimens because women metabolise some medications differently, and hormone fluctuations vary across the lifespan and eventually result in significant risk of bone loss and loss of muscle mass in post-menopausal women (Tilstra et al 2020). Indigenous women in particular suffer a disproportionate burden of diseases, including those related to pregnancy and childbirth (Ministry of Health and Minister of Health 2020). In their later years, women also experience a higher burden of dementia and other cognitive disorders, primarily because of their longevity (AIHW 2021c).

Another disadvantage arises from the fact that women's medical treatments often show marked differences from the way men's health is managed. Women's screening for illnesses is also different to men's and women are less likely to be treated according to guideline-indicated therapies, such as cardiac rehabilitation programs, despite evidence indicating the advantages of such programs (Tarricone & Riecher-Rössler 2019). These disparities have been linked to medical practitioners' differential interpretation of guidelines, the gender of the practitioner and attentiveness to the gender of the patient (Tarricone & Riecher-Rössler 2019). Women in rural areas can also be disadvantaged by the lack of specialist practitioners to help in dealing with family planning or pregnancy issues, and are more frequently exposed to interpersonal violence but less likely to be screened by their primary provider (Turshen 2020).

Some practitioners have little understanding of the cross-cultural differences in women's experience of health. For example, a study in New Zealand found that when an alert system was implemented in general practice, designed to flag if a patient was at risk of harm due to a preexisting medical condition or current medication, clinicians took less action for women, with the authors attributing this to the status of women in society (Leitch et al 2021). Because many Indigenous cultures tend to see 'women's business' as private, issues such as menstrual health and hygiene and menopause frequently go unnoticed or unreported (Krusz et al 2019). One in 12 young women in New Zealand miss school due to period poverty, or the inability to afford menstrual products (Artz 2021). Non-attendance at school impacts educational outcomes, disadvantaging young women due to factors beyond their control. As a result, New Zealand introduced free sanitary products in schools in 2021 and Australia removed the goods and services tax from menstrual hygiene products in an attempt to rectify this inequity. Women's mental health also suffers from the combination of lack of understanding and inability to access a range of treatments. In some cases, Indigenous women are under-diagnosed with mental ill health due to the high acuity and prevalence of conditions such as postnatal depression being considered as normal in their population.

KEY POINT

Women's global disadvantage

- Unequal power relationships
- Social norms impinging on their opportunities
- Focus on reproductive roles
- Physical, sexual, emotional violence

Globally, human trafficking, lack of education, poverty, war, refugee status and cultural norms such as female genital mutilation (FGM) have a profound impact on the health of women. Women are also more vulnerable to the effects of climate change as they are more likely to live in poverty, are less able to relocate when their community is imperilled by weather events or disasters and face systemic violence that increases during periods of instability (Lee et al 2021, McCarthy 2020). The irony is that women have been identified as important participants and leaders in addressing climate change but the narrative around women and climate change continues to portray them as victims (Lee et al 2021, Lewis 2016). Gender inequity remains one of the most important contributors to global health and must remain a key focus in our endeavours to improve wellbeing (Horton 2019). As health practitioners, we can advocate for women to be involved at all levels of climate change mitigation and support work towards achieving the sustainable development goals (see Chapters 2 and 3). We can also be aware of the particular experiences of refugee and migrant women who may be experiencing severe trauma from their lives previous to arriving in Australia or New Zealand including FGM and posttraumatic stress disorder. Such women may be more prone to family violence due to the challenges of settling into a new country with a new culture and away from traditional family support systems. As health practitioners, our obligation to these women is to work with other members of the healthcare team to help them through the multiple transitions, supporting the women and their families in achieving health and wellbeing at as high a standard as possible. Community nurses encounter these women in the context of home visiting, child and school health centres, neighbourhood or community groups, or in specialised community centres for victims of torture and trauma, including women who have been trafficked. Nurses must be wary of imposing Western ideals of healthcare, parenting and maternity on migrant mothers. Ways in which nurses traditionally provide care to the individual may paradoxically disempower migrant women whose collective ideals may differ from those of their care providers (DeSouza 2013). Cultural adaptation of an intervention where it is modified to become more suitable to a migrant population can be a successful way of improving outcomes for migrant women. Adaptation of the Healthy Beginnings early obesity prevention program for Arabic and Chinese mothers in Australia is one example where cultural adaptation has been used to modify an existing program, with the adapted program drawing on experiences of migrant women to ensure the program is culturally safe for participants and avoids imposing Western approaches to healthcare (Marshall et al 2021).

Where to find out more on ...

Refugee and migrant women

Australia

- Forced Migration Research Network: www.unsw.edu.au/arts-design-architecture/our-schools/social-sciences/our-research/research-networks/forced-migration-research-network
- Refugee Health Network of Australia: www.refugeehealthaustralia.org
- Refugee Council of Australia: www.refugeecouncil.org.au/getfacts/settlement/livinghere/health

New Zealand

- Auckland Regional Public Health Service Refugee Health Service: www.refugeehealth.govt.nz
- Refugee Council of New Zealand: http://rc.org.nz

A lack of education is a major risk to women's health. In every region of the world, educating girls is the single most powerful way to promote equitable personal opportunities, and pathways to health and wellbeing. It is also good for the economy, with a flow-on effect for building social cohesion. Women with access to education tend to marry later than uneducated women. They have smaller families, make better use of antenatal and delivery care and understand how to use family planning methods. They seek medical care sooner in the event of illness, maintain higher nutritional standards and raise their daughters to receive sufficient education to keep the cycle of health improvements moving in a positive direction (Schrader-King 2021). Educated women typically have the level of health literacy to retain control over their reproductive function. They understand the issues involved, the presence of risk and the steps that need to be taken to ensure health and safety for them and their babies. It is also widely accepted that education prepares mothers in developing early, enhanced child-rearing practices, which affects their children's lifelong potential. However, education alone cannot completely prevent a gender gap in terms of women's professional lives and levels of pay (see earlier).

KEY POINT

Educating girls is the single most powerful way to promote equitable personal opportunities and pathways to health and wellbeing in any country.

MEN'S HEALTH ISSUES

Like women's health, men's health is created in the context of the SDH. Sometimes these determinants go unrecognised, especially when it comes to the socially determined differences between men and women. It is far easier for most people to relate to men's and women's health in terms of biological factors, categorising health and health needs in terms of their respective reproductive systems or body parts, instead of socially constructed patterns of behaviours. Images of health and wellbeing are also socially engineered by the media. These images disguise reality, by portraying biologically perfect specimens doing exciting things or, in complete contrast, images of young people engaged in a wide range of antisocial acts. Little wonder that those on the verge of developing their gender identity are uncertain of where to find role models.

KEY POINT

Men's behaviours are due to a combination of social and cultural expectations regarding expectations of the 'male ideal'.

Basically put, men have poorer health status than women. In both Australia and New Zealand, men are more likely to engage in risky behaviours and die sooner than women. Since the 1970s, reasons for this disparity beyond biological or physiological explanations have revolved around gender roles, ideologies and norms (Ashraf et al 2021, Courtenay 2000, Salgado et al 2019). Courtenay (2000) argues that social and institutional structures help to sustain and reproduce men's health risks and the social construction of men as the stronger sex. These structures reproduce a *hegemonic* view of gender; that is, that men are dominant over women in society due to the historical social and institutional structures that placed men in a position of power over women. Gender, as an SDH, is one of the most significant influences on health-related behaviour for men, as well as for women, yet common perceptions of gender as a social determinant revolve around women's health. The way men negotiate gender roles actually creates *higher* health risks for many men as compared to women. Their elevated risk of some of the most prevalent conditions, such as cardiovascular disease, type 2 diabetes and mental illness, is linked to a cluster of unhealthy lifestyle behaviours that many men see as synonymous with masculinity. These are the deadly risks of smoking, drinking and driving, unhealthy diets, avoiding exercise and emotional help or screening for various conditions. However, recent research shows that masculinity can also result in health protective behaviours and that health-related interventions that focus on men's emotional expressiveness, address heterosexist and sexist attitudes and account for aspects of masculinity may be helpful (Salgado et al 2019).

Besides notions of the 'male ideal', men's lifestyles are also determined by their SEP on the social gradient. Rurality or remoteness, limited help-seeking behaviours and poor health literacy contribute further to the premature mortality, injury and disease incidence and prevalence among men (AIHW 2019b). COVID-19 threw into stark contrast the difference between men's and women's health outcomes with men 2.4 times more likely to die from COVID-19 than females irrespective of age or comorbidities (Baker 2020, Carson 2020). The likely causes of the disparity include immunological differences in response to the virus, underlying comorbidities, greater prevalence of smoking and the possibility that men were less concerned about the pandemic than women and potentially more prone to associated risk-taking behaviours (Baker 2020, Carson 2020).

To some extent, men's unhealthy behaviours are due to the greater social pressure to conform, relative to women. Conforming to the male ideal means a man sees himself as not only strong, but independent, in control, self-reliant, robust and tough (Salgado et al 2019). Although some behaviours are shaped by ethnicity, social class and sexuality, most men also take unnecessary risks to assert their masculine side. They brag about resisting the need for sick leave from work, boast that drinking does not impair their driving and dismiss the need for preventative healthcare, all aimed at maintaining their ranking among other men (Salgado et al 2019). Illness is not masculine, so they tend to ignore anything that does not seem to be life-threatening.

The social construction of masculinity does not negate biological differences, but there are several other important social and cultural determinants of men's health. Men have more intentional and non-intentional injuries than women, particularly Indigenous men. They die younger than women, with three times as many young men (four times as many young Indigenous men) dying from suicide than women (AIHW 2021a, 2021b). Like women, the main cause of death among Australian and New Zealand men is cardiovascular disease (AIHW 2019b, Ministry of Health and Minister of Health 2020). The cluster of major risk factors for men's ill health includes obesity, physical inactivity, alcohol and substance abuse, tobacco smoking, injuries and violence. These risk factors, combined with hereditary predisposition and social disadvantage, lead to high rates of type 2 diabetes (especially in those over the age of 55), cardiovascular disease, cancers and depression (AIHW 2019b, Ministry of Health and Minister of Health 2020). Men are also disproportionately represented in workplace injury statistics, especially in construction, mining and, in New Zealand, forestry.

Psychological health is also a different experience for men and women. Depression is a problem for

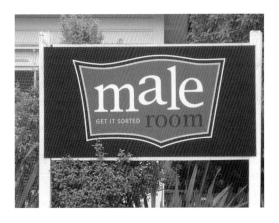

Figure 9.1 The Male Room is a drop-in centre for men, providing counselling and other mental health services.

Source: Photo courtesy of Jill Clendon.

many young people, but girls tend to seek help more readily than young males do. Men are more likely to use illicit drugs than women are—in particular methamphetamine (AIHW 2019b). For indicators of psychological health, such as self-esteem, men tend to be favoured, but in the web of factors comprising mental health, men's risks are greater. (See Fig 9.1.)

The social pressures of masculinity, especially in socially dictated norms and roles, create conditions that see many men disadvantaged in relationships. Men hesitate to talk about sensitive issues which are often seen as damaging to their identity (Herron et al 2020, Salgado et al 2019). Their hesitancy to disclose stress or other psychological problems is a major problem for rural men, who have few sources of community support. Men in rural and remote areas are at significant risk of suicide (Herron et al 2020).

Depression is the major risk factor for suicide and, in men, it is often less likely to be diagnosed (Armstrong et al 2020). Depression can manifest in aggressive behaviour, obsession about work, substance abuse, destructive thoughts and refusal to seek help. Behind these behaviours may be vulnerabilities that are not well understood, including experience of postnatal depression

(Wynter et al 2019). This context of mental ill health has thus far been virtually ignored in the healthcare system. Similarly, attention to the psychological and physical health of single fathers has been overlooked, yet the same factors of low income, unemployment, social isolation and childcare affect both men and women as single heads of the household. Men's psychological health is further jeopardised by a lack of appropriate counselling services, especially those that could address the constellation of determinants that shape men's lives. Whereas women-only services have been developed to help women feel comfortable in treatment and screening, equivalent services for men have yet to emerge and, where they do exist, they are often provided to address deficiencies, such as sexual dysfunction clinics. The exception is 'Men's Sheds', which have evolved in tandem with the men's health movement to encourage safe spaces for men to interact and share emotional as well as physical issues, with demonstrable improvements in social inclusion, health promotion and mental health among men who attend (Culph et al 2015, Wilson et al 2019).

KEY POINT

Depression may manifest itself among men in different ways to women. Health practitioners need to be able to recognise male-specific symptoms and risk situations in order to be able to provide appropriate care.

Men's and women's health policies

Australia has developed both men's and women's health policies to ensure the health needs of both groups are addressed. Both have a core focus on the SDH and addressing immediate and future health challenges. Addressing health inequities is also key. New Zealand does not have policies specific to men's or women's health. The country does, however, have a Ministry for Women. The Ministry for Women, Manatū Wāhine, has a key role in providing policy advice on improving outcomes for women in New Zealand. There is no men's equivalent. One of the most important elements of any health policy is to ensure it is making a difference for the people it is intended to help. Health policy evaluation is discussed in detail in Chapter 2.

Where to find out more on …

Health policy and research

- Australian Men's health policy: www.health. gov.au/resources/publications/national-mens-health-policy-2010#
- Australian Men's health research: www. tentomen.org.au
- Australian Women's health policy: www. health.gov.au/resources/publications/national-womens-health-policy-2010
- Australian Women's health research: https:// alswh.org.au
- New Zealand women: http://women.govt.nz

Gender issues among sexually diverse populations

Lesbian, gay, bisexual, transgender/transsexual, queer, intersex, asexual, takatāpui, fa'afafine (LGBTQIA+) populations face a variety of healthcare disparities, frequently because they are marginalised in many Western societies such as our own, by discrimination and social exclusion. Although each of these groups have distinctive and specific needs unique to that group, as a whole, they have an additional illness burden related to their sexual identities and expressions. The socially patterned discrimination and heteronormative structures that dominate society lead to heightened risks of violence, harassment, suicide, emotional distress, chronic stress, decreased physical and mental health, social invisibility and marginalisation (Eisenberg et al 2019, Siverskog & Bromseth 2019). Population studies in the United Kingdom, the United States, Australia and New Zealand indicate that LGBTQIA+ people have higher rates of certain chronic illnesses, cancers, mental health issues, alcohol, tobacco and other drug abuse, body dysmorphia, disordered eating practices and sexually transmitted infections such as human immunodeficiency virus (HIV) (Donald & Ehrenfeld 2015, Perales 2019). The minority stress model contends that stigmatism, discrimination and prejudice explain many of these differences in health and wellbeing (Perales 2019). Health conditions are also exacerbated by lower levels of access to health services that are appropriate and culturally and gender sensitive (Alba et al 2020, Donald & Ehrenfeld 2015). Members of the community often choose not to disclose their gender identity or sexual orientation to avoid being stereotyped, stigmatised or treated in a prejudicial or discriminatory manner (Grant & Walker 2020). Lack of recognition of the fluidity of gender identity and sexual attraction can also create barriers to comprehensive, individualised care. Worse still, in some cases, members of sexual minorities are refused care, or have their needs dismissed by health practitioners, which creates a lack of trust in the health system and perpetuates the disparities that they have experienced throughout their lives (Kuzma et al 2019).

The past few years have seen growing acceptance of gender difference within many communities and that acceptance is becoming increasingly visible. For example, people's email signatures that include their identifying pronouns are becoming increasingly common. More widely adopted language to describe gender and sexual identity such as asexual, pansexual and cisgender are becoming commonplace. These conversations encourage acceptance and inclusion of LGBTQIA+ individuals and families within communities. There is still much to be done to overcome the health effects of long-term stigmatisation and discrimination among this group, but a start has been made.

Where to find out more on …

Gender definitions

- www.transstudent.org/definitions/

School nurses are an important source of support and empowerment for children and young people who identify as LGBTQIA+ or whose parents identify as such. The children of sexually diverse parents can also experience discrimination regardless of their own sexual orientation and gender identity. Many do not identify as LGBTQIA+, but spend their lives concealing the sexual orientation or gender identity of their parents as a way of preventing bullying or overt discrimination. School nurses can help children and young people maintain perspective and mental health. They also play an important role in encouraging inclusiveness in the wider school environment and helping non-diverse peers recognise the value of diversity within a school.

Where to find out more on …

The health and wellbeing of gender-diverse people in Australia

- http://lgbtihealth.org.au

Supporting LGBTQIA+ young people in New Zealand

- https://insideout.org.nz

Mental health issues have a major impact on the lives of sexually diverse people. Institutionalised and interpersonal discrimination increases vulnerability to mental illness and distress and the LGBTQIA+ populations experience some of the poorest mental health outcomes of any group (Eisenberg et al 2019). Because sexually diverse people have not previously been recognised as an identifiable population group for healthcare, their health needs are virtually ignored in mainstream service planning. Intersex people are visibly marginalised as soon as a person is asked to identify their gender. For those who identify as intersex, which box do they tick—male or female? Some researchers are adding 'prefer not to say' to surveys but this approach is also problematic—it still does not identify those who identify as intersex and may skew gender analyses. As a group, sexually diverse people underutilise health services, often because of a lack of confidence and systemic discrimination, which leaves some with substandard care. Because of typical patterns of medical history taking, their gender identity, sexual orientation and health-related behaviour or circumstances are often overlooked. This leaves health problems undiagnosed, misdiagnosed or untreated, especially where risky sexual practices have not been identified. Because health services are generally based on the expectation that most clients are heterosexual, it is important that health practitioners use inclusive language, and that questions regarding gender identity and sexual orientation are included in assessment processes.

INTIMATE PARTNER VIOLENCE

Intimate partner violence (IPV) is usually about one partner in a relationship controlling another. Although we have addressed family violence in the context of family relations in Chapter 7, it is addressed here as one of the most gender-specific causes of women's disempowerment. Violence against women is a pervasive global problem. In Australia and New Zealand, between 17% and 35% of women have experienced some form of violence against them (AIHW 2019a, Fanslow et al 2021).

Besides physical injuries, the outcomes of violence against women can include stress, poor mental health, self-harm, substance abuse, difficulty accessing services and poor sexual and reproductive outcomes (AIHW 2019a). The threat of having children removed from a violent home can act as a deterrent to disclosure and lead women to escape the domestic situation for the sake of their children. Some then become homeless, which starts a vicious cycle of disempowerment for them and their children. The social context of homelessness can leave them enmeshed in a network of alcohol and substance abusers as well as ongoing vulnerability to further violence on the streets. Young homeless women and women who have been victim to trafficking are particularly vulnerable to sexual coercion simply to survive. In some cases, women who have fallen into this type of cycle become further victimised by health and social services, especially where personnel have been ill prepared to understand the depth or breadth of their distress or the physical effects of sex work, which can include sexually transmissible infections and other illnesses (Treloar et al 2021).

The effects of IPV also have profound harmful effects on the children witnessing abuse in any context. Young children in detention centres are often exposed to gender norms of violence that may be culturally acceptable but not appropriate in terms of the gendered behaviours they will observe in their host country post-migration, which are usually more gender balanced. Their time in detention can therefore leave them at risk of a distorted view of gender relations. In other living environments children may be caught between violent parents or partners role modelling violence on a regular basis, or intermittently at the time of transitions between staying with one or another parent. Their exposure is a serious problem in both the immediate and long term and has widespread

repercussions as children who witness abuse are more likely to be abused themselves, to have behaviour problems and increased exposure to other adversities such as alcohol and drug abuse, crime and other antisocial coping strategies (AIHW 2019a). The risk factors for violence against women and their children vary across cultures and, to date, there remains no definitive pattern for predicting which factors will lead a man to abuse a woman. Figure 9.2 shows the range of factors associated with IPV towards women.

The frequency of violence against women inspired the WHO Global Campaign for Violence Prevention and development of the global plan of action (WHO 2016). The global plan of action calls for member states to strengthen health systems to focus on preventing violence against women and children through multisectoral actions. Addressing the risk

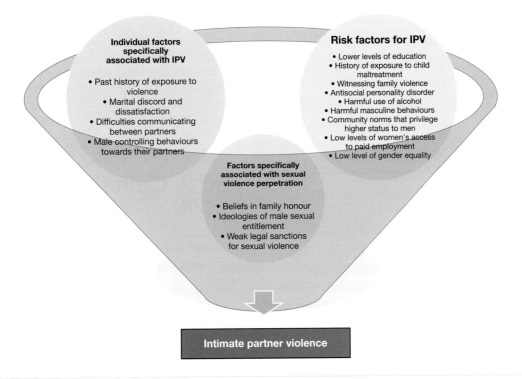

Figure 9.2 Factors associated with intimate partner violence and sexual violence against women

Source: Adapted from World Health Organization (WHO), 2021b. Violence against women. Online. Available: www.who.int/news-room/fact-sheets/detail/violence-against-women.

factors associated with family violence (see Fig 9.2) is the ideal approach to preventing violence. Nurses, midwives, paramedics and other health practitioners who work in communities and frequently see people in their own homes are often best positioned to respond with assistance and support. Many are leading advocates for championing the rights of women and addressing IPV and its effects on health and wellbeing. Screening for violence in health settings and home visits by maternal, child and family nurses is also gaining momentum, particularly with research studies indicating that women appreciate being asked about abuse (Withiel et al 2020). New Zealand and Australian screening protocols are based on empowerment and safety. Of utmost importance is ensuring health practitioners receive appropriate training and have the confidence to screen for IPV and respond appropriately (Hooker et al 2021b, 2021a).

KEY POINT

Screening for interpersonal violence is an effective means of reaching women who may be at risk of violence. It also offers the opportunity to provide support, safety and validation of the woman's experience.

GOALS FOR GENDER-INCLUSIVE COMMUNITIES

- Eliminating all forms of gender bias
- Public awareness of the need for gender sensitivity in health
- Health literacy, targeting the fundamental issues related to gender equality, such as poverty and social exclusion
- Equal access to fair conditions and fair remuneration in the workplace
- Gender equality in power and decision-making in the family
- Eliminating all forms of discrimination and violation of human rights

- Heightening awareness of the gender bias inherent in globalisation
- Gendering the social and political debates on childcare, gun control, crime prevention, transportation, education and other forums for intersectoral collaboration
- Heightening awareness of linkages between health, healthcare, cultural norms and human rights
- Promoting the health and safety of all family members, free from violence in the home
- National childcare strategies accommodating the needs of different family types
- Healthy, just and equitable public policies

We now turn our attention towards culture and inclusiveness. While our predominant focus is on Indigenous culture, refugee and migrant communities and, in particular, Pacific communities, also warrant further attention. As noted earlier the most compelling mark of an inclusive society is the respect conferred on its Indigenous people. The gross social and health inequities experienced by Indigenous people in Australia and New Zealand are a result of colonisation, disempowerment, individual and institutional racism, alienation from land and culture and social exclusion that extends back generations. How these are addressed moving forward is an area all health practitioners should be concerned with.

Part 2: Culture and health

Indigenous people in Australia and New Zealand have different histories and experiences. As population groups, what they have in common is a history of colonisation and dispossession that has not yet been fully redressed by non-Indigenous people in either country. New Zealand has made greater progress than Australia in valuing its Indigenous people, particularly since the Treaty of Waitangi and its mandate for recognition of all New Zealanders as equal before the law. Although Australia has yet to develop a treaty with Indigenous people, there is a renewal of political attention to the need for reconciliation between Australia's Indigenous and non-Indigenous people. This was enshrined in the national public apology to Indigenous people by Australia's Prime Minister in 2008, but much remains to be done in re-shaping Australia as an inclusive society. State, Territory and Commonwealth government initiatives to 'control' Indigenous affairs, and therefore Indigenous people's health, have polarised public opinion. Some condone heavy-handed measures to intervene in the way some Indigenous communities live their lives, while others are outraged that non-Indigenous norms and expectations would be placed on Indigenous communities. Australian public opinion is also divided on the plight of refugees from other countries, with some citizens advocating a greater human rights orientation, and others arguing for 'fairness' in the way migrants are processed and/or allowed into the country. This is one area where New Zealand political will is decidedly clear, supporting a compassionate basis for decision-making.

The relevance of political decisions governing migrants and Indigenous people is of major importance to nurses and other health practitioners working towards community health and wellness. As a basis for any type of intervention, the professions need to be fully informed of how both historical factors and current realities interact to keep Indigenous or other cultural groups socially disadvantaged. Understanding Indigenous ways of knowing, and the worldviews of other cultures, should lead to change, but it does not always achieve this. The challenge is to advance this knowledge as a basis for informing community awareness, then provide a rationale for policy and practice with the ultimate goal of social justice and inclusion.

We are both members of the non-Indigenous cultures of our respective countries, and we write this section drawing on a wide range of Indigenous and non-Indigenous literature, in consultation with members of Indigenous cultures, and on our respective experiences of the health and political environments in which we live and work. From this base of knowledge, we can work together, seeking common solutions that redress past and current barriers to health and wellness. We can then work towards helping Indigenous people negotiate retention of their culture, and promote equitable, inclusive environments for health and wellbeing.

CULTURE

Cultural groups are bound together by a tapestry of historically inherited ideas, beliefs, values, knowledge and traditions, art, customs, habits, language, roles, rules and shared meanings about the world. *Culture* is therefore multidimensional. Cultural influences are often tacit in people's behaviours, as unconscious, shared predispositions, rather than deliberate attempts to be distinctive. Although there are commonalities that bind members of a particular cultural group, individual expressions of culture vary according to a person's characteristics and experiences.

Diversity in expressions of culture is also a product of how people relate to their environments. Culture is integral to a person's social life, part of his or her ecological relationship with the world, which is dynamic and adaptive. In ecological terms, as people in any cultural group interact with their environments, there is a reciprocal effect on the environments and the people themselves. Culture is also experienced differently at different ages and stages of life, as people self-reflect, develop their own identities and respond to circumstances and self-reflection. Their cultural behaviours are therefore shaped by a range of experiences besides the cultural norms of language, lifestyle habits and family expectations. Although cultural traditions can bind people together, it is inappropriate to consider members of one or another culture as homogeneous, as within cultural groups there is often wide variability.

A critical view of culture seeks to overcome the *monolithic* view that all members are relatively similar. Instead, understanding individuals comes from exploring their history, behaviour and particular view of the world as it is embedded in their culture, but distinctive in their patterns of attitude and behaviour. Conducting an assessment of a person's needs therefore has to include both unique and common strengths and needs. Like other cultural groups, Indigenous 'culture' is not something that can be made explicit, and health services need to be designed using localised evidence obtained through culturally appropriate methods, guidelines and culturally safe care

(Hokowhitu et al 2020, Mitchell et al 2021). Trying to define a certain culture as a cultural outsider is difficult and can lead to stereotyping. To be authentically inclusive, health practitioners have to understand the history and structural factors that have been part of a person's experience, in the context of diversity within and external to the group (Power et al 2020). This non-stereotypical approach provides insight into people's worldview and their history, their declaration of what they value and the barriers and strengths that can lead to empowerment and self-determined decision-making. These choices are embedded in family and community and the human right to achieve social and cultural capital (see Fig 9.3). We have previously defined social capital in terms of trust, civic engagement, participation and belonging. Cultural capital refers to the source of power and resources that can help people maintain social capital in a way that will be beneficial and validate their ways of knowing and understanding.

> **KEY POINT**
> ....
> - **Social capital:** The values of trust, reciprocity, participation and belonging.
> - **Cultural capital:** The power and resources that help people maintain social capital in a way that values cultural understandings.

CULTURE CONFLICT

In some cases, the ecological interactions (the way in which people interact with each other and with their physical environments) between people, their culture and other cultural groups is mutually beneficial. People of different cultures settling together in a new land often learn from one another. Over time, their long-term contact with one another can result in the type of *acculturation* where two cultural groups become integrated; or relatively

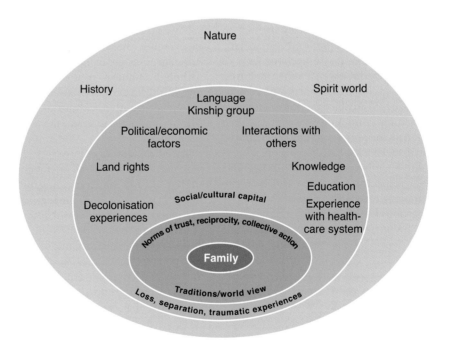

Figure 9.3 Family, culture and social capital

similar (Liu et al 2020). However, attempts at acculturating two groups can also be fraught with conflict. Much of the acculturation literature draws on Berry (1995) who describes four different reactions to acculturation. The first is *assimilation*, where one culture group abandons their culture in favour of the new or host culture. *Integration* is the creative blending of the two cultures. *Rejection* is a reaction in which the new culture replaces the heritage culture, and *marginalisation* occurs where neither the new nor the old culture is accepted. Clearly, the most desirable option is integration, with marginalisation the least desirable. It is important to recognise that acculturation is neither a lineal nor a universal process (Liu et al 2020).

KEY POINTS

....

- **Assimilation**—abandoning culture
- **Integration**—blending cultures
- **Rejection**—replacing culture
- **Marginalisation**—non-acceptance of culture

Culture conflict typically occurs where people are not committed to similar goals or ambitions and where societal decision-making is based on dissimilar principles and philosophies. In its extreme form, culture conflict can be enacted within racialised social structures, such as occurs when all groups are defined and their behaviours measured according to white Western beliefs. Racialised social structures often pervade Indigenous cultures in countries like Australia, Canada, New Zealand and the United States, where discriminatory and often racist attitudes promulgated by media stereotypes portray Indigenous people as a 'problem' rather than showing balanced, positive images of successful Indigenous people and families. Problematising their lives can subjugate Indigenous knowledge, beliefs and values in a way that disempowers members of Indigenous cultures by establishing standards and expectations against which differences, or deviations from the norm, are measured, valued and often demeaned. For example,

the high rate of smoking among pregnant Māori women in New Zealand is frequently seen as an individual choice and women are blamed and condemned for this behaviour (Houkamau et al 2016). What this fails to account for is the reasons Māori women smoke in the first place, such as institutional racism that results in fewer occupational, social and educational opportunities, poverty, chronic stress and a lack of psychological resources to support efforts to quit (Houkamau et al 2016).

At the community level, culture conflict erodes social and cultural capital by causing disharmony. When this occurs, members of the conflicting groups close ranks and withdraw from each other, rather than cooperating to build a system of mutual community support. On the other hand, when people from different cultures live with realistic possibilities for the future, they are more likely to work within a type of *cultural relativism*; acceptance and respect for difference where a person's beliefs, values and practices are understood based on that person's own culture and not judged against the criteria of another (Khan Academy 2021). Cultural relativism lies at the centre of tolerance and social inclusiveness. For two cultures to work together, no one culture needs to abandon its traditions or philosophies, but each suspends judgment of the other's beliefs and practices. In this process, each makes a conscious decision to proceed on the basis of their willingness to recognise and respect the beliefs and practices of others, and to continually question their own views and presumptions (Tremblay et al 2020). This is also the first step in maintaining cultural safety.

CULTURAL SAFETY

A culturally safe environment safeguards the authenticity and acceptability of diversity in people's beliefs, behaviours and social constructs. Appreciation of this concept has become an integral component of community health practice. It requires all health practitioners to reflect on their own cultural identity in order to understand and acknowledge how their mores influence their interactions and healthcare practice with clients (Tremblay et al 2020). The same holds true for organisations who need to reflect on how their policies, procedures, systems and structures may embed institutional bias and systemic racism. Cultural safety is the lynchpin in achieving equity for those impacted by colonisation, marginalisation, racism and oppression.

KEY POINT

....

Culturally safe practice

1 Acknowledge that the healthcare relationship is power-laden, with the healthcare professional holding the majority of power.

2 Reflect on your impact on the 'other'.

3 Commit to achieving equity for those disadvantaged through colonisation, racism, marginalisation and oppression.

Cultural safety is a term that grew out of the colonial history of Aotearoa (New Zealand). It was first described in 1988 by Māori nursing students expressing their concern about safeguarding their culture as they were socialised into the world of nursing education and ensuring the safety of Māori culture among those they would be helping in practice (Eckermann et al 2010). Their concerns were recorded by Irihapeti Ramsden, a Māori nurse, educationalist, philosopher and writer who spearheaded the cultural safety movement in Aotearoa, ensuring that cultural safety found its way into curricula and nursing practice (Hunter et al 2021). Ramsden's legacy has extended beyond Aotearoa and now underpins approaches to recognising, respecting and transforming healthcare practices with Indigenous cultures globally (Tremblay et al 2020). Further, cultural safety is seen as inclusive of all cultures and all healthcare recipients whose culture differs from their healthcare provider in any way (Westenra 2019). Cultural safety is concerned with how culture shapes power relations within the social world of the community. It is designed to enable safe spaces for the interaction of all cultural groups, and their understanding of cultural identity.

It is absent in the face of actions that assault, diminish, demean or disempower the cultural identity and wellbeing of any individual (Nursing Council of New Zealand 2012).

Cultural safety includes recognising the fact that any healthcare relationship is unique, power-laden and culturally dyadic. In other words, there is always the potential for one person (the health provider) to hold power over the other person (someone seeking to access services). Cultural safety requires people to engage in reflection and self-exploration of their own life experience and realities, and the impact this may have on others– particularly in the context of healthcare provision. Being culturally safe means maintaining a conscious commitment to ensuring preservation and protection of others' cultures. Cultural safety is therefore a type of advocacy informed by a recognition of self, the rights of others and the legitimacy of difference (Nursing Council of New Zealand 2011). It is aimed at unveiling the unconscious and unspoken assumptions of power of health practitioners with a view towards transferring some of this power to those seeking care by using an inclusive approach, receptive to new ways of knowing and understanding (Curtis et al 2019). Nurses in New Zealand are required to demonstrate how they practise in a culturally safe manner as part of maintaining their nursing registration (Nursing Council of New Zealand 2016). In the process of being inclusive of others' voices, they gain an authentic understanding of health issues as a basis for planning care.

Equally as important is the need for culturally safe healthcare systems and organisations that value diversity and focus on achieving equity (Curtis et al 2019). Developing organisations to embed cultural safety as fundamental to their approach to addressing equity is a paradigm shift that requires commitment, critical awareness and the ability to critique existing power structures within the organisation. Box 9.1 outlines the requirements for culturally safe organisations and healthcare systems.

MULTICULTURALISM

The intent of *multiculturalism* is that ethnic group differences should be appreciated and celebrated

BOX 9.1

CULTURALLY SAFE HEALTH SYSTEMS AND ORGANISATIONS

- Focus on achieving health equity with a clear action plan and measurable progress.
- Acknowledge and encourage diversity within the organisation.
- Mandate cultural safety and unconscious bias training as part of ongoing professional development for ALL staff.
- Include evidence of cultural safety (of organisations and practitioners) as a requirement for accreditation.
- Systematically monitor and assess inequities in the health workforce and in health outcomes.
- Provide culturally appropriate care recognising that cultural safety extends beyond acquiring knowledge about different cultures.
- Enable self-determination and reciprocity.

Source: Adapted from Curtis, E., Jones, R., Tipene-Leach, D., et al, 2019. Why cultural safety rather than cultural competency is required to achieve health equity: A literature review and recommended definition. Int. J. Equity Health, 18 (1). Online. Available: https://doi.org/10.1186/s12939-019-1082-3.

and that different groups make unique and valued contributions to society (Vorauer & Quesnel 2017). However, multiculturalism is a value-laden term that has sometimes been used as a panacea for intolerance. The term has been used to camouflage feelings of superiority of one culture over another. It has also been used to salve the consciences of many people, believing that because they live in a community containing many cultures, the community must be inclusive, when this may be disputed by the realities of daily life.

Although small steps have been made towards heightening public awareness of the role of culture in health, these have been only marginally effective in improving health outcomes. To advance multiculturalism, societies need to institutionalise understanding and tolerance of one another's cultural beliefs and practices in the context of daily living as well as in the healthcare system, and in planning for a future in which all cultures will be sustained. Not many societies achieve this level of equity, but it is seen to be an aspiration worthy of just and civil societies.

ETHNOCENTRISM, RACISM, UNCONSCIOUS BIAS AND DIFFERENTIAL HEALTHCARE

Ethnocentrism is an individual-level and multidimensional attitudinal construct characterised by a strong preoccupation with the importance of one's own ethnic group (Bizumic et al 2020). With the rise of far right wing politics in the late 2010s and early 2020s, ethnocentrism as a phenomenon has seen a global resurgence. It is a negative construct characterised by: devotion to one's own ethnic group; group cohesion at the expense of individual freedom; preference or an attitude of preferring and liking one's own ethnic group over others; superiority over other groups; purity or an attitude in favour of one's own ethnic group; and exploitativeness or an attitude in favour of giving greater importance to ethnic ingroup interests over outgroup interests (Bizumic et al 2020). Ethnocentrism contributes to prejudice, stereotyping, racism and discrimination. Although each of us views the world through the cultural lens with which we have been socialised, this lens should not inhibit our ability to see beyond our own culture. This is why it takes a conscious effort to really 'see' other cultures. When people develop an aversion to the very notion of tolerating other cultures, they are described as *xenophobic*: fearing and despising those who differ. Xenophobia is often used synonymously with *racism*, which is a belief in the distinctiveness of human races, usually involving the idea that one's birth-ascribed race or skin colour is superior to another (Australian Human Rights Commission 2018, Markwick et al 2019). Maintaining feelings of superiority about another race, or another group, is called *stereotyping*. These feelings can lead to *prejudicial attitudes*, which, when acted upon, result in *discrimination*. Discrimination is shown by speaking against the other person or group, excluding or segregating them, committing acts of violence against them or, at its extreme, exterminating them as has occurred in World War II and other wars and conflicts.

Institutional racism operates at the level of legal, political and economic organisation in a society (Talamaivao et al 2020) creating the impression that, because power dominance is exerted by essential and respected forces in society, it is somehow tacitly acceptable. Institutional racism is a significant contributor to creating and sustaining racial and ethnic inequalities in health outcomes (Talamaivao et al 2020). *Systemic bias* allows one group to dominate another through the predominant social order, where organisational and communication skills, financial resources and commitment of those involved in running a system are able to exclude others, making them dependent on the powerful group rather than allowing them full participation (Markwick et al 2019). In some cases, this type of power imbalance occurs because of a lack of knowledge and awareness rather than an intention to dominate. For example, *culture blindness*, where, inadvertently, someone who believes they are working within an ethos of social justice develops universalism, or an approach to health and social care where an individual proclaims to 'treat everyone the same' (Curtis et al 2019). The issue here is that some people have greater needs than others, so a universal approach will not help achieve equal opportunities and therefore may perpetuate disparities for disadvantaged cultural groups (Marmot 2016). *Unconscious bias* is related to cultural blindness and occurs automatically as the brain makes rapid judgments about people and situations based on their own personal background, experiences and environment (Kuzma et al 2019). Our perceptions cause responses that we are consciously unaware of. As a result, we are likely to favour groups we perceive as similar to our own group and display discrimination against groups that are dissimilar without being aware of it (Houkamau & Clarke 2016). These actions directly result in systemic bias and institutional racism which in turn cause healthcare disparities and inequitable outcomes (Fitzgerald & Hurst 2017, Houkamau & Clarke 2016, Marcelin et al 2019).

> ### KEY POINT
>
> Systemic bias is:
>
> - benchmarking Indigenous health against non-Indigenous population norms
> - using a universal or 'one-size-fits-all' approach to healthcare
> - attributing needs to culture instead of structural and social determinants of health.

The other manifestations of systemic bias are evident when the health of Indigenous people is analysed according to benchmarks established for non-Indigenous populations, or when the blame for social and health problems is attributed to cultural characteristics instead of inequities in the healthcare system. There is now a body of evidence showing that Indigenous people in Australia and New Zealand have inadequate access to health services and lower rates of medical interventions when they are hospitalised (Came et al 2018, de-Vitry Smith 2016, Houkamau & Clarke 2016, Talamaivao et al 2020, Zambas & Wright 2016). Stereotyping anyone's health needs can be detrimental to health. For example, there are cases where a person's refusal of treatment is described as a lack of adherence, when it could be due to communication difficulties.

We frequently focus on the disparities in health and the state of inequity that exists as a result of these inequities. And rightly so as this identifies the issues and enables us to focus on interventions that may help address these. However, by focusing solely on the disparities and poor state of health of Indigenous people in both Australia and New Zealand, we fail to recognise the strength and resiliency that individuals, families and communities bring to addressing their own health needs. To understand this strength and resiliency, we need to understand more about each of these groups.

ABORIGINALITY, CULTURE AND HEALTH

The term '*Aboriginal*' refers to the initial, or earliest, inhabitants of a place. They are also described as

First Nations, or *Indigenous*, people. The earliest inhabitants of Aotearoa New Zealand are Māori and in Australia it is Aboriginal and Torres Strait Islander people. Aboriginal and Torres Strait Islander people are often also referred to as Indigenous Australians. Not all Aboriginal and Torres Strait Islanders like the term as they consider it too generic (Australian Institute of Aboriginal and Torres Strait Islander Studies [AIATSIS] 2021). It is therefore important to find out what individuals prefer to be called rather than making assumptions given the diverse subcultures and worldviews that exist within Indigenous societies. In this text we respectfully use the term Indigenous based on the United Nations understanding of Indigenous that does not define the term but base it on the fundamental human right of self-identification (Chakrabarti 2006).

Members of different Indigenous groups have different influences on their lives, many as a result of their environment. The influences on their health are shaped by different determinants beyond biology, age, gender, education, socioeconomic status, family membership or neighbourhood. In some groups, cultural knowledge may prescribe everything from diet and eating habits to child-rearing practices; from reactions to pain, stress and death to which behaviours may violate cultural norms. Cultural knowledge may also dictate a palpable sense of past, present and future, the impact of community and economic structures and the different ways people respond to healthcare services and practitioners. Figure 9.4 shows child health nurse Tshpiso Mojapelo (Daisy) with some of the Indigenous children she supports as part of her role in Wurrimiyanga, Northern Territory.

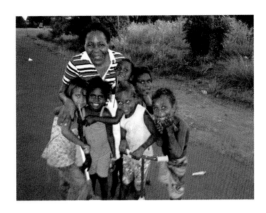

Figure 9.4 Tshepiso Mojapelo (Daisy), child health nurse in Wurrumiyanga (Bathurst Island), Tiwi Islands, Northern Territory

Source: Photo courtesy of Tshepiso Mojapelo.

physical, mental, cultural and spiritual dimensions of health, and the harmonised interrelationships between these and environmental, ideological, political, social and economic conditions (Gall et al 2021). At the centre of Indigenous people's relationship with each dimension of health is a fundamental spiritual connection with land, symbolising their responsibility as inhabitants of the land, to take care of it and preserve it for the next generations (Gall et al 2021). This is integral to their ecological connection between health and place.

INDIGENOUS PEOPLE'S RELATIONSHIPS BETWEEN HEALTH AND PLACE

The spiritual relationship with land is a metaphysical connection, governing all other interrelationships. The land is typically described by Indigenous Australians as 'Country', which is the place that gives and receives life and is part of the support cycle of life-death-life (Pol 2021). Indigenous Australians talk about Country in the same way that they would talk about a person. Country refers to everything including land, air and water and Indigenous Australians have a spiritual connection to the land built over thousands of generations (Pol 2021). This is a different concept of land from the non-Indigenous

KEY POINT

Indigenous understandings of health and wellbeing are manifest within holistic, symbolic, spiritual and ecological perspectives.

The most distinctive feature of Indigenous cultures is a holistic, ecological, spiritual view of health and wellbeing. This perspective encompasses understanding, where land is considered an empty space to be 'tamed' or worked (Kingsley et al 2013). What we do know is that a stronger connection to Country has a positive effect on general health for Indigenous children in Australia (Dockery 2020). We also know that Indigenous mothers who birth on Country feel more supported and have their needs more fully met than those who didn't (Dragon 2019, Marriott et al 2019). New Zealand Māori articulate a similar connection with the land to the Aboriginal understanding. The land historically provided the sustenance necessary for life, but it is also the spiritual, cultural and ancestral home for Māori. This relationship is based on the worldview that Ranginui (Sky Father) and Papatūānuku (Earth Mother) are the primal parents from whom all Māori descend. Māori refer to themselves as tangata whenua (people of the land), which captures the spirit of this kin relationship making the people and the land inseparable. Platforms for Māori health are considered to be 'constructed from land, language, and whānau; from marae and hapū; from Rangi and Papa; from the ashes of colonisation; from adequate opportunity for cultural expression; and from being able to participate fully within society' (Durie 2003, pp. 35–36).

The close connection with land is what distinguishes the Indigenous 'holistic' view from other common perceptions of holism (Dragon 2019). The uncritical way non-Indigenous policymakers and health planners understand Indigenous 'holism' is problematic when it is seen as a biomedical concept and translated into strategies for health and health services without deeper understandings of this holistic worldview (Creamer & Hall 2019). Locally relevant interventions need to reflect local knowledge from place-based communities whose members have developed the skills to articulate their needs from the holistic interpretations that resonate with the community (Creamer & Hall 2019, Mackean et al 2020).

THE HEALTH OF INDIGENOUS AUSTRALIAN PEOPLE AND NEW ZEALAND MĀORI

It is well known that there are gross inequities in health outcomes for both the Indigenous people of Australia and New Zealand Māori. Life expectancy

---

BOX 9.2

....

THE HEALTH OF AUSTRALIAN INDIGENOUS PEOPLE AND NEW ZEALAND MĀORI

....

Indigenous health in Australia

- Support and information for those working in the Aboriginal and Torres Strait Islander health sector: www.healthinfonet.ecu.edu.au/about
- Information and research on Aboriginal Australians: www.aihw.gov.au/reports-data/population-groups/indigenous-australians/overview

Māori health in New Zealand

- Information and research on Māori health: www.health.govt.nz/our-work/populations/maori-health
- Māori health promotion information: http://hauora.co.nz/maori-health-promotion/
- Health data and statistics: www.health.govt.nz/nz-health-statistics/health-statistics-and-data-sets/maori-health-data-and-stats?mega=Health%20statistics&title=M%C4%81ori%20health

---

for both groups is substantially less than that of the non-Indigenous populations in either country. Health outcomes across most measures are also worse. Further information on where to find more on the specific statistics and health issues that face both groups can be found through the links in Box 9.2. Because work is under way in both countries to address these inequities, we choose here to focus on the strengths and efforts that are being made to address inequities rather than on the deficits. We focus closely on mental health and healing.

HEALTH AND HEALING

Therapeutic approaches to healing must be based on understanding the cultural meanings of kinship, the land, spirituality and heritage of Indigenous people (Kopua et al 2020, NiaNia et al 2016). Working with Indigenous people to improve health

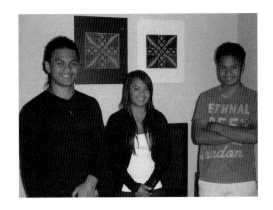

Figure 9.5 Young Māori thriving

Source: Photo courtesy of the Powell whānau.

is a circular process of holistic, spiritual and cultural understandings of the contextual realities of a person's life, family context and past experiences (NiaNia et al 2016, 2019) (see Fig 9.5).

Assessing an Indigenous person's wellbeing must be done in a way that is sensitive to the way mental health is conceptualised. For example, some Indigenous Australian groups may believe they are being 'sung' by an aggrieved party, married the 'wrong way', 'caught out' by the law or 'crying for Country'. The last example illustrates the interrelatedness of health and place, acknowledging Indigenous people's close connection to Country.

The Whare Tapa Wha Māori Model of Health developed by Mason Durie in New Zealand articulates a concept of holism that has been adopted by many Māori and non-Māori, as a means of understanding the way in which Māori conceptualise health. The four cornerstones of the Whare Tapa Wha model are Hinengaro (mental wellbeing), Tinana (physical wellbeing), Whānau (family wellbeing) and Wairua (spiritual wellbeing). Each cornerstone is interlinked, and health may not be achieved without a balance between all four cornerstones (Durie 2004).

As a spiritual journey, healing requires time and a culturally safe, capacity-strengthening approach to assist in the recovery from past traumas, addictions or other problems. The 'by Māori for Māori' or *Kaupapa Māori* health services in New Zealand are one approach to addressing many of the cultural needs of Māori as they seek to address their health needs. These services are based in both traditional settings, such as hospitals, and in non-traditional settings, such as on marae (Māori meeting ground).

Importantly, past traumas, such as those experienced by the Stolen Generations, cannot be resolved until there is government and societal acknowledgment of the source of these problems. Long-term grief and trauma can become transgenerational, and can lead to dysfunctional family life, including violence, self-harm and suicide. In Australia, Indigenous suicide rates range from 1.4 to 2.3 times that of non-Indigenous Australians (AIHW 2021a).

Where to find out more on ...

Health promotion programs developed to address young Indigenous people's mental health which include cultural healing and counselling

- Resourceful Adolescent Program: www.rap.qut.edu.au
- The Healing Foundation: https://healingfoundation.org.au

The oppression of Indigenous people is indisputable, and it creates enormous challenges for nurses, midwives, paramedics, health workers, medical practitioners, teachers, police and other practitioners working in Indigenous communities. For all of these health advocates the objective is to work out ways of helping people retrieve their sense of self, family, culture, community and society (see Fig 9.3). This can begin through delving into the root causes of a set of behaviours such as alcohol or substance misuse that create cycles of risk, then working with individuals and families to see what can be done to reset the pattern for a more optimistic future.

GOALS FOR INDIGENOUS HEALTH

- Eliminate racism and all forms of discrimination against Indigenous people.

- Address the social determinants of disadvantage and inequity for Indigenous people.
- Improve child and youth health and wellbeing through perinatal and early childhood intervention and prevention strategies.
- Recognise the uniqueness and importance of Indigenous family and extended family networks.
- Promote public acceptance of the unique needs and sensitivities of Indigenous people.
- Improve the cultural safety of mainstream services through better transparency and accountability, and develop specific services tailored to cultural needs.
- Develop a well-resourced evidence base for best practice in Indigenous health.
- Recognise the impact of environmental degradation on Indigenous people, and create genuine opportunities for affected communities to participate in decision-making for environmental restoration.
- Acknowledge the uniqueness of Indigenous systems of knowledge in caring for Country.
- Maintain the health of Indigenous people as the highest priority for health planning.
- Support the development of economic, social and cultural capital to foster self-determinism, and strategies for culturally appropriate, sufficiently resourced education and skill development.
- Adopt strategies for intersectoral collaboration in all policies and planning strategies at all levels.
- Ensure cultural safety in all service provision for all people.
- Enshrine diversity and culture in the laws and social processes of the country.

INCLUSIVE MIGRANT COMMUNITIES—THE PACIFIC EXPERIENCE IN NEW ZEALAND

Pacific people comprise approximately 7.4% of the New Zealand population and come from over 22 different Pacific nations. Each Pacific community has its own distinctive culture, language, history and health status. The largest Pacific groups are the Samoan, Cook Island, Tongan and Niuean communities. Just under 65% of the Pacific people living in New Zealand live in the Auckland area (Stats NZ 2018). Auckland (along with Sydney, Australia) is now recognised as one of the most culturally diverse cities in the world, but Pacific people in New Zealand experience poorer health outcomes than other New Zealanders across a range of health and disability indicators (Ministry of Health 2020).

New Zealand has made a significant and long-term commitment to addressing the inequities experienced by Pacific people, working closely with the Pacific community to develop a range of policies designed to improve health. The current action plan for addressing Pacific health, Ola Manuia Pacific Health and Wellbeing Action Plan 2020–2025 (Ministry of Health 2020) identifies a range of outcomes to be achieved for Pacific people. These include ensuring Pacific people lead independent and resilient lives, live longer in good health and have equitable health outcomes. These outcomes are underpinned by a set of system enablers that must be in place to ensure the outcomes are achieved. The system enablers include ensuring Pacific leadership is prominent and accountable at all levels of the health system, that the health and disability workforce is culturally safe and competent, that workforce development programs are in place to support recruitment and retention of Pacific people in health roles, that there is effective and efficient organisational and infrastructural capacity to support Pacific health and development, and that funding and investment focuses on the needs of Pacific communities (Ministry of Health 2020). A range of actions and outcome measures are also identified to ensure accountability for achieving the goals of the plan. Ola Manuia was developed in collaboration with a range of clinical and community leaders in an effort to ensure the policy goals and actions are in line with the expectations of the community. Such inclusive approaches to policy development are essential to achieving health equity for Indigenous people and for migrant and refugee groups.

Conclusion

We discuss the various experiences of refugee, migrant, Indigenous and other minority and gender groups throughout this book with the ultimate goal of health, equity, social justice and inclusiveness for all. Social inclusion is a social determinant of health equity. Achieving equity and, therefore, social justice begins with acknowledging the interrelatedness of health, place and economic viability. Creating a strong sense of identity among Indigenous people, addressing Māori health through approaches such as whānau ora, fostering community, place-based initiatives, empowering communities through engagement and co-design and building human capital through education, parenting skills and work experience skills will all engender inclusiveness. Health practitioners must get involved in communities' self-defined priorities for health and wellbeing. Advocacy, maintaining current knowledge of the decisions that are being taken at the political level, maintaining cultural safety and seeking the views of local Indigenous people on how actions may affect their capacity for self-determination are all essential in achieving these goals. Equally as important is developing the Indigenous and minority health workforce to ensure Indigenous and minority groups have access to health practitioners of their choice. Inclusive communities emerge from conditions where everyone has an equal opportunity in their daily lives. We will now reflect on the big issues identified throughout the chapter before examining issues of inclusiveness for the Smith and Mason families.

Where to find out more on ...

Whānau Ora

Whānau Ora is an approach designed to reduce health and social wellbeing disparities among vulnerable families by supporting families to achieve their maximum health and wellbeing: www.tpk.govt.nz/en/whakamahia/whanau-ora

Reflecting on the Big Issues

- Social inclusion and social exclusion are two points on a continuum of social equity.

- Our society remains unequal, with pockets of systematic discrimination and oppression on the basis of gender, race, ethnicity and sexual diversity.

- Women and men have different health issues and some common issues related to a combination of biological, behavioural and social factors.

- Intimate partner violence is caused by one person's need to exert power and control over another.

- Migrant, refugee and LGBTQIA+ groups have multiple layers of disadvantage through discrimination and stereotyped societal responses to their needs.

- The reasons for the lower health status and shorter lifespan of Indigenous people compared with non-Indigenous people include socioeconomic disparities, deprivation, unequal treatment, racism, discrimination and unhealthy environments.

- Societies cannot be inclusive until historical traumas against Indigenous people are dealt with by the wider society.

- Cultural safety and respect for Indigenous culture underpin our approach to addressing inequities.

Inclusiveness and the Smith and Mason families

The mining site where Colin works has encouraged the employment of Indigenous men through the Australia One initiative. The Indigenous mining training program has proven successful in creating employment for local Indigenous people. The management group and health and safety group have done some public awareness work on the company's social inclusion agenda in all aspects of the mining operations.

Rebecca has been supporting a group of young mothers in her community to advocate for safe breastfeeding spaces in public places. A number of the young women had been made to feel uncomfortable about breastfeeding in public and, with the support of some of the older mothers in the community, were working with local businesses to make breastfeeding accepted.

Huia is very connected to her Māori culture and is determined that her children remain engaged in Māori culture, so she makes the effort to send them to the nearest Māori immersion school (Te Kura Kaupapa Māori) and preschool (Kohanga Reo). While having her mother come to live in the family home is challenging, Huia finds the relationship and connections between her mother and her children rewarding.

Jason is working with his company to develop an inclusive workplace policy aimed at creating a safe workplace for LGBTQIA+ workers. This has included creating gender-neutral bathrooms and signage. The new policy has been challenging for some in the workplace but has been welcomed by others.

Reflective questions: How would I use this knowledge in practice?

1 What indicators of social exclusion exist in your community?

2 What are the most prevalent issues confronting women in today's workplace?

3 Identify the chain of factors related to colonisation that predispose Indigenous people to ill health.

4 Outline a strategy for promoting health literacy among middle-aged Indigenous residents of a rural or remote community with a view towards managing chronic illness.

5 Explain how you would develop a plan for a domestic violence prevention session to include Indigenous and non-Indigenous workers at the mining site.

6 What primary health care initiatives would you include in a program to develop a socially inclusive Health Promoting School in either Maddington or Papakura?

7 Construct a set of guidelines or prompts that you might use to ensure your interactions are culturally safe, irrespective of your client group.

References

Alba, B., Lyons, A., Waling, A., et al, 2020. Health, well-being, and social support in older Australian lesbian and gay care-givers. Health Soc. Care Community, 28 (1), 204–215. Online. Available: https://doi.org/10.1111/hsc.12854.

Armstrong, G., Haregu, T., Caine, E.D., et al, 2020. High prevalence of health and social risk behaviours among men experiencing suicidal thoughts and behaviour: The imperative to undertake holistic assessments. Aust. N. Z. J. Psychiatry, 54 (8), 797–807. Online. Available: https://doi.org/10.1177/0004867420924098.

Artz, J., 2021. Period poverty: New Zealand announces free menstrual products for all students. Global Citizen. Online. Available: www.globalcitizen.org/en/content/period-poverty-new-zealand-free-products/.

Ashraf, K., Ng, C.J., Goh, K.L., 2021. Theories, models and frameworks in men's health studies: A scoping review. J. Men's Health, 17 (2), 15–24. Online. Available: https://doi.org/10.31083/jomh.2021.006.

Australian Human Rights Commission, 2018. What is racism? Australian Human Rights Commission. Online. Available: https://humanrights.gov.au/sites/default/files/whatisracism.pdf.

Australian Institute of Aboriginal and Torres Strait Islander Studies (AIATSIS), 2021. Indigenous Australians: Aboriginal and Torres Strait Islander people. Explore. AIATSIS. Online. Available: https://aiatsis.gov.au/explore/indigenous-australians-aboriginal-and-torres-strait-islander-people.

Australian Institute of Health and Welfare (AIHW), 2019a. Family, domestic and sexual violence in Australia continuing the national story 2019. AIHW. Online. Available: www.aihw.gov.au/getmedia/b0037b2d-a651-4abf-9f7b-00a85e3de528/aihw-fdv3-FDSV-in-Australia-2019.pdf.aspx?inline=true.

Australian Institute of Health and Welfare (AIHW), 2019b. The health of Australia's males. AIHW, Canberra. Online. Available: www.aihw.gov.au/getmedia/fbe37c6b-869a-45f0-8930-db08e028701a/The-health-of-Australia-s-males.pdf.aspx?inline=true.

Australian Institute of Health and Welfare (AIHW), 2021a. Deaths by suicide amongst Indigenous Australians. Suicide and self-harm monitoring. AIHW, Canberra. Online. Available: www.aihw.gov.au/suicide-self-harm-monitoring/data/populations-age-groups/suicide-indigenous-australians.

Australian Institute of Health and Welfare (AIHW), 2021b. Deaths by suicide over time. Suicide and self-harm monitoring. AIHW, Canberra. Online. Available: www.aihw.gov.au/suicide-self-harm-monitoring/data/deaths-by-suicide-in-australia/suicide-deaths-over-time.

Australian Institute of Health and Welfare (AIHW), 2021c. Deaths in Australia. AIHW. Online. Available: www.aihw.gov.au/getmedia/743dd325-7e96-4674-bb87-9f77420a7ef5/Deaths-in-Australia.pdf.aspx?inline=true

Ayittey, F.K., Dhar, B.K., Anani, G., et al, 2020. Gendered burdens and impacts of SARS-CoV-2: a review. Health Care Women Int., 41 (11/12), 1210–1225. Online. Available: https://doi.org/10.1080/07399332.2020.1809664.

Baker, P., 2020. Men's health policy: it is time for action. Trends Urol. Men's Health, 11 (6), 11–13. Online. Available: https://doi.org/10.1002/tre.774.

Berry, J., 1995. Psychology of Acculturation. In: Goldberg, N., Veroff, J. (Eds), The culture and psychology reader. New York University Press, pp. 457–488.

Bizumic, B., Monaghan, C., Priest, D., 2020. The return of ethnocentrism. Polit. Psychol. Online. Available: https://doi.org/10.1111/pops.12710.

Boniol, M., McIsaac, M., Xu, L., et al, 2019. Gender equity in the health workforce: Analysis of 104 countries. World Health Organization, Geneva, 1–8 March. Online. Available: https://apps.who.int/iris/handle/10665/311314.

Came, H., Doole, C., McKenna, B., et al, 2018. Institutional racism in public health contracting: Findings of a nationwide survey from New Zealand. Soc. Sci. Med., 199, 132–139. Online. Available: https://doi.org/10.1016/j.socscimed.2017.06.002.

Carson, C.C., 2020. Why men's health? Postgrad. Med., 132 (sup4), 1–3. Online. Available: https://doi.org/10.1080/00325481.2020.1805867.

Chakrabarti, O., 2006. Who are indigenous peoples? In: Indigenous peoples, Indigenous voices (pp. 1–3). United Nations. Online. Available: www.un.org/esa/socdev/unpfii/documents/5session_factsheet1.pdf.

Courtenay, W.H., 2000. Constructions of masculinity and their influence on men's wellbeing: a theory of gender and health. Soc. Sci. Med., 50 (10), 1385–1401. Online. Available: https://doi.org/10.1016/S0277-9536(99)00390-1.

Creamer, S., Hall, N.L., 2019. Receiving essential health services on country: Indigenous Australians, native title and the United Nations Declaration. Public Health (Elsevier), 176, 15–20. Online. Available: https://doi.org/10.1016/j.puhe.2019.08.024.

Culph, J., Wilson, N., Cordier, R., et al, 2015. Men's Sheds and the experience of depression in older Australian men. Aust. Occup. Ther. J., 62 (5), 306.

Curtis, E., Jones, R., Tipene-Leach, D., et al, 2019. Why cultural safety rather than cultural competency is required to achieve health equity: a literature review and recommended definition. Int. J. Equity Health, 18 (1). Online. Available: https://doi.org/10.1186/s12939-019-1082-3.

de-Vitry Smith, S., 2016. Strategies to improve maternal health for Indigenous women and children. Aust. Nurs. Midwifery J., 23 (8), 43. Online. Available: https://pubmed.ncbi.nlm.nih.gov/27132397/.

DeSouza, R., 2013. Regulating migrant maternity: nursing and midwifery's emancipatory aims and assimilatory practices. Nurs. Inq., 20 (4), 293.

Dockery, A.M., 2020. Inter-generational transmission of Indigenous culture and children's wellbeing: Evidence from Australia. Int. J. Intercult. Relat., 74, January, 80–93. Online. Available: https://doi.org/10.1016/j.ijintrel.2019.11.001.

Donald, C., Ehrenfeld, J., 2015. The opportunity for medical systems to reduce health disparities among lesbian, gay, bisexual, transgender and intersex patients. J. Med. Syst., 39 (11), 178.

Dragon, N., 2019. Birthing on country: Improving Aboriginal and Torres Strait Islander infant and maternal health. Aust. Nurs. Midwifery J., 26 (5), 18–20. Online. Available: https://anmj.org.au/birthing-on-country-improving-indigenous-health/.

Durie, M., 2004. An Indigenous model of health promotion. Health Promot. J. Austr., 15 (3), 181–185.

Durie, M., 2003. Ngā kāhui pou launching Māori futures. Huia Publishers.

Eckermann, A., Dowd, T., Chong, E., et al, 2010. Binan Goonj: bridging cultures in aboriginal health (Vol. 3). Elsevier.

Eisenberg, M.E., Gower, A.L., Rider, G.N., et al, 2019. At the intersection of sexual orientation and gender identity: variations in emotional distress and bullying experience in a large population-based sample of US adolescents. J. LGBT Youth, 16 (3), 235–254. Online. Available: https://doi.org/10.1080/19361653.2019.1567435.

Fanslow, J., Hashemi, L., Malihi, Z., et al., 2021. Change in prevalence rates of physical and sexual intimate partner violence against women: Data from two cross-sectional studies in New Zealand, 2003 and 2019. BMJ Open, 11 (3), 1–14. Online. Available: https://doi.org/10.1136/bmjopen-2020-044907.

Faulkner, N., Zhao, K., Kneebone, S., et al, 2019. The Inclusive Australia Inclusion Index: 2019 Report. Inclusive Australia. Online. Available: https://inclusive-australia.s3.amazonaws.com/files/Inclusive-Australia-Social-Inclusion-Index-WEB.pdf.

Fitzgerald, C., Hurst, S., 2017. Implicit bias in healthcare professionals: A systematic review. BMC Med. Ethics, 18 (1). Online. Available: https://doi.org/10.1186/s12910-017-0179-8.

Gall, A., Anderson, K., Howard, K., et al, 2021. Wellbeing of Indigenous peoples in Canada, Aotearoa (New Zealand) and

the United States: A systematic review. Int. J. Environ. Res. Public Health, 18 (11), 5832. Online. Available: https://doi.org/10.3390/ijerph18115832.

Grant, R., Walker, B., 2020. Older Lesbians' experiences of ageing in place in rural Tasmania, Australia: An exploratory qualitative investigation. Health Soc. Care Community, 28 (6), 2199–2207. Online. Available: https://doi.org/10.1111/hsc.13032.

Herron, R.V., Ahmadu, M., Allan, J.A., et al, 2020. 'Talk about it:' changing masculinities and mental health in rural places? Soc. Sci. Med., 258. Online. Available: https://doi.org/10.1016/j.socscimed.2020.113099.

Hokowhitu, B., Oetzel, J.G., Simpson, M.L., et al, 2020. Kaumātua Mana Motuhake Pōi: A study protocol for enhancing wellbeing, social connectedness and cultural identity for Māori elders. BMC Geriatr., 20, 1–15. Online. Available: https://doi.org/10.1186/s12877-020-01740-3.

Hooker, L., Nicholson, J., Hegarty, K., et al, 2021a. Maternal and Child Health nurse's preparedness to respond to women and children experiencing intimate partner violence: A cross-sectional study. Nurse Educ. Today, 96. Online. Available: https://doi.org/10.1016/j.nedt.2020.104625.

Hooker, L., Nicholson, J., Hegarty, K., et al, 2021b. Victorian maternal and child health nurses' family violence practices and training needs: A cross-sectional analysis of routine data. Aust. J. Prim. Health, 27 (1), 43–49. Online. Available: https://doi.org/10.1071/PY20043.

Horton, R., 2019. Offline: Gender and global health—an inexcusable global failure. Lancet, 393 Britis(10171), 511. Online. Available: https://doi.org/10.1016/S0140-6736(19)30311-3.

Houkamau, C.A., Clarke, K., 2016. Why are those most in need of Sudden Unexplained Infant Death (SUDI) Prevention information the least likely to receive it? A comment on unconscious bias and Māori health. N. Z. Med. J., 129 (1440), 114–119. Online. Available: https://assets-global.website-files.com/5e332a62c703f653182faf47/5e332a62c703f630ed2f d16b_Houkamau Final.pdf.

Houkamau, C., Tipene-Leach, D., Clarke, K., 2016. The high price of being labelled 'high risk': Social context as a health determinant for sudden unexpected infant death in Māori communities. J. N. Z. Coll. Midwives, 52, 56–61. Online. Available: https://doi.org/10.12784/nzcomjnl52.2016.9.56-61.

Hunter, K., Roberts, J., Foster, M., et al, 2021. Dr Irihapeti Ramsden's powerful petition for cultural safety: Kawa Whakaruruhau. Nurs. Prax. Aotearoa N. Z., 37 (1), 25–28. Online. Available: https://doi.org/10.36951/27034542.2021.007.

Khan Academy, 2021. How is culture defined? Cultural Relativism. Online. Available: www.khanacademy.org/test-prep/mcat/society-and-culture/culture/a/cultural-relativism-article.

Kingsley, J., Townsend, M., Henderson-Wilson, C., et al, 2013. Developing an exploratory framework linking Australian Aboriginal peoples' connection to Country and concepts of wellbeing. Int. J. Environ. Res. Public Health, 10 (2), 678–698. Online. Available: https://search.proquest.com/docview/1346610464?accountid=14782.

Krusz, E., Hall, N., Barrington, D.J., et al, 2019. Menstrual health and hygiene among Indigenous Australian girls and women: barriers and opportunities. BMC Women's Health, 19 (1), 1–6. Online. Available: https://doi.org/10.1186/s12905-019-0846-7.

Kopua, D.M., Kopua, M.A., Bracken, P.J., 2020. Mahi a Atua: A Māori approach to mental health. Transcult. Psychiatry, 57 (2), 375–383. Online. Available: https://doi.org/10.1177/1363461519851606.

Kuzma, E., Pardee, M., Darling-Fisher, C., 2019. Lesbian, gay, bisexual, and transgender health: Creating safe spaces and caring for patients with cultural humility. J. Am. Assoc. Nurse Pract., 31 (3), 167–174. Online. Available: https://doi.org/10.1097/JXX.0000000000000131.

Lee, Y.S., Behn, M., Rexrode, K.M., 2021. Women's health in times of emergency: We must take action. J. Women's Health, 30 (3), 289–292. Online. Available: https://doi.org/10.1089/jwh.2020.8600.

Leitch, S., Zeng, J., Smith, A., et al, 2021. Medication risk management and health equity in New Zealand general practice: a retrospective cross-sectional study. Int. J. Equity Health, 20 (1), 1–8. Online. Available: https://doi.org/10.1186/s12939-021-01461-y.

Lewis, N.D., 2016. Sustainable development through a gendered lens: climate change adaptation and disaster risk reduction. Rev. Environ. Health, 31 (1), 97–102. Online. Available: https://doi.org/http://dx.doi.org/10.1515/reveh-2015-0077.

Liu, S., Dane, S., Gallois, C., et al, 2020. The dynamics of acculturation among older immigrants in Australia. J. Cross Cult. Psychol., 51 (6), 424–441. Online. Available: https://doi.org/10.1177/0022022120927461.

Mackean, T., Fisher, M., Friel, S., et al, 2020. A framework to assess cultural safety in Australian public policy. Health Promot. Int., 35 (2), 340–351. Online. Available: https://doi.org/10.1093/heapro/daz011.

Marcelin, J.R., Siraj, D.S., Victor, R., et al, 2019. The impact of unconscious bias in healthcare: How to recognize and mitigate it. J. Infect. Dis., 220 (Suppl 2), S62–S73. Online. Available: https://doi.org/10.1093/infdis/jiz214.

Markwick, A., Ansari, Z., Clinch, D., et al, 2019. Experiences of racism among Aboriginal and Torres Strait Islander adults living in the Australian state of Victoria: A cross-sectional population-based study. BMC Public Health, 19 (1), 1–14. Online. Available: https://doi.org/10.1186/s12889-019-6614-7.

Marmot, M.G., 2016. Empowering communities. Am. J. Public Health, 106 (2), 230–231. Online. Available: https://doi.org/10.2105/AJPH.2015.302991.

Marriott, R., Reibel, T., Coffin, J., et al, 2019. 'Our culture, how it is to be us'—Listening to Aboriginal women about on Country urban birthing. Women & Birth, 32 (5), 391–403. Online. Available: https://doi.org/10.1016/j.wombi.2019.06.017.

Marshall, S., Taki, S., Love, P., et al, 2021. The process of culturally adapting the Healthy Beginnings early obesity prevention program for Arabic and Chinese mothers in Australia. BMC Public Health, 21 (1), 1–16. Online. Available: https://doi.org/10.1186/s12889-021-10270-5.

McCarthy, J., 2020. Understanding why climate change impacts women more than men. Global Citizen. Online. Available: www.globalcitizen.org/en/content/how-climate-change-affects-women/?template=next.

Ministry of Health, 2020. Ola Manuia: Pacific health and wellbeing action plan 2020–2025. Ministry of Health, New Zealand Government. Online. Available: www.health.govt.nz/system/files/documents/publications/ola_manuia-phwap-22june.pdf.

Ministry of Health and Minister of Health, 2020. Health and independence report 2019. Ministry of Health, New Zealand.

Mitchell, A.G., Diddo, J., James, A.D., et al, 2021. Using community-led development to build health communication about rheumatic heart disease in Aboriginal children: A developmental evaluation. Aust. N. Z. J. Public Health, 45 (3), 212–219. Online. Available: https://doi.org/10.1111/1753-6405.13100.

New Zealand Ministry of Health, 2019. Mortality 2017 data tables. Online. Available: www.health.govt.nz/publication/mortality-2017-data-tables.

NiaNia, W., Bush, A., Epston, D., 2016. Collaborative and Indigenous mental health therapy: Tataihono—stories of Māori healing and psychiatry. Routledge.

NiaNia, W., Bush, A., Epston, D., 2019. He korowai o ngā tīpuna: Voice hearing and communication from ancestors. Australas. Psychiatry, 27 (4), 345–347. Online. Available: https://doi.org/10.1177/1039856219833792.

Nursing Council of New Zealand, 2011. Guidelines for cultural safety, the Treaty of Waitangi and Māori health in nursing education and practice. Nursing Council of New Zealand. Online. Available: www.nursingcouncil.org.nz.

Nursing Council of New Zealand, 2012. Code of conduct for Nurses. Nursing Council of New Zealand.

Nursing Council of New Zealand, 2016. Competencies for registered nurses. Nursing Council of New Zealand.

Perales, F., 2019. The health and wellbeing of Australian lesbian, gay and bisexual people: a systematic assessment using a longitudinal national sample. Aust NZ. J Public Health, 43 (3), 281–288. Online. Available: https://doi.org/10.1111/1753-6405.12855.

Pol, G. (2021). What is Country? Online. Available: www.commonground.org.au/learn/what-is-country.

Power, T., Lucas, C., Hayes, C., et al, 2020. 'With my heart and eyes open': Nursing students' reflections on placements in Australian, urban Aboriginal organisations. Nurse Educ. Pract., 49. Online. Available: https://doi.org/10.1016/j.nepr.2020.102904.

Ramsden, I., 1992. Teaching cultural safety. New Zealand Nursing Journal, 85 (5), 21–23.

Rees, S., Wells, R., 2020. Bushfires, COVID-19 and the urgent need for an Australian Task Force on gender, mental health and disaster. Aust. N. Z. J. Psychiatry, 54 (11), 1135–1136. Online. Available: https://doi.org/10.1177/0004867420954276.

Salgado, D.M., Knowlton, A.L., Johnson, B.L., 2019. Men's health-risk and protective behaviors: The effects of masculinity and masculine norms. Psychol. Men Masc., 20 (2), 266–275. Online. Available: https://doi.org/10.1037/men0000211.

Schrader-King, K., 2021. Girl's education. The World Bank. Online. Available: www.worldbank.org/en/topic/girlseducation.

Seeta Prabhu, K., Iyer, S.S., 2019. Gender and human development. In: Seeta Prabhu, K., Iyer, S.S. (Eds), Human development in an unequal world, first ed. Oxford University Press, pp. 230–269.

Sin, I., Stillman, S., Fabling, R., 2018. What drives the gender wage gap? September. Motu Economic and Public Policy Research. Online. Available: www.motu.nz/assets/Documents/our-work/population-and-labour/individual-and-group-outcomes/Gender-Wage-Gap-Executive-Summary.pdf.

Siverskog, A., Bromseth, J., 2019. Subcultural spaces: LGBTQ aging in a Swedish context. Int. J. Aging Hum. Dev., 88 (4), 325–340. Online. Available: https://doi.org/10.1177/0091415019836923.

Sorrentino, J., Augoustinos, M., Le Couteur, A., 2019. '[It] does not explain everything ... , nor does it explain nothing ... it explains some things': Australia's first female Prime Minister and the dilemma of gender. Fem. Psychol., 29 (1), 19–39. Online. Available: https://doi.org/10.1177/0959353518790595.

Stats NZ, 2018. Pacific People's ethnic group. 2018 Census ethnic group summaries. Online. Available: www.stats.govt.nz/tools/2018-census-ethnic-group-summaries/pacific-peoples.

Talamaivao, N., Harris, R., Cormack, D., et al, 2020. Racism and health in Aotearoa New Zealand: a systematic review of quantitative studies. N. Z. Med. J., 133 (1521), 55–68. Online.

Available: https://assets-global.website-files.com/5e332a62c703f653182faf47/5f5008b324cdb0d434b3ebae_Talamaivao FINAL.pdf.

Tarricone, I., Riecher-Rössler, A., 2019. Health and gender resilience and vulnerability factors for women's health in the contemporary society. Springer International Publishing. Online. Available: https://doi.org/10.1007/978-3-030-15038-9.

Tilstra, S.A., Kwolek, D., Mitchell, J.L., et al, 2020. Sex- and gender-based women's health: A practical guide for primary care. Springer International Publishing. Online. Available: https://doi.org/10.1007/978-3-030-50695-7.

Treloar, C., Stardust, Z., Cama, E., et al, 2021. Rethinking the relationship between sex work, mental health and stigma: A qualitative study of sex workers in Australia. Soc. Sci. Med., 268. Online. Available: https://doi.org/10.1016/j.socscimed.2020.113468.

Tremblay, M.-C., Graham, J., Porgo, T.V., et al, 2020. Improving cultural safety of diabetes care in indigenous populations of Canada, Australia, New Zealand and the United States: A systematic rapid review. Can. J. Diabetes, 44 (7), 670–678. Online. Available: https://doi.org/10.1016/j.jcjd.2019.11.006.

Turshen, M., 2020. Women's health movements: A global force for change, second ed.. Springer Singapore. Online. Available: https://doi.org/10.1007/978-981-13-9467-6.

Vorauer, J.D., Quesnel, M.S., 2017. Salient multiculturalism enhances minority group members' feelings of power. Pers. Soc. Psychol. Bull., 43 (2), 259–271. Online. Available: https://doi.org/10.1177/0146167216679981.

Westenra, B., 2019. A framework for cultural safety in paramedic practice. Whitireia Nurs. Health J., 26, 11–17. Online. Available: https://search.informit.org/doi/10.3316/informit.972385942431350.

Wilson, N.J., Cordier, R., Parsons, R., et al, 2019. An examination of health promotion and social inclusion activities: A cross-sectional survey of Australian community Men's Sheds. Health Promot. J. Austr., 30 (3), 371–380. Online. Available: https://doi.org/10.1002/hpja.217.

Withiel, T.D., Allen, B., Evans, K., et al, 2020. Assisting clients experiencing family violence: Clinician and client survey responses in a child and family health service. J. Clin. Nurs., 29 (21/22), 4076–4089. Online. Available: https://doi.org/10.1111/jocn.15434.

Workplace Gender Equality Agency, 2020. Women's economic security in retirement. Australian Government. Online. Available: www.wgea.gov.au/sites/default/files/documents/Women%27s_economic_security_in_retirement.pdf.

World Health Organization (WHO), 2016. Global Plan of Action. WHO, Geneva. Online. Available: www.who.int/reproductivehealth/publications/violence/global-plan-of-action/en/.

World Health Organization (WHO), 2021a. Gender and Health. WHO, Geneva. Online. Available: www.who.int/health-topics/gender#tab=tab_1.

World Health Organization (WHO), 2021b. Violence against women. WHO, Geneva. Online. Available: www.who.int/news-room/fact-sheets/detail/violence-against-women.

Wynter, K., Wilson, N., Thean, P., et al, 2019. Psychological distress, alcohol use, fatigue, sleepiness, and sleep quality: An exploratory study among men whose partners are admitted to a residential early parenting service. Aust. Psychol., 54 (2), 143–150. Online. Available: https://doi.org/10.1111/ap.12348.

Zambas, S.I., Wright, J., 2016. Impact of colonialism on Māori and Aboriginal healthcare access: a discussion paper. Contemp. Nurse, 52 (4), 398–409. Online. Available: https://doi.org/10.1080/10376178.2016.1195238.

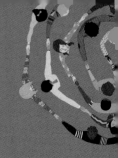

Introduction

Planning to support the health of individuals, families and communities relies on quality information regarding what is effective, efficient in terms of resource use and appropriate to the people whose lives will be affected. Effectiveness, efficiency and appropriateness are important variables to study in relation to healthcare systems and how health services and programs are implemented in communities. What is effective, efficient or appropriate can vary for particular individuals and groups across different settings and circumstances. Because of this variability, and the fact that people's lives are constantly changing, the research agenda is continually evolving. It will always be necessary to gather information on community needs, strengths and resources to identify what is transferable across settings, and what is unique to a particular community. For example, we know that a multidimensional health promotion strategy that is inclusive of environmental as well as behavioural factors will be more effective in helping people quit smoking than a single-factor intervention. However, the way a quit-smoking intervention is introduced, planned and received by various members of the community can vary widely.

Planning an effective intervention for smoking cessation, or any other initiative, depends not only on aggregated, population-level information from programs that have worked, but on the strengths of the community and characteristics of the group for whom the intervention is intended. These characteristics can be demographic features, such as age, stage or gender, or clinical factors, such as

OBJECTIVES

By the end of this chapter you will be able to:

1 describe the importance of translating research evidence into better community health and wellbeing

2 identify a range of research approaches that may be useful in a primary health care setting

3 explain the major issues in undertaking culturally safe research

4 develop a research question grounded in the conceptual foundations of primary health care to respond to a specific community health issue

5 outline the most important ethical issues associated with primary health care research and practice.

whether or not the impetus for smoking cessation has come from an illness, impairment or, in some cases, the influence of a significant other. Other important issues lie in situational factors such as people's preferences, their receptiveness or readiness to make a change, their level of health literacy, how they view the constraints and/or facilitating factors that affect their health choices and what supports are available to them to sustain the change. So although the findings from a body of research can sometimes be translated into practice across settings, there remains a need for contextual information, to study effectiveness and acceptability at the local level. This is the essence of most community health research. It is often evaluative; focusing on gathering and analysing data from within and external to the community, to identify what works, for whom, where, why, with what costs and outcomes, including acceptability by local residents.

Primary studies that collect evidence on the effect of certain interventions can be useful in studying population-level outcomes as a basis for benchmarking. This is a process of comparing outcomes across populations to forecast the likelihood of success in other populations. However, research is also needed on the differential needs and effects for various groups, and how certain interventions were experienced by people whose lives were changed. Although scientific evidence is important to indicate what works from a statistical point of view, community health research also requires explanations of why it did, or did not. This type of contextual information can help health planners understand what structural features of the community contributed to the health outcomes, and whether certain initiatives or processes could be tried in other contexts and with other people.

Besides identifying needs, structures, processes and outcomes, the research agenda also needs to include the type of studies that are aimed at developing conceptual frameworks for community health. These studies advance the field of community health by building a scaffold for knowledge development that can attract scholars and researchers to investigate the broader dimensions of community health. There is a need to study examples of good and best practice by

nurses and others who promote the health of a community through health education, advocacy or specific interventions. The research agenda should also include studies that link community health practice outcomes with the level or type of practitioners' educational preparation, experience, expertise and scope of practice. Attention to these issues is fundamental to informing our professional knowledge development and mapping our progress in developing and adapting new understandings.

Undertaking research should be a partnership, where information is seen to be the property of those providing it, often in the spirit of generating mutual understanding and benefits. Despite different methods, designs and philosophical approaches, the common goal of research is to inform improvements to the health of the population or the community itself, either through small incremental contributions to knowledge, or through studies of such magnitude as to create system change. This chapter provides an overview of issues and progress related to community health research, and suggests a number of research challenges and strategies that could be used to inform the creation and maintenance of community health.

KEY POINT

Why we research

- To advance knowledge
- To practise effectively, from an understanding of what works, for whom, in what context, why, with what costs and outcomes
- To compare or 'benchmark' knowledge with others to develop guidelines for best practice

KEY POINT

Community health research needs both scientific evidence to support outcomes *and* explanations of why an intervention may or may not have worked.

Researching the social determinants of health—globally, nationally and locally

Research is a core competency of nursing practice around the world (International Council of Nurses 2016, Nursing and Midwifery Board of Australia 2016, Nursing Council of New Zealand 2016). Communities are part of a global network working towards the common goal of social justice. Ideally, research studies that underpin the social justice agenda would build a body of knowledge to inform health promotion strategies, policies and practices to respond to global problems that also have implications at the local level. These problems include poverty, inequity in resource allocation, disparities in health and education, discrimination and disadvantage on the basis of gender, culture, race, age or geography, infectious diseases among those without access to treatment and environmental issues such as climate change and its impact on the health of communities. However, the global research agenda continues to be disadvantaged by the lack of large, interlinked databases, inadequate funding and, in some cases, the lack of political will to secure effective mechanisms for research collaborations.

Research studies are expensive. They require funding for researchers, investment in support structures (including the type of databases that could help integrate findings), personnel and, in many cases, specialised equipment. Clinicians, academics, policymakers and technical staff with research skills often have work demands other than research, which means that without financial support, their research becomes relegated to a low priority. Funding can help ensure that data are gathered and analysed appropriately, and that researchers have time and resources to promote collegial deliberation and dissemination of findings. Like other activities that have resource implications, research is inherently political. This means that at the national, regional and institutional levels, there are competing agendas for budget allocations. Decisions about funding research can be made on the basis of local issues, researcher interests or the needs of policymakers and politicians to demonstrate a short-term impact. When short-term, local goals are the focus, the broader global social justice agenda is likely to be given little attention. As health practitioners, it is important to advance local agendas and be responsive to the need for local research, but at the same time, maintain a commitment to the wider agenda of collecting data and translating findings into better healthcare for the global population.

KEY POINT

Think global in translating local findings into better healthcare for the global population, especially those investigating the social determinants of health (SDH).

KEY POINT

The global research agenda includes:

- poverty
- equity
- disparities in health and education
- discrimination and social exclusion
- lack of access to treatments
- environmental issues.

The most salient community issues at all levels are generally those related to the SDH. Research into the SDH is increasing. In 2006, 523 papers were indexed in PubMed using the term 'social determinants'. In 2016, this had increased to 2398 and by 2021 there were 375,563! Despite these increases, underresearched issues remain. These include questions that investigate models of empowerment for various groups differentiated by gender, culture and ethnicity, mechanisms for education and health literacy, climate change and the impact on Indigenous populations and environmental supports for healthy childhoods and lifelong wellbeing, including healthy ageing. These are complex issues, and research addressing these social determinants involves long-term, multidisciplinary studies of multiple factors across various settings and groups. There are limited opportunities for large-scale, comprehensive, longitudinal studies that would gather data from diverse groups in different countries over sufficient time to provide definitive answers to research questions. These studies are costly and rely on ongoing funding—often over decades. However, the findings from such studies provide much of the evidence for how the SDH impact on people's lives and will provide the future evidence for how interventions we develop now will work. For these reasons, it is imperative such studies continue. Box 10.1 describes the Nurses'

BOX 10.1

....

THE NURSES' HEALTH STUDY

....

The Nurses' Health Study (NHS) started in 1976 and is now into its third generation of nurses. It is one of the largest prospective investigations into the risk factors for chronic disease among women. Over 280 000 participants have taken part since its inception. Regular follow-up of study participants and repeated assessments of health and lifestyle factors have played a key role in shaping public health recommendations over many decades. Examples include:

- uncovering early links between smoking and cardiovascular disease
- determining links between postmenopausal obesity and breast cancer
- identifying a range of links between physical activity and health including how moderate physical activity reduces the risk of cognitive impairment
- identifying links between anxiety, posttraumatic stress disorder, childhood violence, caregiver burden and job insecurity and increased risk of coronary heart disease and diabetes (Trudel-Fitzgerald et al 2016).

Further information on the Nurses' Health Study can be found at www.nurseshealthstudy.org.

Health Study as an example of the findings of longitudinal studies and their contribution to the SDH.

The theoretical basis of studies examining the SDH has also increased as researchers attempt to explain the dynamics of the relationship between the SDH and disease. The life course theory proposes that socioeconomic disadvantage originating in childhood accumulates over the life course to disadvantage health in older age and vice versa (Cockerham et al 2017, Pacquiao & Douglas 2019). This theory underpins much of the discourse in Australian and New Zealand policy around the SDH. The fundamental cause theory suggests that, for a social variable to cause disease and mortality, it must: (1) influence multiple diseases; (2) affect those diseases through multiple pathways of risk; (3) be reproduced over time; and (4) involve access to resources that can minimise or avoid the risks and consequences of the disease (Cockerham et al 2017). An example would be socioeconomic status and the impact of income (or lack of) on various pathways to health and ill health. A third explanatory theory of the SDH is the health lifestyle theory that suggests structural variables such as class circumstances (age, gender, ethnicity), social networks and living conditions provide the social context for socialisation and the types of experiences that influence life choices (Cockerham et al 2017). Particularly important to understand in this theory is that health lifestyles are not the individualised decisions of a single person but are personal routines that merge into an aggregated characteristic of specific groups and classes (Cockerham et al 2017). These growing theories underpin the development of the SDH research agenda and our growing knowledge of the increasing number of factors that interact to create health and how we can strengthen these. However, challenges remain.

Golden and Wendel (2020) argue that traditional, epidemiological and biomedical approaches to public health are no longer sufficient to address the determinants of health or improve health inequities. Instead, they propose shifting towards diverse, knowledge-producing practices that allow for subjectivity and irreducibility (Golden & Wendel 2020). Adopting critical theory, hermeneutics and design thinking into the way we explore and understand the SDH will stimulate curiosity and innovation in a way that doesn't limit our understanding of phenomena to traditional Western biomedical approaches to the study of health (Golden & Wendel 2020).

Another constraint on the evidence-based agenda is the lack of coherence in the topics studied in different countries and between different cultures. To drive major change, research studies need to be collaborative, right from the stage of establishing the research agenda to identifying and evaluating solutions. The logistics of international or cross-institutional collaboration is sometimes prohibitive in terms of time or commitment of individual researchers, or when collaborators have different organisational pressures. Some of these pressures revolve around the lack of understanding by policymakers and research-granting agencies of the need for different perspectives in investigating a problem. Funding bodies often favour studies that are highly scientific, such as systematic reviews of existing research, especially clinical trials, rather than evaluative studies based on community perspectives. Community-based research studies must be collaborative—locally with community members, and nationally and internationally with those committed to generating the evidence to address equity.

The current trend towards translational research involves generating evidence, combining findings from multiple studies in a systematic review or integrative review, and translating the collective findings into clinical guidelines and change management strategies. An example of how research can lead to changes in policy, development of guidelines and ultimately improved health outcomes is the work undertaken to address sudden infant death syndrome (SIDS) also known as sudden unexplained death of an infant (SUDI) among Indigenous groups.

Evidence, to education, to child health practice in preventing SIDS/SUDI— case study

Australian and New Zealand child health professionals have spent the past two decades researching sudden unexpected infant deaths. In partnership with public health policymakers, clinicians and community members, their work is directed towards ensuring translation of research into policy and then into the best possible practice. Significant work is being done to address the high rate of SIDS/SUDI among Indigenous groups in both Australia and New Zealand, and recent falls in rates in New Zealand are demonstrating that the partnership approach between researchers, policymakers and practitioners is working (Tipene-Leach & Abel 2019). A 'blitz' approach to SUDI education, the targeted provision of portable infant safe sleeping devices (such as the Pēpi-Pod® and wahakura) and the development of safe sleeping policy across district health boards are seen as combining to create the reduction in incidence of SUDI (Tipene-Leach & Abel 2019).

The Pēpi-Pod® program comprises the provision of a portable infant sleeping device, safe sleeping parent education and safety briefing, and a family commitment to share safe sleeping messages within social networks (Young et al 2017). Māori researchers have also examined the efficacy of the *wahakura*. A wahakura is a hand-woven flax basket rather than the plastic Pēpi-Pod® that the baby is put to sleep in. The wahakura with baby in it then stays in the bed so that the baby is close to mum but has its own sleeping space. Researchers have found the wahakura is culturally acceptable, just as safe as a bassinet and has other benefits including improved breastfeeding rates among women who use it for their infants (Baddock et al 2017). These outcomes demonstrate the value of embedding Indigenous tradition alongside evidence of other preventive initiatives for SUDI (Tipene-Leach & Abel 2019). But despite many years of research and declining rates of SIDS/SUDI in the total population, rates for Aboriginal and Torres Strait Islanders in Australia have not reduced at the same rate as non-Indigenous, with rates remaining approximately three times higher for SIDS and four times higher for SUDI (Freemantle & Ellis 2018). Investigation by Cole and colleagues (2020) found that only 13% of families routinely practise all six of the Australian Red Nose safe sleeping recommendations. Unfortunately very few Aboriginal or Torres Strait Islanders participated in the study (1.9% or 62 individuals) and analysis on specific outcomes for this group were not included. However, another study examining the differences in the prevalence of risk factors for SUDI between Aboriginal and Torres Strait Islanders and non-Indigenous infants found bed/surface sharing and smoking were significant contributors to the rate of SUDI in this group and recommended culturally responsive prevention efforts targeting both (Shipstone et al 2020). The Pēpi-Pod® program has been successful in New Zealand and was trialled successfully in Queensland with the Aboriginal and Torres Strait Islander population (Young et al 2018; see Fig 10.1) but clearly more work is required.

KEY POINT

....

The evidence-based recommendations for safe sleeping are:

- sleep the baby on its back
- keep the baby's head and face uncovered
- keep the baby smoke-free before and after birth
- provide a safe sleeping environment night and day
- give the baby their own sleeping place in the adult caregivers' room for 6–12 months
- breastfeed the baby
- keep their immunisations up to date.

Evidence-based practice

Since the 1970s the evidence-based practice (EBP) movement has worked towards involving health professionals throughout the world in evidence-based health planning and evidence-informed practice. The objective of EBP at the global level is to help societies achieve efficiency, effectiveness, equity and improved global health. At the local level many EBP initiatives are intended to achieve similar goals and, in the process, to advance knowledge that can be used to develop capacity for ongoing developments. The SIDS/SUDI case study is an excellent example of EBP.

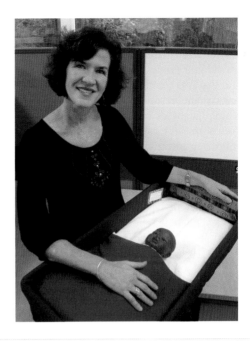

Figure 10.1 Professor Jeanine Young demonstrating a safe sleeping pod

Source: Photo courtesy of Professor Jeanine Young

EBP is often described in relation to evidence-based medicine (EBM), which was originally devised to inform a medical practitioner's intention to treat or intervene in a person's care. EBP is the integration of three things: the best available research evidence; the clinician's knowledge and expertise; and the individual patients' preferences, needs and values. All of these inform decision-making regarding care and treatment (Greenhalgh et al 2020). Establishing a research culture of EBP in any health service or community promotes an attitude of inquiry among health practitioners. A further benefit is that evidence can play a role in maintaining accountability for health resources by guiding decision makers to plan appropriately (Hoffman et al 2020). The process of EBP involves five steps. First, convert the need for information into an answerable research question. Some of the most important research questions for community health pose questions about how to promote health literacy or participation among certain groups, how outcomes may be moderated by various approaches to health promotion or the context of care or the effectiveness of interventions across cultural groups or across the life course. The second step is to search for the best existing evidence to answer the research question, which involves searching databases or scholarly journals or other sources of research such as local reports or reviews. The third step is to critically appraise existing evidence for its validity, impact and applicability. This step is made easier by the fact that in recent years helpful guidelines have been developed to help researchers appraise different types of studies. The EQUATOR Network (Enhancing the QUAlity and Transparency Of health Research) is one of the most useful of these guidelines (www.equator-network.org). The fourth step in EBP is integration of the evidence with the researcher's existing knowledge, contextual information about the group or community circumstances and preferences, and any other situational information that may help inform practice. The fifth step is concerned with quality in that it involves evaluation and self-reflection on the thoroughness and accuracy of steps 1 to 4 (Hoffman et al 2020).

> **KEY POINT**
>
> Evidence for practice is the best available research evidence, the clinician's knowledge and expertise and the individual patient's views and preferences.

In most cases, researchers begin by posing their question, then refining it to reduce ambiguity, to clarify what data they will collect, and to guide the literature search. It is helpful to collect and review the literature around the PICO mnemonic. That is, search for studies of the Population (children, adults, etc.), the Intervention (e.g. smoking cessation), Comparisons (group versus individual health education and supports) and Outcomes (e.g. smoke-free days). In the process of searching the literature, researchers usually use synonyms and variant words and expressions, often in databases like CINAHL, MEDLINE, PubMed or PROQUEST with which they are familiar, or in

journals where similar studies have been published in the area of interest. In some cases, the research project *is* the literature review, either as a systematic review, an integrative review or a meta-analysis.

> **KEY POINT**
>
> The steps in EBP are:
>
> 1 researchable question
>
> 2 literature review
>
> 3 critical appraisal of studies
>
> 4 integrate knowledge with contextual information
>
> 5 evaluate and re-check accuracy of steps above.

SYSTEMATIC REVIEWS, LITERATURE REVIEWS, INTEGRATIVE REVIEWS AND META-ANALYSES

A systematic review establishes the parameters for adequate or best available research evidence using preset criteria, derived primarily from randomised controlled clinical trials (RCTs) and other high-quality primary research studies. The original intention of systematic reviews for EBM was to provide the basis for treatment recommendations (Bero & Rennie 1995). In community health the 'best treatment' often means the best strategies for health promotion. The advantage of a systematic review is that it uses an explicit and auditable protocol. Common protocols are available from the resources of the Cochrane Collaboration (www.cochrane.org) or the Joanna Briggs Institute (https://jbi.global/). Using a protocol ensures breadth and consistency in terms of appraising the participants, interventions and outcomes. The systematic review involves a clear definition of eligibility criteria for a study, a comprehensive search of all relevant studies available at the time of the review, explicit, reproducible and uniformly applied criteria in selecting studies for the review, rigorous appraisal of potential bias in the studies reviewed and a synthesis of study results (Bennett et al 2020). A *meta-analysis* takes the review to another level by combining and statistically analysing the evidence from a number of studies on a similar topic to enhance the validity of findings in relation to the outcomes of the study or the *effect size*. This statistical computation can provide a better estimate of a clinical effect than simply analysing the results from individual studies (Shaikh & Jha 2020). In cases where the studies selected cannot be combined statistically, the review can consist of a narrative analysis.

Diabetes is one area of community health that has attracted a proliferation of systematic reviews in recent times, which reflects its importance to clinicians and policymakers. Systematic reviews have been conducted on the links between lifestyle changes and glycaemic control (García-Molina et al 2020) and progression to type 2 diabetes in women with a known history of gestational diabetes (Vounzoulaki et al 2020). Other systematic reviews have been conducted on different populations in relation to the uptake of programs and benefits of physical activity and/or good nutrition (Muley et al 2021, Xia et al 2020). Others focus on the systemic changes that might be required to improve diabetes care. For example, Zhou and colleagues (2020) evaluated the cost-effectiveness of interventions designed to prevent type 2 diabetes among both high-risk individuals and whole populations. They found that both lifestyle and metformin interventions in high-risk individuals were cost-effective from a health system or societal perspective and taxing sugar-sweetened beverages as a

population-based intervention was cost saving from both the healthcare system and governmental perspectives (Zhou et al 2020). However, Zhou and colleagues caution that the conclusions from the review still need to be viewed with caution as many of the studies, and in particular the population-based strategies, utilise simulation modelling as it is difficult to truly ascertain the cost-effectiveness beyond a study trial period. Systematic reviews always conclude with statements about the limitations of the analysis in terms of disparate methods, the failure of some researchers to identify the theoretical foundations of their research, the difficulties in comparing different population groups and the need for more studies on a particular topic. These criticisms are typical of most systematic reviews, particularly where the reviewers try to draw definitive conclusions on appropriate intervention strategies or clinical guidelines from different research approaches. Box 10.2 provides a cautionary tale on how a systematic review can be taken to extremes.

Some researchers argue that all research should be preceded by a systematic review; however, there are many aspects of community health for which systematic reviews are not available, so researchers setting out to conduct a study often review the literature available using alternative strategies such as *integrative reviews*. Integrative reviews also review the literature pertaining to a certain topic, but they are broader reviews than systematic reviews in that they include experimental and non-experimental studies (Toronto & Remington 2020). An integrative review can also be designed to define concepts, review theories, review evidence and analyse methodological issues (Toronto &

Because of the myriad factors influencing community health, formulaic research strategies are not always appropriate. Community problems and issues require different paradigms that encourage researchers to articulate the range of problems and solutions in the context of the community or group. A persuasive argument for a multidimensional approach to research is cleverly presented in a study of parachute use to prevent death and major trauma related to gravitational challenge (Smith & Pell 2003). The authors' objective was to determine whether parachutes are effective in preventing major trauma. Predictably, they found no RCTs in their systematic review, and concluded that the effectiveness of parachutes has not been subjected to rigorous evaluation. They suggested that the most radical proponents of EBP, those who criticise observational studies, might want to conduct a double blind, randomised, placebo-controlled, crossover trial of jumping out of a plane without a parachute!

The main advantage of an integrative review is that combining and summarising several types of literature, including theoretical literature, can provide a more complete picture of a phenomenon or healthcare problem (Toronto & Remington 2020). Others have used a *scoping review*, which is broader than a review of a single problem or issue in that it is intended to scope a broad topic. Beks and colleagues' (2020) scoping review for evidence of mobile primary health care clinics implemented specifically for Indigenous populations in Canada, Australia, New Zealand and the United States found both geographical gaps in the implementation and a paucity of evaluation of such clinics. The reviewers recommend mixed methods evaluations inclusive of Indigenous views and perspectives to gain greater insight into the value and potential of these clinics (Beks et al 2020).

Another useful type of review is the *concept analysis*, which can help build a common theoretical foundation for future studies from a consistent set of understandings. Literature retrieval and appraisal can be time-consuming and requires a high level of skill. Because not all community practitioners have the time or support from management to develop and use these skills in practice, access to quality systematic reviews can be achieved through journals whose sole purpose is to collate and share systematic reviews. These include the *International Journal of Evidence-based Healthcare* and *Evidence-Based Nursing*.

RANDOMISED CONTROLLED TRIALS

Randomised controlled trials (RCTs) are described as the 'gold standard' in research, because they use an experimental study design, which allows the researcher the greatest control over the research (Conway & Duff 2020). Some studies are 'quasi-experimental' in that the researcher may not have the degree of control expected of a scientific experiment, such as when they are unable to randomise subjects. Over the past two decades researchers have refined the techniques involved in conducting RCTs with a set of guidelines, the Consolidated Standards of Reporting Trials (CONSORT), which are widely used throughout

Remington 2020). As care provision shifts from hospitals into primary health care settings, a number of useful integrative reviews have helped identify issues for nurses transitioning to work in primary health care. For example, Zambas and colleagues (2020) examined the factors affecting retention and success of Māori undergraduate nursing students. They identified three key factors that play a role in Māori student success and retention: Māori student identity, institutional support factors and program factors. Recommendations included reframing teaching strategies and curricula and developing strategies that align with Māori values and beliefs (Zambas et al 2020).

the world to ensure consistency in reporting findings (see www.consort-statement.org). At a basic level, the RCT uses a population sample and randomly allocates approximately half to an experimental group and the other half to a control group. The experimental group receives an intervention, while the control group typically has 'usual care' or no intervention. The outcome of interest is measured in both groups before (pre-test) and after (post-test) the intervention. Changes that occur in the experimental group between the pre-test and the post-test are reasonably attributed to the intervention (Conway & Duff 2020). This attribution relies on the condition that all other influences are controlled, which can be difficult for educational interventions. So, for example, if a researcher was introducing a program to teach parents about nutrition it would be necessary that the intervention group had no outside influences other than the education provided as part of the program. This would be a challenge as some parents may have preexisting knowledge, others may have little access to the recommended foods and others may have a child who was a fussy eater. In these cases, the challenge would be to eliminate extraneous influences by selecting participants with exactly the same knowledge level, similar access to the nutritious foods and infants with similar temperaments. Some researchers would find this level of control impossible and they may revert to a more qualitative evaluation of their educational program.

Clearly, RCTs are important for developing well-verified, objective research studies, but in reducing the factors studied within tightly defined criteria they often fail to reveal the complexity within which people maintain health (de Jong et al 2015). Another criticism of RCTs is that the controlled conditions of a clinical trial are rarely available in communities. It would be unethical and not useful to allocate people to an RCT, giving one group the intervention and withholding it from the other. On the other hand, a meta-analysis that combines the findings from a group of studies can be useful, especially if the findings and conclusions of the studies are synthesised into new ways of looking at the community or planning for community change.

Evidence for practice: home visiting

We have noted throughout this book that home visiting is an important practice strategy for nurses and others working in primary health care settings. It is used as an intervention across the spectrum from prior to birth through to old age and palliative care. David Olds and colleagues were among the original researchers to examine the positive outcomes among children and their mothers where the mothers had received intensive nurse home visiting in the first 2 years of the child's life (Kitzman et al 2010). More recently, Beatson and colleagues (2021) undertook a systematic review of RCTs into nurse home visiting programs and identified seven core components of program effectiveness: antenatal commencement, support to age 2 years, at least 19 scheduled visits, experienced or highly qualified nurses with specific training, caseloads of approximately 25 families, regular supervision and multidisciplinary support. In summary, the research has shown nurse home visiting programs have a range of significant outcomes for mothers, children and governments including decreased spending on social welfare, longer partner relationships, decreased role impairment from drugs or alcohol at 12 years post intervention (Kitzman et al 2010) and increased safety, increased warm parenting, increased home parental involvement and more regular bedtimes at 2 years (Goldfeld et al 2019).

Other research into home visiting programs in the early childhood period has, however, had more mixed results. In a local example, a nine-year follow-up study of children and families who had received intensive home visiting as part of the Early Start program in New Zealand found that while some outcomes were encouraging, others were less so. The positive outcomes included significantly reduced risk of hospital attendance for unintentional injury, lower risk of parent-reported harsh punishment, lower levels of physical punishment, higher parenting competence scores and more positive child behavioural adjustment scores. However, there were no significant differences in a range of measures of parental behaviour and family outcomes such as maternal depression, parental substance use, intimate partner violence, adverse economic outcomes and life stress (Fergusson et al 2013). A more recent quasi-experimental study of a similar program in New Zealand called Family Start had similar findings showing good outcomes in some areas (e.g. post neonatal infant mortality and SUDI) but less positive results in other areas (e.g. child maltreatment) (Vaithianathan et al 2016).

So how does the evidence guide our practice when there are such variable outcomes? While a systematic review gives us a useful overview of outcomes, it is also important to consider the context within which interventions are designed and implemented, and the research question that guides the review. The evidence suggests that home visitation programs are most effective when they focus on children through providing parents with new skills, knowledge and approaches to parenting, but less successful when targeted at changing long-standing parent or family issues and challenges. It is important that home visitation programs have clear goals and that nurses and others engaged in them are realistic about the outcomes that can be achieved.

Big data

Big data is the term used to refer to the massive data sets that are being generated from a range of sources, including electronic medical records, mobile devices, laboratory studies and administrative claims data (Remus & Donelle 2019). Researchers are starting to explore how these data can be analysed on a mass basis to identify patterns, causes and outcomes of disease, improve the understanding of health behaviour, provide the basis for more personalised medicine and enable nurses and other clinicians the ability to analyse data instantly to make good clinical and managerial decisions (Remus & Donelle 2019). Very little nursing data is analysed in these data sets currently and there is a growing imperative to ensure nurse leaders have the informatics skills to be able to mine large data sets for the information required to make good decisions (Remus & Donelle 2019). It is also essential that nurses in practice understand the value of big data and how it can contribute to patient care. Nurses, general practitioners and practice managers interviewed in Victoria, Australia identified the

value of data accessed from general practice electronic medical records but also had concerns regarding privacy, the risk of data breaches and patient consent (Monaghan et al 2020). These are legitimate concerns and must be addressed openly and transparently to foster trust in the use of big data. However, other risks exist, not least that when we use data, machine learning, artificial intelligence and other numerically focused data sources, we risk losing contextual information about individuals and communities. If we do not understand the experience of people and communities, our efforts to support them may be futile. So although big data provides new and exciting opportunities for understanding the world, it is only one source of information about people and communities.

Paradigms

From the early days of EBP, 'evidence' was considered as quantifiable data situated within the paradigm of logical positivism. A paradigm is a set of beliefs or perspectives that creates a pattern for scholarly inquiry. Paradigms therefore encompass the philosophical assumptions that underpin the way we view natural phenomena (Sweet & Davis 2020). The *positivist paradigm* is used in quantitative studies, where the research is based on rigid rules of logic and measurement, truth, absolute principles and prediction (Sweet & Davis 2020). RCTs and systematic reviews are part of the positivist paradigm. In contrast, the *interpretive paradigm* focuses on the meanings people ascribe to their actions and interactions and is one of the approaches used in qualitative studies. Interpretive research is undertaken on the assumption that reality is socially constructed through the use of language and shared meanings, so researchers seek to understand phenomena by listening to people or observing their actions (Sweet & Davis 2020). Another paradigm or philosophical perspective is the *critical perspective*, sometimes called the *critical social theory* paradigm, which addresses social institutions and issues of power and alienation as well as new opportunities (Sweet & Davis 2020). Critical perspectives are based on the assumption that knowledge is value-laden, and shaped by historical, social, political, gender and economic conditions that, for some people, can be oppressive. Critical approaches endeavour to encourage empowerment and equality for participants, as well as generate knowledge that can be used as a basis for change (Sweet & Davis 2020).

These existing approaches provide the basis for what may become the next paradigm of thought that will come to bear on nursing. New technologies, including artificial intelligence, cyborgs, biotechnologies and other information technologies, such as big data, blur the boundaries between what is human and what is artificial. Nurses traditionally span the borders between technology and the person, but these borders are narrowing. Our research endeavours will be challenged as we seek to balance person-centred care approaches with new technologies and what they mean for the way people live their lives and respond to healthcare. Teixeira de Almeida Vieira Monteiro (2016) proposes that nursing research must now be built on these previous paradigms but will take a different shape and meaning as we begin to grasp the impact of technology on human life as we know it today.

KEY POINT

A paradigm is an understanding or viewpoint of the world. Three common paradigms are positivist, interpretive and critical. The impact of artificial intelligence, cyborg technology, genomics and big data on human life will see the advent of a new paradigm of thought we have yet to fully conceptualise.

The multidimensional nature of communities requires us to include the cultural, spiritual and environmental dimensions of community life when we undertake research within this domain. The type of knowing we gain from this approach is multifaceted and likely to provide richer knowledge than that obtained from systematic assessments of prior research findings. It is often described as *naturalistic inquiry*, as information is gleaned from the natural setting and interpreted using various

interpretive, rather than *statistical*, techniques. Naturalistic data can include informant interviews, focus groups (sometimes called 'yarning' groups, particularly in Indigenous populations), observational data and document analysis (Whitehead & Disler 2020). The knowledge gained from this type of research is an important element in informing policy and practice changes, especially when more than one type of inquiry is used in combination. Interpretive methods can be a useful approach to gathering and analysing data on the realities of community life for different groups of people. Three of the most common interpretive methods that are based on naturalistic inquiry are phenomenology, ethnography and grounded theory. Case study research is also becoming increasingly common in community settings. The EQUATOR Network outlined earlier in the chapter also provides criteria for reporting qualitative research known as COREQ. These criteria help us appraise the quality of qualitative research.

Where to find out more on ...

Qualitative research approaches

- Qualitative Research Guidelines Project: www.qualres.org/index.html

Translational research: knowledge translation and knowledge transfer (KT)

Translating research into policy and/or practice is a complex social process involving multiple interactions and linkages between producers and users of research. Knowledge transfer, or knowledge translation as this process is known, includes not only disseminating or distributing knowledge but using carefully planned strategies to identify target audiences and delivering messages in ways that are understandable, actionable, accommodating and cost-effective (Lockwood et al 2020). In translating program knowledge to practice, partnerships with community members are integral to success,

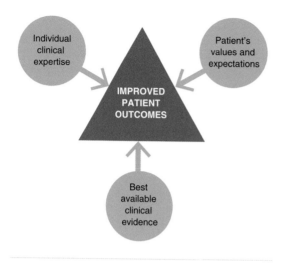

Figure 10.2 Translating evidence to practice

ensuring the acceptability of implementation strategies. Figure 10.2 shows the interactions required to translate evidence into practice.

One of the trends guiding research in nursing and other health disciplines is the move towards community-based research partnerships. Community-based research provides an ideal opportunity to inform policies from the ground up as well as supporting communities to implement the findings of the research back into their communities. It is also a way of providing feedback to policymakers of the applicability of policies on the ground, where people live, work, study or play. Funding bodies often support community partners such as government departments, hospitals or health districts, as collaborators in research studies, knowing that the information that will emerge will be more authentic than it would be if the researcher was working alone to investigate a community problem. Local partnerships are also considered to have *ecological validity*; that is, real-world relevance.

Partnering with communities in planning and implementing research creates many kinds of knowledge. These include *propositional* knowledge gained from identifying the research question(s), *practical knowledge*, from developing the skills and competencies of research, *experiential knowledge* from participating in the research and *presentational knowledge* from sharing information that will address the research question. Generating these types of

knowledge through ongoing interaction between researchers and the many levels of stakeholders is crucial to translating evidence to practice for evidence-informed decision-making. A study by Chowdhury and colleagues (2021) identified multiple different types of knowledge translation activities to engage with community members including community meetings, information or education sessions, community forums and engaging with community members throughout the research process such as in planning and conceptualisation of the study, data collection, interpretation, dissemination or implementation. Dissemination and implementation approaches need to be culturally appropriate and draw on Indigenous preferences. Such preferences may include culturally appropriate flyers or posters, local radio or the provision of food at community meetings to discuss research findings (Blue Bird Jernigan et al 2020). Engaging community members in the process also builds capacity, not only in knowledge development but in fostering skills and confidence among community members for empowerment and long-term commitment (Nykiforuk 2021). Some other types of research that involve community members closely in the research process include community-based participatory research and action research.

Researchers have also come to realise that clinical guidelines are a crucial aspect of promoting knowledge transfer (KT). Techniques for developing clinical guidelines are rapidly evolving with the development of protocols for grading evidence and rating the strength of recommendations from research studies. The Cochrane Collaboration and other organisations maintain a repository of protocols or 'guidelines for developing guidelines'.

Relevant to the way in which knowledge transfer takes place is implementation science or the scientific study of methods to promote the uptake of research or evidence-based practices into routine practice and improve the quality of healthcare (McCluskey & O'Connor 2020).

COMMUNITY-BASED PARTICIPATORY RESEARCH (CBPR)

CBPR is a collaborative research approach that specifically focuses on the equitable involvement of community partners in the research process (Israel 2013, Springer & Skolarus 2019). CBPR should always begin with a research topic of importance to the community and be based on the principles of co-learning and community partnerships in investigating inequities, which is intended to address health from both positive and ecological processes and promote sharing of findings (Brush et al 2020, Israel et al 2001, Israel 2013). CBPR is a culturally sensitive approach to community health research in that the researcher adopts an attitude of 'cultural humility', which is intended to redress power imbalances and maintain mutually respectful, dynamic community partnerships (Springer & Skolarus 2019). The key principles of CBPR are listed in Box 10.3, and Box 10.4 describes

---

BOX 10.3

KEY PRINCIPLES OF CBPR

1 Acknowledges community as the unit of identity
2 Builds on community strengths and resources
3 Facilitates collaborative, equitable involvement of all partners in all research phases involving an empowering and power-sharing process that attends to social inequalities
4 Promotes co-learning and capacity building among all partners
5 Integrates knowledge and action for mutual benefit
6 Focuses on the local relevance of public health problems and emphasises an ecological approach to health
7 Involves systems development using a cyclical and iterative process
8 Disseminates findings and knowledge to all partners
9 Involves a long-term process and commitment to sustainability

Source: Israel, B., Eng, E., Schulz, A., Parker, E., 2012. Introduction to methods for community-based participatory research for health. In: B. Israel, E. Eng, A. Schulz, E. Parker (Eds), Methods for community-based participatory research for health (second ed., pp. 3–37). John Wiley & Sons, Inc.

BOX 10.4

CBPR IN ACTION: THE ROLE OF ELDERS IN THE WELLBEING OF A CONTEMPORARY AUSTRALIAN INDIGENOUS COMMUNITY

CBPR is a useful approach to working with Indigenous communities as it engages with the community prior to, during and after the research. This engagement ensures the research is grounded in the reality of people's lives and will have meaningful outcomes for those whose lives may be impacted by the results. Busija and colleagues (2020) undertook a CBPR project with a regional Indigenous community in Queensland, Australia, to develop a conceptual model of the role of Elders in the community. Even before the study started, the researchers and community held a yarning circle to discuss the proposed research and potential impact of the findings on the community. The yarning circle established a working relationship between researchers and the community, identified issues of importance to the community and refined the aims of the research to ensure relevance to the community. Data collection, data structuring, interpretation of results and generation of a concept map all included community participants. The study developed a seven-cluster concept map of the role of Elders including community relations, passing down the knowledge, dealing with racism and oppression, building a better-resourced community, intergenerational connectedness, safeguarding our identity and caring for our youth. The results were strongly endorsed by the Elders. The outcomes of the study provide knowledge regarding the strengths Elders bring to their communities and the importance of their involvement in the development of local solutions and governmental policy to increase community wellbeing.

an example of CBPR in action. We also discuss CBPR in Chapter 4.

ACTION RESEARCH

Action research revolves around flexible planning through iterative (repetitive) cycles, wherein the researchers and their partners in the community consider a research problem, then together engage in cycles of planning, proposed action, evaluation and further cycles of planning and action (Whitehead & Halcomb 2020). Action research studies are conducted within the critical paradigm with the aim of decreasing the gap between research and implementation (Whitehead & Halcomb 2020). Action research actively engages those who would normally be considered subjects of research and is a particularly useful method for changing clinical practice (Hannes & Bennett 2020). Action research adopts a partnership approach similar to CBPR, in which all partners are considered co-researchers in exploring solutions to an issue of concern. As in CBPR, the researcher's role is to create a trusting environment, and to help keep the analysis on track with careful documentation, while helping others develop analytical skills and capacity. One of the most salient issues relevant to community health research is the capacity of action research studies to help people clarify their meanings, behaviours and interactions in the cultural contexts of their lives. Action research is an umbrella term that captures a range of different research processes including appreciative inquiry, participatory action research, community action research, co-operative inquiry and emancipatory action research.

Mixed methods research

While this chapter cannot report on all the differing types of research that exist, the types mentioned are particularly appropriate for use when working with communities. The final type we cover here is mixed methods research. Mixed methods research is an approach that combines qualitative and quantitative data, different qualitative approaches to explore a single phenomenon or different quantitative approaches to examine a single factor (Whitehead & Halcomb 2020). Incorporating contextual and cultural elements to the traditional designs of RCTs or quasi-experimental studies can help improve both theoretical and practical understandings that lie at the heart of community interventions. Similarly, discovering people's perspectives on health and wellbeing by listening to their stories or interview responses can lead to hypotheses that can be tested in the controlled conditions of quantitative research (Whitehead & Halcomb 2020).

Questions that require a mixed-method design are: those that cannot be explained by only one type of data; issues that require considerable breadth and depth; problems where there is a need to confirm or enhance findings with a second type of data; or studies where a research instrument is being developed from comprehensive information about the topic (Whitehead & Halcomb 2020). Mixed method research provides deeper insight into the area under study and is ideal when working in the complex field of community health where people's experiences and views are as important as the statistics underlying community health issues.

Researching culture

Over the past decades, research into cultural issues has grown steadily. This agenda is starting to be extended to provide insights into the features of inclusive societies, intergenerational interactions in different cultures and how expressions of culture affect health and wellbeing. Investigating cultural issues as a basis for practice is essential to successfully confront the needs of migrant groups during transitions to their new life, to anticipate influences on differing cultural groups' health and health service preferences throughout ageing, to understand how Indigenous cultures experience health and wellbeing and to explore how families negotiate, change and work within the context of their cultural and social lives.

Naturalistic research, on its own or in combination with other methods, is an ideal approach to begin a program of culturally oriented research, especially if the nascent ideas for the study arise from the cultural community itself. This often occurs in a round table or discussion forum, where ideas can evolve into CBPR. One approach that has gained popularity with different cultural groups is *appreciative inquiry*, which is conducted within the interpretive or naturalistic paradigm. An appreciative inquiry is similar to participatory action research and participatory evaluation in that the objective is to ensure inclusive, empowering research processes that build hope, trust, respect and, ultimately, capacity for change. The focus in appreciative inquiry is on what is working well and how this can be enhanced rather than identifying a problem to be solved, with the researcher bringing people together to 'discover, dream, design and deliver' innovations for change (Burns et al 2020). This can begin from a storytelling group, as is often the case in understanding cultural aspects of social life from individuals' oral histories. Research approaches such as photovoice could be considered as a form of appreciative inquiry, or an adjunct to ethnographic studies. (See Fig 10.3.) Appreciative inquiry can be used as a form of evaluation that focuses on the strengths of an approach rather than weaknesses which is often the focus of traditional evaluation. In Chapter 5 we discuss evaluation more closely in relation to project planning.

Ethnography focuses on the descriptive study of cultures and the different ways cultural groups view relationships and the world around them (Whitehead & Disler 2020). This means that all data must be culturally contextualised with special attention to cultural relevance of language and meaning at the individual, group and community level (Molloy et al 2021). Research studies that do not attend to these cultural aspects may be well intentioned, but they can potentially negate the sociocultural reality of a vulnerable population (Sheridan & Geia 2020, Wilson & Neville 2009). Ethnographers explore the artefacts, structures and

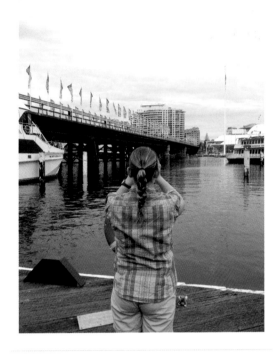

Figure 10.3 Photos capture many stories and perspectives that may differ from the written word.

Source: Photo courtesy of Jill Clendon.

dimensions of a culture that create people's life worlds, including their knowledge.

In any context, researching people's experiences of health and wellbeing can be strengthened with a trajectory perspective, particularly over the life course. Trajectory research is a succinct and useful way to describe changes over time to identify assets and risks as a basis for planning how, when and for whom nursing and other interventions and self-care are most effective. For example, a study of the developmental trajectories of suicidal ideation among a sample of 521 early to middle adolescents found suicidal ideation varies according to age, meaning the best time for intervention is in early adolescence, particularly around school transitions (Adrian et al 2016).

Researching with Indigenous people

Indigenous people have been the focus of many studies in Australia and New Zealand, and some of this research has not advanced the type of knowledge that contributes to their empowerment or self-determination. In some cases, researchers have forged relationships that have unearthed important features of Indigenous people's health, but in other cases, research reports have shown stereotypical perspectives of the researchers, rather than the researched. Some studies have actually damaged relationships, resulted in significant loss of trust and violated the principles of cultural safety (Bobba 2019, Wilson & Neville 2009). This oversight has not been an intended goal of the research, but rather a lack of understanding of the cultural and structural constraints on gathering meaningful data. As Bandler (2015, p. 187) asserted:

> The progression of research, particularly health research, and research ethics in work with Aboriginal Australians, parallels the progression of Australian history, from protection and biological assimilation through cultural assimilation to political activism and self-determination.

CULTURALLY SAFE RESEARCH

Researchers involved in research with Indigenous people must approach any project from a position of humility and cultural safety. Research is never done *on* people but *with* people, acknowledging their rights, recognising their sovereignty and respecting their perspective. There are a number of guiding documents for researchers seeking to work with Indigenous populations in Australia or New Zealand. A list of these can be found in Box 10.5. Most importantly, for culturally safe research, there is a need for non-Indigenous researchers to eliminate their propensity to draw comparisons between Indigenous and non-Indigenous populations, and instead study phenomena or events in Indigenous groups over time, ideally using Indigenous methodologies, focusing on strengths and reclaiming heritage (Sheridan & Geia 2020).

BOX 10.5

GUIDING DOCUMENTS FOR RESEARCHERS WORKING WITH INDIGENOUS POPULATIONS IN AUSTRALIA AND NEW ZEALAND

Te Ara Tika Guidelines for Māori Research Ethics: A framework for researchers and ethics committee members (Hudson et al 2010)

Ngā Pou Rangahau The Strategic Plan for Māori Health Research 2010–2015 (Health Research Council of New Zealand 2010)

Ethical conduct in research with Aboriginal and Torres Strait Islander peoples and communities: Guidelines for researchers and stakeholders (NHMRC 2018a)

National statement on ethical conduct in human research, 2007 (Updated 2018) (National Health and Medical Research Council 2018b)

Because of the deep relationship between Indigenous culture and land, health research must consider the connection between health and place. Other important aspects for researchers to consider include the use of language appropriate to the context, the engagement of Elders or Kaumatua in the research process and the place of kinship and ancestors within Indigenous ways of knowing (Sheridan & Geia 2020). Research must reflect Indigenous interests and not only produce locally relevant knowledge but also develop their research capacity. Such research offers the opportunity to focus on strengths with the premise of creating social change through empowerment, especially in reinforcing Indigenous identity (Gray & Oprescu 2016). Academics can be part of these networks, framing cultural communities as learning communities where all members are co-producers of knowledge. A major task for the researcher is to create safe spaces for dialogue and negotiation, so the group can determine the extent and nature of their involvement. Bulloch and colleagues' (2019) exploration of strength-based, bottom-up approaches to Aboriginal health and wellbeing services found community-driven, holistic, person-centred approaches that balanced the strengths within their communities with awareness of the constraints of functioning within a post-colonial and neoliberal environments were key to successfully achieving positive outcomes. One of the key elements in each of the communities included in the study was the use of 'yarning circles' to engage with community members (Bulloch et al 2019). Yarning is a culturally appropriate way of encouraging dialogue with Aboriginal and Torres Strait Islander people and involves the sharing of stories between a storyteller and a story listener (Marriott et al 2019). Yarning enables Indigenous people to talk freely and as a research approach can help eliminate the structural disadvantage that can occur when externally imposed research contributes to the process of decolonisation (Sharmil et al 2021).

In New Zealand, concern and distrust over the way in which research on Māori has been practised and by whom has led to a growth in research using an approach called Kaupapa Māori research (Rolleston et al 2016, Tipa 2019). Kaupapa Māori is a term used by Māori to describe the practice and philosophy of living a life that is informed by Māori culture (Rolleston et al 2016). Kaupapa Māori research (by Māori, for Māori, of Māori) describes research that is collectivist, acknowledges Māori aspirations for research and is largely conceived, developed and frequently carried out by Māori with the end outcome of benefit to Māori (Rolleston et al 2016, Tipa 2019). Although the approach was first developed in education research, it has become commonly used in health and other areas. Hapeta and colleagues (2019) use a Kaupapa Māori case study approach and Indigenous forms of storytelling (pūrākau, whakataukī) to explore how the inclusion of Māori forms of knowledge influenced the sense of identity, leadership and wellbeing on and off the field of a men's provincial rugby team in Aotearoa New Zealand. The study found that research and practice informed by Indigenous knowledge and values can improve the wellbeing of Indigenous people at the individual and collective level (Hapeta et al 2019).

One of the most important elements of planning Indigenous research is for the researcher to assume a reflexive attitude as a first step in ensuring cultural safety. For a non-Indigenous researcher, this involves reflecting on how their worldview might influence the research, and the processes of analysis and dissemination of findings (Sharmil et al 2021, Sheridan & Geia 2020). Another important element is to actively pursue ethical approval for the research from Indigenous-controlled ethics committees, to ensure that Indigenous interests are represented in all processes. These include committees such as the Māori Health Committee of the Health Research Council of New Zealand, the Queensland Aboriginal and Islander Health Forum and the Western Australian Aboriginal Health Ethics Committee. In other states of Australia, besides Western Australia and Queensland, separate arrangements are made for ethical review through Aboriginal peak bodies at state and territory level. What all have in common is adherence to the values and principles mandated by the National Health and Medical Research Councils of Australia and New Zealand, to ensure culturally appropriate research. The Australian principles include *spirit and integrity* (respecting the ongoing connection between Aboriginal and Torres Strait Islander peoples' past, current and future generations and the credibility of intent in the process of negotiations with Aboriginal and Torres Strait Islander communities), *cultural continuity* (maintaining the bonds and relationships between people and between people and their environment), *equity* (commitment to showing fairness and justice), *reciprocity* (equitable and respectful engagement and inclusion), *respect* (transparent acknowledgment of Indigenous beliefs and practices) and *responsibility* (establishing processes to ensure researcher accountability and responsibility to do no harm) (National Health and Medical Research Council [NHMRC] 2018a). The Aotearoa New Zealand principles include *Whakapapa* (relationships), *Tika* (research design including Mainstream, Māori-centred and Kaupapa Māori approaches), *Manaakitanga* (cultural and social responsibility) and *Mana* (justice and equity) (Hudson et al 2010).

Researching the future

Although the research agenda for community health is growing, many areas remain inadequately researched for a number of reasons. In most cases, the length of time required to investigate a web of factors or situations is prohibitive. Research may also be hampered by a lack of funding, due to the rigidity of many granting agencies to support broadly based studies. Dilution of interventions in large sites sometimes leads to a lack of clarity in the findings, which can be complicated by time trend effects. This occurs when the circumstances of the community change over time, or where the true costs of engaging with a community at each step of the process are underestimated.

Another difficulty is that there are varying cultural norms and expectations evident in community health research, which makes sharing the experience between different groups somewhat of a challenge. In action research studies, changes in health outcomes as a result of interventions are often not detectable for many years, which may create tensions on those waiting for results, including funding agencies. This is a particular problem if the effect of an intervention falls outside the political planning timeframe. A further issue is related to the challenges of measuring place-based improvements at the neighbourhood or community level, especially if the research team has not enlisted team members who have cultural and statistical expertise. So, although the optimal approach is to investigate multidimensional studies of community health and wellness, the cautionary tale is that current funding agencies tend to seek out and fund research with short, sharp, measurable outcomes, within the parameters of their reporting requirements and political needs. Fortunately, both Australia and New Zealand are starting to see changes in this space— particularly with increasing funding for Indigenous research that is often best completed in community settings as discussed above.

What remains for the future is to develop incremental, expanded programs of community health research that will highlight the aspects of community culture and social life, in a way that can be readily used for policymakers, health service managers and practitioners and the community itself. This agenda includes the trajectory research mentioned earlier in the chapter, to assess change over time, including the effectiveness of interventions with individuals, families, groups or populations as they experience health and illness across settings and across the life span. The research to policy agenda will always have gaps to be filled with research into ways of shaping healthcare systems to provide appropriate, accessible, acceptable, effective, efficient and equitable care. It will also reflect trends and vested interests, particularly with budget constraints on health and research funding bodies. For those who are not working within large networks of researchers or organised programs of research, numerous research topics arise out of everyday practice with communities. Many practitioners at the cutting edge of practice have an ideal opportunity through research to make significant inroads into healthcare improvements or to manage care and interactions with greater efficiency and effectiveness.

Demographic changes are occurring in the community in tandem with the evolution of sophisticated research strategies that will enable greater clarity in investigating issues such as chronic conditions within a primary health care, social justice ethos. It is crucial that Australian and New Zealand nurses add our voices to those of primary health care nurses internationally to connect care, prevention and attention to the SDH at the grassroots level through to global health policy. Population ageing, exponential increase in chronic illness and lifestyle-related problems such as obesity and mental health problems have heightened the need to research strategies for health literacy, empowerment and various versions of client-centred care. Research studies need to include the rapidly growing cohort of baby boomers, who, as we have mentioned previously, may want personalised accessible services with well-informed choices. Their needs and preferences may see the nursing role transformed into that of knowledge broker, culture broker and collaborative problem-solver partner. The recent COVID-19 pandemic provides further opportunities for primary health care nurses who have often been at the epicentre of the pandemic to undertake research into people's experiences of the pandemic and the ways in which it was managed.

Although there are few audits of nursing research in Australia and New Zealand, a review of published studies in professional journals globally reveals some interesting trends. The *Journal of Community Health Nursing* publishes a wide range of community research, some of which is focused on behaviour change and chronic illness management, but research reports also include studies that advance knowledge; for example, by framing various interventions within a socio-ecological perspective of community life. *Family and Community Health* is another journal which reports studies on health promotion interventions for community residents, as well as social and environmental issues. These include studies of community environments that support injury prevention strategies, healthy adolescence and ageing and reports of various specific nursing interventions. The journal *Health and Social Care in the Community* reports numerous studies of home care and other contexts for care giving. In the past few years, this journal has published widely on service organisation and the needs of carers. Studies also include those addressing the SDH: housing and homelessness, poverty, health inequalities and social inclusion. The *Australian Journal of Rural Health* contains reports of nursing research, but its major focus is on the rural community, so the reports are more interdisciplinary than some of the other nursing and midwifery journals. With workforce shortages, a large proportion of the research concerns recruitment and retention of health professionals, and professional issues related to attracting staff. The *Journal of Advanced Nursing* and the *Journal of Clinical Nursing* publish more frequently than some of the other nursing journals, and these have a strong mix of examples of EBP and topics addressing community health issues. Some of the more recent studies reported in these journals include research into psychosocial issues in healthcare, models of service delivery and approaches for working with vulnerable groups.

KEY POINT

....

Databases such as ProQuest, CINAHL, MEDLINE, PubMed, PsycINFO and Scopus provide extraordinary resources to support research.

Australian journals such as *Contemporary Nurse*, *Collegian* and the *Australian Journal of Advanced Practice* also address a balanced mix of nursing and midwifery research that focuses on interventions, professional development and the needs of communities. All publish international nursing studies. In some cases, the journals develop special issues dedicated to a certain topic which can be particularly helpful to nurses and midwives working in the community. *Contemporary Nurse* publishes many special issues, with a strong emphasis on community and family topics, as well as culture and Indigenous health. *Nursing Praxis in New Zealand* publishes a range of nursing research specific to New Zealand and is an excellent source of New Zealand-specific studies. *Kai Tiaki Nursing Research* is a recently established New Zealand peer-reviewed nursing journal that publishes research on a range of topics specific to nursing and is another useful source of research specific to New Zealand. The *Journal of Primary Healthcare* likewise is a New Zealand-specific journal that takes a multidisciplinary approach to research, publishing peer-reviewed, scientific research targeting general practice. The Australian equivalent is the *Australian Journal of Primary Health*.

There are many aspects of community life in Australia and New Zealand that have yet to be sufficiently researched. Our review of journals in which Australian and New Zealand nurses publish their research reveals a dearth of studies that respond to the SDH, although much of this work is published in a range of interdisciplinary journals, especially public health and health promotion journals. However, with the trend towards researching chronic conditions and ageing, numerous other journals publish studies relevant to all aspects of community practice. We have tried throughout this book to outline a wide range of resources from the most community-relevant journals. The best way to extend this work is by accessing further information through the large, comprehensive databases that are available to most scholars and practitioners who have access to the internet. When all else fails, there is always Google! Some of the burning questions that remain are listed in Box 10.6.

The research questions found in Box 10.6 could be used to guide an entire program of research.

BOX 10.6

COMMUNITY HEALTH
RESEARCH QUESTIONS

- What community support mechanisms will create the best opportunities for empowerment and self-determinism among disadvantaged people? How can these be tailored to groups differentiated by race, ethnicity, gender, health status, age or geography?
- What policies and practices will create the best opportunities for enriched parenting? What are the barriers to good parenting for different age, stage and socioeconomic groups? How can communities support parenting?
- What are the most helpful strategies in reducing alcohol and tobacco use/overuse for particular groups? How are these embedded in social and environmental factors?
- Which interventions have shown the most promise in fostering the combination of healthy nutrition and physical activity across the lifespan? What environmental influences facilitate healthy lifestyles for which groups?
- What are the moderators of workplace stress in promoting family health and happiness? Which occupational supports can help alleviate workplace stress for different types of workers?
- How can nurses enhance access to effective neighbourhood or community-based strategies for supporting families experiencing disruptions and transitions? Where and how are they most effective?
- What is good and best practice, or good and best process in maintaining mental health for different age groups? How are these practices implemented in rural and remote areas?
- How can schools support urban and rural adolescents through the crucial time of emerging identities?
- Which technologies are most helpful to develop health assets and meeting health needs for different age groups?
- How can health practitioners participate in creating sustainable neighbourhoods to support healthy ageing?
- To what extent do emerging technologies, particularly telecommunications, provide health benefits for older rural residents?
- What are the barriers and facilitators involved in nurses becoming active advocates for social policies to protect human rights?
- In what ways can collaborative practice enhance health outcomes for communities?
- How do nurses understand the SDH and how do they integrate this understanding into their practice?
- In what way did the COVID-19 pandemic impact on the practice of nurses, midwives or allied health professionals in the community? What role did these health professionals play in the pandemic and how did they work with communities to alleviate the impact on those most vulnerable?
- What are the most effective models of nursing care for chronic condition management, for health promotion, for community capacity building?

However, the most important element in any investigation is the need to pose a manageable question; one that can be addressed in the timeframe allowed, using a defined pool of resources. Although other aspects of the research process are important, the method is ultimately driven by the research question. Information on writing a study proposal and tips for arguing for the study to a granting body are available online at the Elsevier site associated with this book. These tips are offered in the hope that we have persuaded all readers of this text to participate in generating and/or using the evidence base that will help communities become healthy, happy, vibrant and sustainable.

Conclusion

Nurses and other health practitioners at the cutting edge of practice often identify problems or issues that need to be researched. In this chapter we have covered a wide range of approaches to research and how these can be used in the community context. While it may not always be practicable for frontline practitioners to do the research themselves, knowledge of the research process, where to find good quality research and how to contribute to research within communities are essential skills. We encourage you to use research wisely, identify and recommend research to be undertaken in the communities you work with and read widely. These skills will help develop your community practice and strengthen your work with individuals, families and communities. Community health and wellness can be achieved through a combination of knowledge generation, practical application of that knowledge in communities and an approach to working with people and the communities within which they live that recognises their strengths and capabilities. Thinking globally and acting locally has never been more important. We finish this book by first reflecting on the big issues and then turning to the last of our case studies with the Mason and Smith families. We hope you have enjoyed their company while you have journeyed through this book.

Reflecting on the Big Issues

- Research is an important part of practice.
- Researching community health issues requires a broader approach than the traditional evidence-based practice methods.
- Mixed-method research can help provide the community perspective as well as specific investigation of designated variables.
- Research is time and resource intensive.
- Interdisciplinary studies can give a greater breadth to studies of community health.
- Special considerations must be given to researching with Indigenous people, to ensure their cultural safety.

- Community-based participatory research, especially participatory action research, is well suited to studies of the community.
- The research questions should dictate the research method, which then follows appropriate conventions for data collection, analysis and dissemination of findings.
- Translational studies are designed to transfer or translate knowledge into practice.
- The community research agenda has many gaps that indicate the need for ongoing research by nurses, particularly addressing the SDH.
- Research is something that all nurses working in communities can and should be involved in.

CASE STUDY

EBP to assist the Mason and Smith families

Nurses working in the mine site and in the home communities of both families are conscious of the need for EBP. A number of research findings have already affected the families, including global studies on sustainable environments and studies on family life and child health. For example, Huia has enrolled Jake in a research study to examine the effectiveness of nurse-led asthma clinics in managing childhood asthma. School health nurses in Perth are evaluating healthy school initiatives in relation to children's coping strategies and public health researchers are working with nurses to identify the range of issues associated with fly-in fly-out (FIFO) family life to develop support programs.

Reflective questions: How would I use this knowledge in practice?

1 Identify one research question for each family unit involved in the case study throughout the previous chapters.

2 Explain how you would investigate each of these questions.

3 How would the results of each study inform primary health care in your practice?

4 There are innumerable topics that nurses can and do research. Working in pairs, identify a topic area that interests you. Why is it important that nurses undertake research in this area? Argue your case for undertaking nursing research in this area to the wider group.

We hope you have enjoyed this book as much as we have enjoyed writing it for you. A book is a labour of love and we hope you will find within it the tools you need to work successfully with communities and contribute in some small way to improving the lives of those you work with. Ngā mihi mahana kia koutou.

Jill Clendon

As an author, academic and community child and adolescent health nurse at Curtin University in Western Australia, I am privileged to be working in Noongar (or Nyungar) Country. Out of respect to the traditional custodians, the Nyungar people and their Elders past, present and future, I would like to say farewell and thank you using 'Boordah' which is a Noongar/Nyungar word that refers to 'later on' or 'in the future'.

Ailsa Munns

References

Adrian, M., Miller, A.B., McCauley, E., et al, 2016. Suicidal ideation in early to middle adolescence: Sex-specific trajectories and predictors. J. Child Psychol. Psychiatry, 57 (5), 645–653. Online. Available: https://doi.org/10.1111/jcpp.12484.

Baddock, S.A., Tipene-Leach, D., Williams, S.M., et al, 2017. Wahakura versus bassinet for safe infant sleep: A randomized trial. Pediatr., 139 (2). Online. Available: https://doi.org/10.1542/peds.2016-0162.

Bandler, L.G., 2015. Beyond Chapter 4.7. Health Promot. J. Austr., 26 (3), 186–190. Online. Available: https://doi.org/10.1071/HE15068.

Beatson, R., Molloy, C., Goldfeld, S., et al, 2021. Systematic review: An exploration of core componentry characterizing effective sustained nurse home visiting programs. J. Adv. Nurs., November 2020, 1–14. Online. Available: https://doi.org/10.1111/jan.14755.

Beks, H., Ewing, G., Charles, J.A., et al, 2020. Mobile primary health care clinics for Indigenous populations in Australia, Canada, New Zealand and the United States: a systematic scoping review. Int. J. Equity, 19 (1). Online. Available: https://doi.org/10.1186/s12939-020-01306-0.

Bennett, S., Hannes, K., O'Connor, D., 2020. Appraising and interpreting systematic reviews. In: Hoffman, T., Bennett, S., Del Mar, C. (Eds), Evidence-based practice across the health professions, third ed. Elsevier, pp. 292–322.

Bero, L., Rennie, D. (1995). The Cochrane Collaboration: Preparing, maintaining and disseminating systematic reviews of the effects of health care. J. Am. Med. Assoc., 274 (24), 1935–1938.

Blue Bird Jernigan, V., D'Amico, E.J., Keawe'aimoku Kaholokula, J., 2020. Prevention research with indigenous communities to expedite dissemination and implementation efforts. Prev. Sci., 21, 74–82. Online. Available: https://doi.org/10.1007/s11121-018-0951-0.

Bobba, S., 2019. Ethics of medical research in Aboriginal and Torres Strait Islander populations. Aust. J. Prim. Health, 25(5), 402–405. Online. Available: https://doi.org/10.1071/PY18049.

Brush, B.L., Mentz, G., Jensen, M., et al, 2020. Success in long-standing community-based participatory research (CBPR) partnerships: A scoping literature review. Health Educ. Behav., 47 (4), 556–568. Online. Available: https://doi.org/10.1177/1090198119882989.

Bulloch, H., Fogarty, W., Bellchambers, K., 2019. Aboriginal Health and Wellbeing Services: Putting community-driven, strengths-based approaches into practice. The Lowitja Institute and the National Centre for Indigenous Studies, The Australian National University.

Burns, E., Triandafilidis, Z., Schmied, V., 2020. Designing a model of breastfeeding support in Australia: An appreciative inquiry approach. Health Soc. Care Community, 28 (5), 1723–1733. Online. Available: https://doi.org/10.1111/hsc.12997.

Busija, L., Cinelli, R., Toombs, M.R., et al, 2020. The role of Elders in the wellbeing of a contemporary Australian Indigenous community. Geront., 60 (3), 513–524. Online. Available: https://doi.org/10.1093/geront/gny140.

Chowdhury, N., Naidu, J., Chowdhury, M.Z.I., et al, 2021. Knowledge translation in health and wellness research focusing on immigrants in Canada. J. Prim. Health Care, 13 (2), 139–156. Online. Available: https://doi.org/10.1071/HC20072.

Cockerham, W.C., Hamby, B.W., Oates, G.R., 2017. The social determinants of chronic disease. Am. J. Prev. Med., 52 (1, Supplement 1), S5–S12. Online. Available: http://dx.doi.org/10.1016/j.amepre.2016.09.010.

Cole, R., Young, J., Kearney, L., et al, 2020. Infant care practices and parent uptake of safe sleep messages: a cross-sectional survey in Queensland, Australia. BMC Pediatrics, 20 (1), 1–13. Online. Available: https://doi.org/10.1186/s12887-020-1917-5.

Conway, A., Duff, J., 2020. Common quantitative methods. In D. Whitehead, C. Ferguson, G. LoBiondo-Wood, J. Haber (Eds), Nursing and midwifery research: Methods and appraisal for evidence-based practice, sixth ed. Elsevier, pp. 98–117.

de Jong, G., Schout, G., Abma, T., 2015. Examining the effects of family group conferencing with randomised controlled trials: The golden standard? Br. J. Soc. Work, 45 (5), 1623–1629. Online. Available: https://academic.oup.com/bjsw/article-abstract/45/5/1623/1628976?redirectedFrom=fulltext.

Fergusson, D.M., Boden, J.M., Horwood, L.J., 2013. Nine-year follow-up of a home-visitation program: A randomized trial. (Report). Pediatr., 131 (2), 297.

Freemantle, J., Ellis, L., 2018. An Australian perpective. In Duncan, J., Byard, R. (Eds), SIDS sudden infant and early childhood death: The past, the present and the future. Adelaide University Press, pp. 349–374.

García-Molina, L., Lewis-Mikhael, A.-M., Riquelme-Gallego, B., et al, 2020. Improving type 2 diabetes mellitus glycaemic control through lifestyle modification implementing diet intervention: a systematic review and meta-analysis. Eur. J. Nutr., 59 (4), 1313–1328. Online. Available: https://doi.org/10.1007/s00394-019-02147-6.

Golden, T.L., Wendel, M.L., 2020. Public health's next step in advancing equity: Re-evaluating epistemological assumptions to move social determinants from theory to Practice. Front. Public Health, 8, 131. Online. Available: https://doi.org/10.3389/fpubh.2020.00131.

Goldfeld, S., Price, A., Smith, C., et al, 2019. Nurse home visiting for families experiencing adversity: A randomized trial. Pediatr., 143 (1). Online. Available: https://pubmed.ncbi.nlm.nih.gov/30591616/.

Gray, M.A., Oprescu, F.I., 2016. Role of non-Indigenous researchers in Indigenous health research in Australia: a review of the literature. Aust. Health Rev., 40 (4), 459–467. Online. Available: https://doi.org/10.1071/AH15103.

Greenhalgh, T., Bidewell, J., Crisp, E., et al, 2020. Understanding research methods for evidence-based practice in health, second ed.. John Wiley & Sons Australia, Ltd.

Hannes, K., Bennett, S., 2020. Understanding evidence from qualitative resesrach. In: Hoffman, T., Bennett, S., Del Mar, C. (Eds), Evidence-based practice across the health professions, third ed. Elsevier, pp. 226–247.

Hapeta, J., Palmer, F., Kuroda, Y., 2019. Cultural identity, leadership and wellbeing: how Indigenous storytelling contributed to wellbeing in a New Zealand provincial rugby team. Public Health, 176, 68–76. Online. Available: https://doi.org/10.1016/j.puhe.2018.12.010.

Health Research Council of New Zealand, 2010. Nga Pou Rangahau The strategic plan for Māori health research 2010–2015. Health Research Council of New Zealand. Online. Available: www.hrc.govt.nz.

Hoffman, T., Bennett, S., Del Mar, C., 2020. Introduction to evidence-based practice. In: Hoffman, T., Bennett, S., Del Mar, C. (Eds), Evidence-based practice across the health professions, third ed. Elsevier, pp. 1–15.

Hudson, M., Milne, M., Reynolds, P., et al, 2010. Te Ara Tika guidelines for Māori research ethics: A framework for researchers and ethics committee members. Health Research Council. Online. Available: www.fmhs.auckland.ac.nz/assets/fmhs/faculty/tkhm/tumuaki/docs/teara.pdf.

International Council of Nurses., 2016. Nurses: A force for change: Improving health systems' resilience. International Council of Nurses, Geneva.

Israel, B.A., 2013. Methods for community-based participatory research for health (second ed.). Jossey-Bass.

Israel, B., Shulz, A., Parker, E., et al, 2001. Community-based participatory research: policy recommendations for promoting a partnership approach in health research. Educ. Health: Change Learn. Pract., 14(2), 182–197. Online. Available: https://pubmed.ncbi.nlm.nih.gov/14742017/.

Kitzman, H.J., Olds, D.L., Cole, R.E., et al, 2010. Enduring effects of prenatal and infancy home visiting by nurses on children: follow-up of a randomized trial among children at age 12 years. Arch. Pediatr. Adolesc. Med., 164(5), 412–418. Online. Available: https://pubmed.ncbi.nlm.nih.gov/20439791/.

Lockwood, C., Graham, I., Hopp, L., 2020. Applying research knowledge: Evidence-based practice development and knowledge translation. In: Whitehead, D., Ferguson, C., LoBiondo-Wood, G., Haber, J. (Eds), Nursing and midwifery research: Methods and appraisal for evidence-based practice, sixth ed. Elsevier, pp. 300–327.

Marriott, R., Reibel, T., Coffin, J., et al, 2019. 'Our culture, how it is to be us'—Listening to Aboriginal women about on Country urban birthing. Women & Birth, 32(5), 391–403. Online. Available: https://doi.org/10.1016/j.wombi.2019.06.017.

McCluskey, A., O'Connor, D., 2020. Implementing evidence. In: Hoffman, T., Bennett, S., Del Mar, C. (Eds), Evidence-based practice across the health professions, third ed. Elsevier, pp. 384–408.

Molloy, L., Guha, M.D., Scott, M.P., et al, 2021. Mental health nursing practice and Aboriginal and Torres Strait Islander people: an integrative review. Contemp. Nurse, 57(1/2), 140–156. Online. Available: https://doi.org/10.1080/10376178.2021.1927773.

Monaghan, T., Manski-Nankervis, J.-A., Canaway, R., 2020. Big data or big risk: general practitioner, practice nurse and practice manager attitudes to providing de-identified patient health data from electronic medical records to researchers. Aust. J. Prim. Health, 26(6), 466–471. Online. Available: https://doi.org/10.1071/PY20153.

Muley, A., Fernandez, R., Ellwood, L., et al, 2021. Effect of tree nuts on glycemic outcomes in adults with type 2 diabetes mellitus: a systematic review. JBI Evid. Synth., 19(5), 966–1002. Online. Available: https://doi.org/10.11124/JBISRIR-D-19-00397.

National Health and Medical Research Council (NHMRC), 2018a. Ethical conduct in research with Aboriginal and Torres Strait Islander peoples and communities: Guidelines for researchers and stakeholders (Issue 63). NHMRC, Australian Government. Online. Available: www.nhmrc.gov.au/about-us/resources/ethical-conduct-research-aboriginal-and-torres-strait-islander-peoples-and-communities#block-views-block-file-attachments-content-block-1.

National Health and Medical Research Council (NHMRC), 2018b. National statement on ethical conduct in human research, 2007 (Updated 2018). NHMRC, Australian Government. Online. Available: www.nhmrc.gov.au/about-us/publications/national-statement-ethical-conduct-human-research-2007-updated-2018#block-views-block-file-attachments-content-block-1.

Nursing and Midwifery Board of Australia, 2016. Registered nurse standards for practice. In Nursing and Midwifery Board of Australia (Issue February). Nursing and Midwifery Board of Australia. Online. Available: www.nursingmidwiferyboard.gov.au/Codes-Guidelines-Statements/Professional-standards.aspx.

Nursing Council of New Zealand, 2016. Competencies for registered nurses. Nursing Council of New Zealand.

Nykiforuk, C.I.J., 2021. Engaging patients in research using photovoice methodology. Can. Med. Assoc. J., 193(27), E1050–E1051. Online. Available: https://doi.org/10.1503/cmaj.210963.

Pacquiao, D.F., Douglas, M., 2019. Social pathways to health vulnerability implications for health professionals, first ed. Springer International Publishing. Online. Available: https://doi.org/10.1007/978-3-319-93326-9.

Remus, S., Donelle, L., 2019. Big data: Why should Canadian nurse leaders care? Nursing Leadership, 32(2), 19–30. Online. Available: https://doi.org/10.12927/cjnl.2019.25964.

Rolleston, A.K., Doughty, R., Poppe, K., 2016. Integration of kaupapa Māori concepts in health research: a way forward for Māori cardiovascular health? J Prim. Health Care, 8 (1), 60–66. CSIRO Publishing. Online. Available: https://doi.org/10.1071/HC15034.

Shaikh, F., Jha, S., 2020. Analysing data in quantitative research. In: Whitehead, D., Ferguson, C., LoBiondo-Wood, G., Haber, J. (Eds), Nursing and midwifery research: methods and appraisal for evidence-based practice, sixth ed. Elsevier, pp. 228–254.

Sharmil, H., Kelly, J., Bowden, M., et al, 2021. Participatory Action Research-Dadirri-Ganma, using Yarning: methodology co-design with Aboriginal community members. Int. J. Equity Health, 20 (1), 1–11. Online. Available: https://doi.org/10.1186/s12939-021-01493-4.

Sheridan, N., Geia, L., 2020. Indigenous peoples and research. In: Whitehead, D., Ferguson, C., LoBiondo-Wood, G., Haber, J. (Eds), Nursing and midwifery research: methods and appraisal for evidence-based practice, sixth ed. Elsevier, pp. 276–299.

Shipstone, R.A., Young, J., Kearney, L., et al, 2020. Prevalence of risk factors for sudden infant death among Indigenous and non-Indigenous people in Australia. Acta Paediatrica, 109 (4). Online. Available: https://doi.org/10.1111/apa.15274.

Smith, C., Pell, J., 2003. Parachute use to prevent death and major trauma related to gravitational challenge: systematic review of randomized controlled trials. Br. Med. J., 327 (7249), 1459–1461. Online. Available: www.ncbi.nlm.nih.gov/pmc/articles/PMC300808/.

Springer, M.V, Skolarus, L.E., 2019. Community-based participatory research. Stroke (1970), 50 (3), e48–e50. Online. Available: https://doi.org/10.1161/STROKEAHA.118.024241.

Sweet, L., Davis, D., 2020. An overview of research theory, process and design. In: Whitehead, D., Ferguson, C., LoBiondo-Wood, G., Haber, J. (Eds), Nursing and midwifery research: methods and appraisal for evidence-based practice, sixth ed. Elsevier, pp. 13–28.

Teixeira de Almeida Vieira Monteiro, A.P., 2016. Cyborgs, biotechnologies, and informatics in health care—new paradigms in nursing sciences. Nurs. Philos., 17(1), 19–27. Online. Available: https://doi.org/10.1111/nup.12088.

Tipa, Z., 2019. The significance of kaupapa Māori research methodology. Kai Tiaki Nursing Research, 10(1), 5–6. Online. Available: www.tandfonline.com/doi/full/10.1080/13645579.2021.1897756.

Tipene-Leach, D., Abel, S., 2019. Innovation to prevent sudden infant death: the wahakura as an Indigenous vision for a safe sleep environment. Aust. J. Prim. Health, 25 (5), 406–409. Online. Available: https://doi.org/10.1071/PY19033.

Toronto, C.E., Remington, R., 2020. A step-by-step guide to conducting an integrative review. Springer International Publishing. Online. Available: https://doi.org/10.1007/978-3-030-37504-1.

Trudel-Fitzgerald, C., Chen, Y., Singh, A., et al, 2016. Psychiatric, psychological, and social determinants of health in the nurses' health study cohorts. Am. J. Public Health, 106 (9), 1644–1649. Online. Available: https://doi.org/10.2105/AJPH.2016.303318.

Vaithianathan, R., Wilson, M., Maloney, T., et al, 2016. The impact of the family start home visiting programme on outcomes for mothers and children: a quasi-experimental study (February issue). Online. Available: www.msd.govt.nz/documents/about-msd-and-our-work/publications-resources/evaluation/family-start-outcomes-study/family-start-impact-study-report.pdf.

Vounzoulaki, E., Khunti, K., Abner, S.C., et al, 2020. Progression to type 2 diabetes in women with a known history of gestational diabetes: systematic review and meta-analysis. Diabetes Prim. Care, 22 (3), 1–11. Online. Available: https://doi.org/10.1136/bmj.m1361.

Whitehead, D., Disler, R., 2020. Common qualitative methods. In: Whitehead, D., Ferguson, C., LoBiondo-Wood, G., Haber, J. (Eds), Nursing and midwifery research: methods and appraisal for evidence-based practice, sixth ed. Elsevier, pp. 156–177.

Whitehead, D., Halcomb, L., 2020. Mixed-methods research. In: Whitehead, D., Ferguson, C., LoBiondo-Wood, G., Haber, J. (Eds), Nursing and midwifery research: methods and appraisal for evidence-based practice, sixth ed. Elsevier, pp. 255–275.

Wilson, D., Neville, S., 2009. Culturally safe research with vulnerable populations. Contemporary Nurse, 33(1), 69–79.

Xia, T., Yang, Y., Li, W., et al, 2020. Meditative movements for patients with type 2 diabetes: A systematic review and meta-analysis. Evid. Based Complement. Alternat. Med., 1–12. Online. Available: https://doi.org/10.1155/2020/5745013.

Young, J., Watson, K., Craigie, L., et al, 2017. Uniting cultural practices and safe sleep environments for vulnerable Indigenous Australian infants. Aust. Nurs. Midwifery J.,

24 (9), 37. Online. Available: https://search.proquest.com/docview/1882375667?accountid=14782.

Young, J., Craigie, L., Cowan, S., et al, 2018. Reducing risk for Aboriginal and Torres Strait Islander babies: trial of a safe sleep enabler to reduce the risk of sudden unexpected deaths in infancy in high-risk environments. Sippy Downs, Australia: University of the Sunshine Coast.

Zambas, S.I., Dutch, S., Gerrard, D., 2020. Factors influencing Māori student nurse retention and success: An integrative literature review. Nurse Educ. Today, 91. Online. Available: https://doi.org/10.1016/j.nedt.2020.104477.

Zhou, X., Siegel, K.R., Ng, B.P., et al, 2020. Cost-effectiveness of diabetes prevention interventions targeting high-risk individuals and whole populations: A systematic review. Diabetes Care, 43 (7), 1593–1616. Online. Available: https://doi.org/10.2337/dci20-0018.

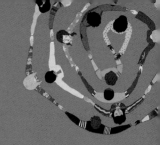

APPENDIX A

The McMurray community assessment framework

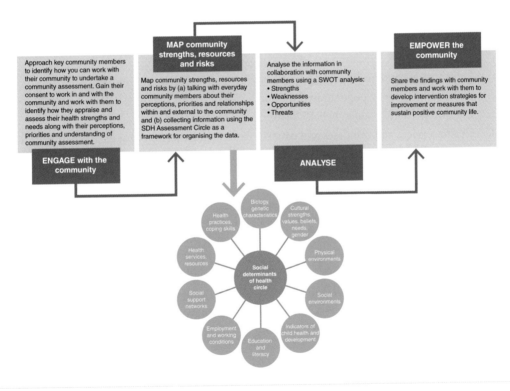

ENGAGE with the community

Approach key community members to identify how you can work with their community to undertake a community assessment. Gain their consent to work in and with the community and work with them to identify how they appraise and assess their health strengths and needs along with their perceptions, priorities and understanding of community assessment.

MAP community strengths, resources and risks

Map community strengths, resources and risks by (a) talking with everyday community members about their perceptions, priorities and relationships within and external to the community and (b) collecting information using the SDH Assessment Circle as a framework for organising the data.

ANALYSE

Analyse the information in collaboration with community members using a SWOT analysis:
• Strengths
• Weaknesses
• Opportunities
• Threats

EMPOWER the community

Share the findings with community members and work with them to develop intervention strategies for improvement or measures that sustain positive community life.

Biology, genetic characteristics

Cultural strengths, values, beliefs, needs, gender

Health practices, coping skills

Physical environments

Health services, resources

Social determinants of health circle

Social environments

Social support networks

Indicators of child health and development

Employment and working conditions

Education and literacy

Figure A.1 McMurray Community Assessment Framework

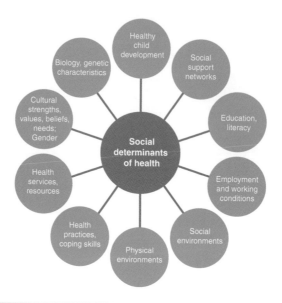

Figure A.2 The SDH community assessment circle

1. Indicators of child health and development
2. Biological or genetic population indicators
3. Cultural strengths, values, beliefs, history and needs; gender
4. Health services and resources and patterns of accessing these by various population groups
5. Health practices, coping skills in the context of recreation and leisure, which may support or compromise health, such as drop-in centres, places that encourage health literacy and capacity, or drug and alcohol misuse
6. Physical environments, including geographical factors such as climate change or transportation barriers to care, or activity-friendly neighbourhoods
7. Social environments, indicators of social inclusion or exclusion
8. Employment and financial status of the population, including unemployment rates, working conditions, types of employers, availability of workplace support
9. Education and literacy indicators
10. Social support networks, access for vulnerable groups, volunteer networks

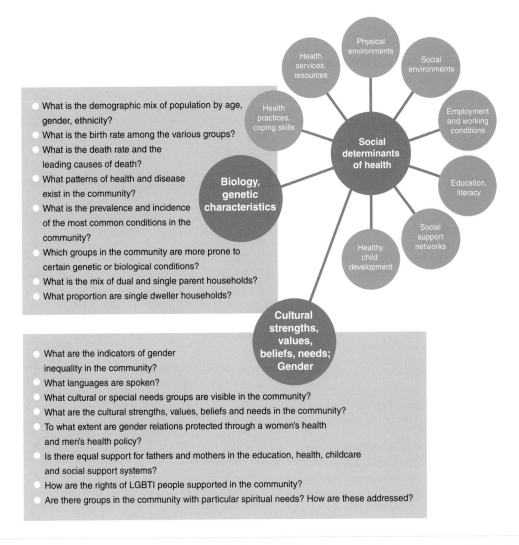

Figure A.3 The SDH community assessment circle—biology/genetic factors and gender/culture

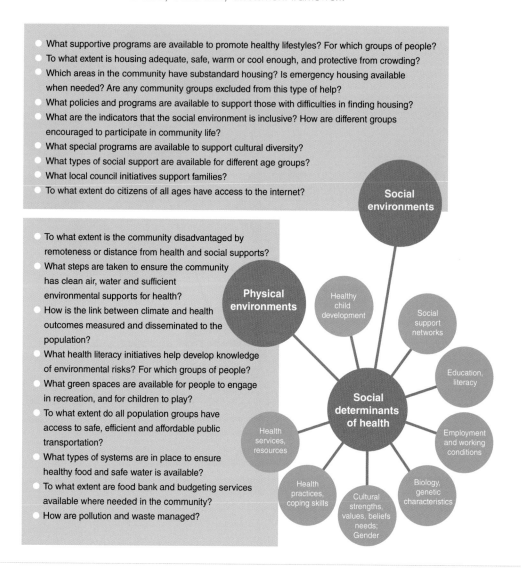

- What supportive programs are available to promote healthy lifestyles? For which groups of people?
- To what extent is housing adequate, safe, warm or cool enough, and protective from crowding?
- Which areas in the community have substandard housing? Is emergency housing available when needed? Are any community groups excluded from this type of help?
- What policies and programs are available to support those with difficulties in finding housing?
- What are the indicators that the social environment is inclusive? How are different groups encouraged to participate in community life?
- What special programs are available to support cultural diversity?
- What types of social support are available for different age groups?
- What local council initiatives support families?
- To what extent do citizens of all ages have access to the internet?

Social environments

- To what extent is the community disadvantaged by remoteness or distance from health and social supports?
- What steps are taken to ensure the community has clean air, water and sufficient environmental supports for health?
- How is the link between climate and health outcomes measured and disseminated to the population?
- What health literacy initiatives help develop knowledge of environmental risks? For which groups of people?
- What green spaces are available for people to engage in recreation, and for children to play?
- To what extent do all population groups have access to safe, efficient and affordable public transportation?
- What types of systems are in place to ensure healthy food and safe water is available?
- To what extent are food bank and budgeting services available where needed in the community?
- How are pollution and waste managed?

Physical environments

Healthy child development

Social support networks

Education, literacy

Social determinants of health

Employment and working conditions

Health services, resources

Health practices, coping skills

Cultural strengths, values, beliefs needs; Gender

Biology, genetic characteristics

Figure A.4 The SDH community assessment circle—physical and social environments

- What is the distribution of publicly subsidised schools in the community? To what extent do these serve all neighbourhoods?
- What initiatives exist to encourage adolescents to complete high school?
- How do schools support the health and wellbeing of children and their families?
- How are schools involved in community life?
- What literacy programs are available for new migrants, non-English-speaking groups?
- What supports are in place for vulnerable and disadvantaged people to undertake education and/or skills retraining?
- How is health literacy addressed in the community? To what extent are health literacy programs inclusive?

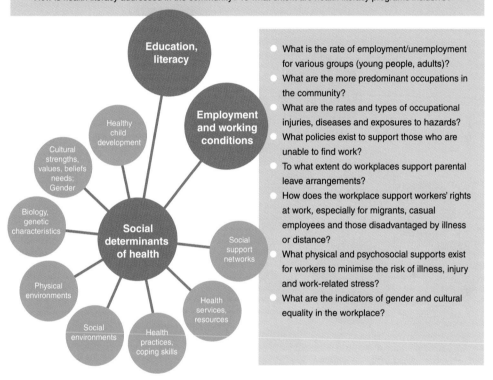

- What is the rate of employment/unemployment for various groups (young people, adults)?
- What are the more predominant occupations in the community?
- What are the rates and types of occupational injuries, diseases and exposures to hazards?
- What policies exist to support those who are unable to find work?
- To what extent do workplaces support parental leave arrangements?
- How does the workplace support workers' rights at work, especially for migrants, casual employees and those disadvantaged by illness or distance?
- What physical and psychosocial supports exist for workers to minimise the risk of illness, injury and work-related stress?
- What are the indicators of gender and cultural equality in the workplace?

Figure A.5 The SDH community assessment circle—education/literacy and employment/ working conditions

- What are the indicators that health and other services are governed by a 'health in all policies' program?
- What is the distribution of acute and community services?
- To what extent are these appropriate for all population groups?
- To what extent does the community provide equal access to affordable care?
- What evidence is there that health services are well governed?
- What evidence-based clinical and management practices are used?
- What is the distribution of culturally appropriate services for indigenous people, and those who have language or communication difficulties?
- What limitations exist on access for older or disabled residents?
- What indicators are there that community services are client-centred, promoting self-care and choice?
- What health promotion initiatives exist to reduce alcohol, tobacco, fat consumption and other hazardous lifestyle factors? What is the prevalence of these lifestyle factors in the community?

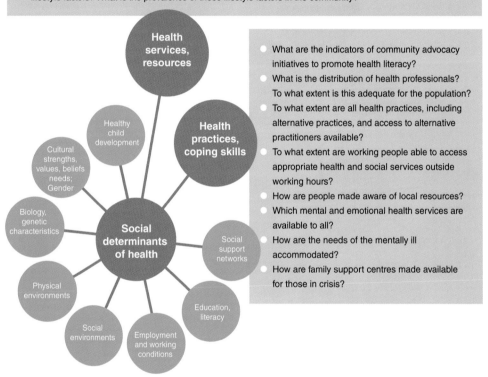

- What are the indicators of community advocacy initiatives to promote health literacy?
- What is the distribution of health professionals? To what extent is this adequate for the population?
- To what extent are all health practices, including alternative practices, and access to alternative practitioners available?
- To what extent are working people able to access appropriate health and social services outside working hours?
- How are people made aware of local resources?
- Which mental and emotional health services are available to all?
- How are the needs of the mentally ill accommodated?
- How are family support centres made available for those in crisis?

Figure A.6 The SDH community assessment circle—health services/resources and health practices/coping skills

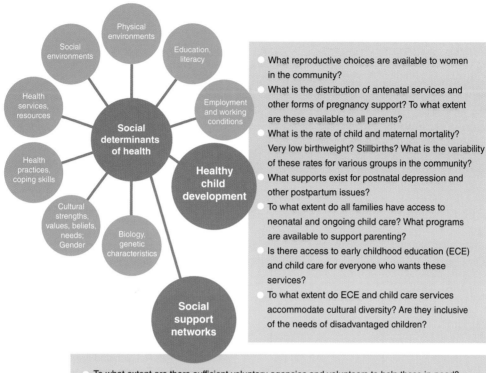

What reproductive choices are available to women in the community?

What is the distribution of antenatal services and other forms of pregnancy support? To what extent are these available to all parents?

What is the rate of child and maternal mortality? Very low birthweight? Stillbirths? What is the variability of these rates for various groups in the community?

What supports exist for postnatal depression and other postpartum issues?

To what extent do all families have access to neonatal and ongoing child care? What programs are available to support parenting?

Is there access to early childhood education (ECE) and child care for everyone who wants these services?

To what extent do ECE and child care services accommodate cultural diversity? Are they inclusive of the needs of disadvantaged children?

To what extent are there sufficient voluntary agencies and volunteers to help those in need?

How does the community support those who are impoverished?

What disability supports are provided for the disabled and their families?

How are community members encouraged to engage in partnerships for health and wellbeing?

How do community organisations reduce social exclusion?

Figure A.7 The SDH community assessment circle—healthy child development and social support networks

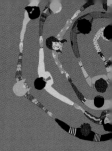

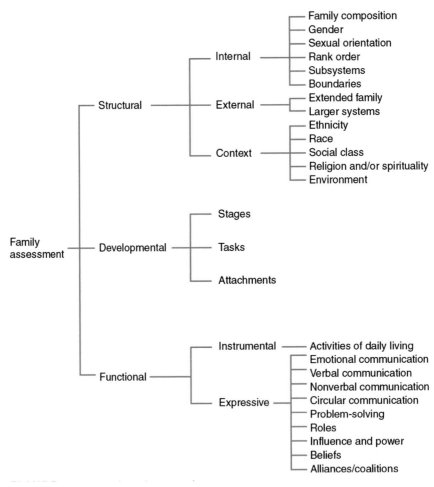

Family assessment

- Structural
  - Internal
    - Family composition
    - Gender
    - Sexual orientation
    - Rank order
    - Subsystems
    - Boundaries
  - External
    - Extended family
    - Larger systems
  - Context
    - Ethnicity
    - Race
    - Social class
    - Religion and/or spirituality
    - Environment
- Developmental
  - Stages
  - Tasks
  - Attachments
- Functional
  - Instrumental
    - Activities of daily living
  - Expressive
    - Emotional communication
    - Verbal communication
    - Nonverbal communication
    - Circular communication
    - Problem-solving
    - Roles
    - Influence and power
    - Beliefs
    - Alliances/coalitions

Pulliam, L.W., Plowfield, L.A., Fuess, S., 1996. Developmental Care: The key to the emergence of the vital older woman. J Obstet Gynecol Neonatal Nurs., 25 (7), 623–628. With permission from Elsevier.

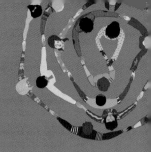

HEEADSSS Assessment Tool for use with Adolescents

A psychosocial assessment of young people is equally as important as a physical assessment. The following tool is based on Goldenring & Cohen's (1988), Goldenring & Rosen's (2004) and Klein et al's (2014) HEEADSSS method of interviewing. HEEADSSS stands for **H**ome, **E**ducation/Employment, **E**ating, peer group **A**ctivities, **D**rugs and Alcohol, **S**exuality, **S**uicide and Depression and **S**afety. We suggest that you also consider exploring the adolescent's level of community involvement as this may be an area of strength for the individual or an area where support can be found.

We recommend you undertake formal training in the use of the HEEADSSS assessment tool prior to use.

The tool

HOME

In the home setting, we cover family, culture and connections, looking for both resiliency and risk issues.

- Where do you live? Who do you live with?
- Ask about extended family links and culture—iwi, hapu, whānau, tribe.
- Where were you born? How long have you been here?
- Do you belong to a church? What activities and length of time have you been involved with the church?
- Tell me about the jobs or responsibilities at your place.

- Who makes the rules? What happens if rules are broken?
- What happens when you fight at your house?
- Is there any violence occurring at your house?
- Who in your family do you get along well with? Not so well?
- Who is the person you talk to most?

EDUCATION

- Tell me about school/training course/work.
- If none—how long have you been out of school/work? Why? Plans? What do you do with your time now?
- If yes—which school? What is good about school? Not so good?
- Do you have friends at school? Is there a teacher you get along well with?
- How do you do in your school work and classes?
- Do you have ideas about what you might like to do when you leave school?
- Do you miss much school? Why?
- Are you bullied at school?

EATING

- What do you like and not like about your body?
- Have there been any recent changes in your diet?

- Have you dieted in the last year? How? How often?
- Have you done anything else to try to manage your weight?
- How much exercise do you get in an average day? Week?
- What do you think would be a healthy diet? How does that compare to your current eating patterns?
- Does your weight or body shape cause you any stress? If so, tell me about it.

ACTIVITIES

Here we cover what you do. for example, with your friends, with your family and in your community.

- What do you and your friends do for fun? (With whom, where and when?)
- What do you and your family do for fun? (With whom, where and when?)
- Do you participate in any sports or other activities?
- Do you regularly attend a church group, club or other organised activity?
- Are you involved in any community activities?
- How do you get money?
- How do you get around? Do you drive sometimes?
- What about sleeping? Do you sleep well?
- Some teenagers tell me they spend much of their time online. What types of things do you use the internet for?
- How many hours do you spend on any given day in front of a screen such as a computer, TV or phone? Do you wish you spent less time on these things?

DRUGS/ALCOHOL

Introduce, for example, 'We know that many young people try alcohol and drugs; is it all right if I ask you some questions about that now?'

- Do young people at your school smoke? Do your friends smoke? Do you smoke?
- Do your friends/parents ever drink alcohol? Do you?

- Have you ever used marijuana? What other drugs/solvents are young people using these days?
- What do you think about that? What have you tried?
- If the young person is using:
  - How much are you using? In what circumstances? What do you like and not like about using?
  - What risks do you take when using? Have you ever considered using less?

SEXUALITY

Introduce, for example, 'We ask everyone about sexuality because that is a very important aspect of young people's lives and can affect their health so much. Is that OK with you? You can "pass" on questions if you want to.'

- Have you had any sexuality education at school? What was that like?
- Do your friends have sexual relationships? Do you?
- Are you attracted to anyone now?
- Are you interested in boys? Girls? Both? Not sure yet?
- What do you know about safe sex?
- What do you do (in terms of keeping sexually safe)? Do you use condoms? How much of the time? (Every time? Just when you can get them? Sometimes?)
- What could you do if you thought you might be pregnant?
- Has anybody ever touched you in a way that you don't like?
- If you ever felt uncomfortable or something unpleasant happened to you, is there anyone that you could tell?
- Are there adults you can go to for advice/help about sex and relationships?
- Do you want to talk about anything else about relationships or sex?

SUICIDE AND DEPRESSION

In this area, we cover issues of mental health and self-harm.

- How would you describe your mood/feelings most of the time? (Scale 1–10)
- Do you have really good/bad times?

If low mood is an issue, review sleeping, eating, energy, concentration, feelings of guilt/worthlessness and safety.

- Do you ever have worries or hassles that bother you?

If yes:

- Do they keep you awake at night?
- Do you have to do anything to keep them under control?
- Do you sometimes feel that life is not worth it?
- Have you ever harmed yourself deliberately?

If no, you may not need to continue this line of questioning.

- Have you ever thought of ending your pain once and for all?
- Do you know anyone who has died from suicide? Who? When?
- How often do you think about doing it? How did you think you would do it?
- How strong are these feelings for you at the moment?
- Do you think you might try?
- What if something went wrong for you? (Relationship break-up, etc.)
- Who could you tell about feeling suicidal?

Regarding previous suicidal behaviour:

- What did they do? How many times? How long ago? What happened?
- How do they feel about the fact that they did not die?
- Do they wish they had died?
- Have things changed since then? What?
- Do they think that they might try again?

SAFETY

- Have you ever been seriously injured? How? How about anyone else you know?

- Do you always wear a seatbelt in the car?
- Have you ever ridden with a driver who was drunk or high? When? How often?
- Do you use safety equipment for sports and/or other physical activities (e.g. helmets for biking or skateboarding)?
- Is there any violence in your home?
- Does the violence ever get physical?
- Is there a lot of violence at your school? In your neighbourhood? Among your friends?
- Have you ever been physically or sexually abused? Have you ever been raped on a date or at any other time?
- Have you ever been in a car or motorbike accident? (What happened?)
- Have you ever been picked on or bullied? Is that still a problem?
- Have you gotten into any physical fights in school or in your neighbourhood? Do you still feel that way?
- Have you ever felt like you needed to carry a knife, gun or other weapon to protect yourself? Do you still feel that way?

Where to find out more on...

HEEADSSS assessment tool

- https://teachmepaediatrics.com/community/holistic-care/headsss-assessment/#:,:text5HEADSSS%20Assessment.%20The%20HEEADSSS%20assessment%20is%20an%20internationally,elf%20harm%20and%20depression%2C%20S%20afety%20and%20abuse
- www.goodfellowunit.org/courses/introduction-heeadsss-assessment

References

Goldenring, J.M., Cohen, E., 1988. Getting into adolescent heads. Contemp. Pediatr., 5 (7), 75–90.

Goldenring, J.M., Rosen, D.S., 2004. Getting into adolescent heads: An essential update. Contemp. Pediatr., 21 (1), 64–90.

Klein, D., Goldenring, J., Adelman, W., 2014. HEEADSSS 3.0: The psychosocial interview for adolescents updated for a new century fuelled by media. Contemp. Pediatr., 31, 16–28.

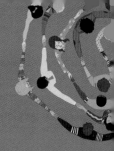

Index

Page numbers followed by 'b' indicate boxes; 'f' figures; 't' tables.